Non-surgical Ablation Therapy for Early-stage Breast Cancer

Takayuki Kinoshita
Editor

Non-surgical Ablation Therapy for Early-stage Breast Cancer

Springer

Editor
Takayuki Kinoshita
Division of Breast Surgery
National Cancer Center Hospital
Tokyo, Japan

ISBN 978-4-431-54462-3 ISBN 978-4-431-54463-0 (eBook)
DOI 10.1007/978-4-431-54463-0

Library of Congress Control Number: 2016941060

Printed on acid-free paper

This Springer imprint is published by Springer Nature
The registered company is Springer Japan KK

Contents

Chapter 1
Introduction

Takayuki Kinoshita

In the surgical treatment of breast cancer, conservative treatment and sentinel lymph node biopsy have already become the standard of care. In addition to being less invasive, treatments are expected to have good aesthetic outcomes. In Japan, the incidence of breast cancer (Fig. 1.1) and the detection rate for early-stage disease have increased due to widespread use of mammography and advances in diagnostic imaging, as is the case in other developed countries. Given this historical background, nonsurgical ablative therapies, noninvasive surgical therapies, have started to attract attention due to patient demand. The nonsurgical ablative therapies used in clinical practice for breast cancer are cryoablation, high-intensity focused ultrasound (HIFU), and radiofrequency ablation (RFA). In Japan, RFA became widespread quickly because of the prevalence and convenience of the device. In this book, an outline of the research on RFA funded by the Japan Agency for Medical Research and Development (AMED), prospects for RFA, and the current status of cryoablation and HIFU are discussed.

Conservative treatment for breast cancer was introduced in Japan in the 1980s as a local treatment for early-stage disease used under cautiously-developed criteria. Its indications have been gradually expanded by, for example, the addition of concomitant preoperative chemotherapy. More than half of breast cancer patients currently benefit from this treatment. Recently, nonsurgical ablative therapies have been tested as definitive conservative therapy. Clinical studies on HIFU and cryoablation began in 2004 and 2006, respectively. Phase I and Phase II multicentre clinical studies of RFA as treatment for early-stage breast cancer were started in 2006 under the Evaluation System of Investigational Medical Care. A prospective Phase III study was started in 2013 under the Advanced Medical Service System.

T. Kinoshita (✉)
Division of Breast Surgery, National Cancer Center Hospital, 5-1-1, Tsukiji, Chuo-ku, Tokyo 104-0045, Japan
e-mail: takinosh@ncc.go.jp

T. Kinoshita (ed.), *Non-surgical Ablation Therapy for Early-stage Breast Cancer*,
DOI 10.1007/978-4-431-54463-0_1

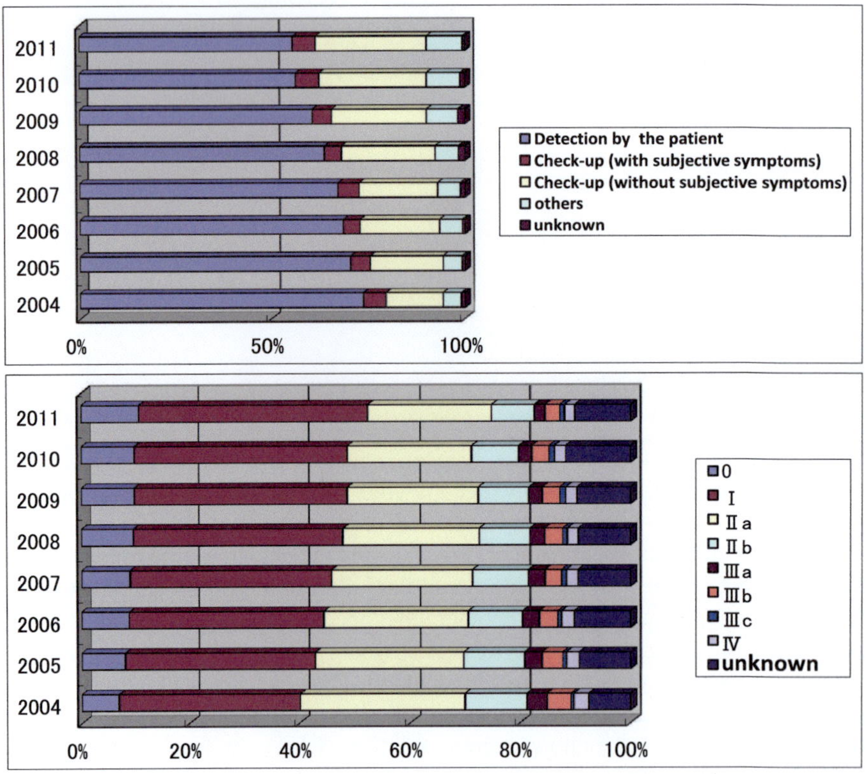

Fig. 1.1 Motives for seeking medical attention and changes in breast cancer stage at diagnosis in Japan

1.1 Current Status of RFA in Japan

In Japan, RFA is used for the treatment of liver cancer. During RFA, alternating electric currents change the ions in the tissue surrounding the electrodes and the heat generated as the result of friction from this change coagulates and necrotises cancer cells. Figure 1.2 illustrates RFA in the liver with the widely used Cool-tip needle (17 G). When the exposure size is 1.5 cm, an area of 3 cm in diameter can be cauterised. This procedure was adopted for the treatment of breast cancer. At first, seven expanding needles were used, as is the case with liver cancer. However, because the tissue of mammary glands is harder than liver tissue and thus it is more difficult to insert needles and control heat propagation to the skin, the Cool-tip FR System (Covidien, Energy-Based Devices, Interventional Oncology, Boulder, CO, USA), which consists of a single needle and allows for easier heat control, is the configuration most commonly used at present for breast cancer.

One advantage of this therapy is that this device has already been widely used for the treatment of liver cancer. At medical institutions that already have the device,

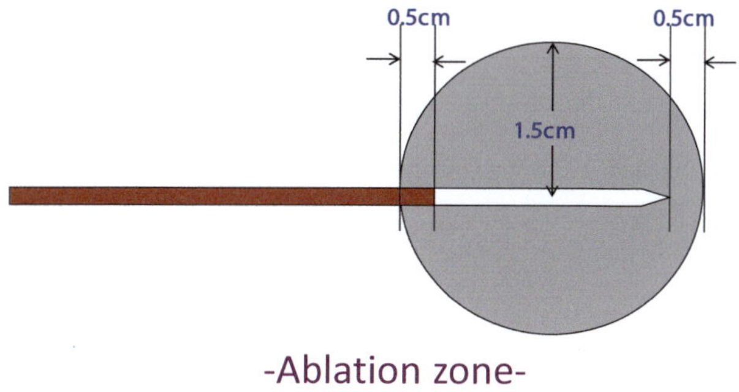

Fig. 1.2 Ablation zone of the cool-tip needle (based on liver tissue data)

only the needles need to be purchased. Therefore, RFA is likely to be prevalent in Japan. The disadvantages of RFA include that general anaesthesia is recommended for the procedure due to severe local pain, observation of the treated area by ultrasonography is difficult due to steam (bubbles) generated in the tissue during the treatment, and the possible development of transient local oedema or induration due to strong local reactions.

According to a survey conducted in fiscal year 2010 by the Japanese Breast Cancer Society, RFA was used to treat breast cancer in 1049 patients at 29 institutions in Japan. However, indications, standard procedures, and management systems varied. At many institutions, RFA was not used within the framework of clinical studies. To respond to this situation, the Japanese Breast Cancer Society requested the use of RFA for breast cancer as a part of clinical studies. Moreover, the Study Group for Minimally Invasive Treatment of Breast Cancer called for examination of the data obtained in the follow-up of patients and their quality of life. It therefore conducted a survey and reported the results at the general meeting of the American Society of Clinical Oncology in 2012. The results confirmed that outcomes for RFA and conservative treatment in Japan were similar for patients with early-stage breast cancer of 2 cm or less in diameter.

1.2 Overseas Studies on RFA

Studies on resection after RFA published from 1999 to date are summarised in Table 1.1 [1–13]. Although there were many studies, all were based at a single institution. The indications and devices used varied. The complete ablation rate ranged from 64% to 100%. The number of subjects in each study was small. None of these studies provided sufficient evidence to support RFA as a standard therapy.

Table 1.1 Studies of RFA followed by surgical excision

Author (year)	No. of Pts.	Disease (T)	Device	Power (W)	Median Treatment Time (min)	Complete Ablation (%)	Complications
Jeffery et al. (1999) [1]	5	T2-3	LeVeen	20–60	30	80	None
Izzo et al. (2001) [2]	26	T1-2	LeVeen	25–80	15	96	Skin burn ×1
Burak et al. (2003) [3]	10	T1	LeVeen	–	13.8	90	None
Singlatary et al. (2003) [4]	29	T1-2	RITA	–	–	86	Skin burn ×1
Hayashi et al. (2003) [5]	22	T1	RITA	–	15	64	Skin burn ×1
							Wound infection ×4
Fornage et al. (2004) [6]	20	T1	RITA	–	15	95	None
Noguchi et al. (2006) [7]	10	T1	RITA	–	15	100	None
Khatri et al. (2007) [8]	15	T1	Cool-tip	7–36	21	93	Skin puckering ×2
							Wound infection ×1
Medina-Franco et al. (2008) [9]	25	T1-2	Elektrotorm	–	11	76	Skin burn ×3
							Wound infection ×1
Garbay et al. (2008) [10]	10	IBTR, ≦3 cm	LeVeen	25–32	11	70	N/A
Imoto et al. (2009) [11]	30	T1	LeVeen	5–42	18	85	Skin burn ×2
							Muscle burn ×7
Kinoshita et al. (2011) [12]	49	T1-2,≦3 cm	Cool-tip	5–118	8.7	63	Skin burn ×2
		T1				89	Muscle burn ×3
Ohtani et al. (2011) [13]	41	T1	Cool-tip	9	9	88	Skin burn ×2

Table 1.2 Studies of cryoablation followed by surgical excision

Author (year)	No. of pts.	Tumour size (cm)	Complete ablation (%)
Pfleidere et al. (2002) [14]	16	0.9–4.0	31
Sabel et al. (2004) [15]	27	0.6–2.0	78
Pfleidere et al. (2005) [16]	29	0.5–1.5	100
Niu et al. (2007) [17]	27	0.8–2.5	85.2
Morin et al. (2007) [18]	25	1.2–6.0	52
Pusztaszeri et al. (2007) [19]	11	0.5–2.6	20
Manenti et al. (2011) [20]	15	0.4–1.2	93

1.3 Cryoablation

Cryoablation for the purpose of achieving haemostasis for ulcerating breast cancer is covered by the national health insurance system in Japan. However, its use as a radical cure of early-stage breast cancer is not covered. In the United States, cryoablation has been used for the treatment of benign tumours (fibroadenoma) for a long time. Cryoablation requires freezing and thawing for definite tumour destruction. At the same time, control of the ice ball is important. Because cryoablation involves freezing, local pain or reactions are minor and it only requires local anesthesia.

Studies on resection after cryoablation published from 2002 to 2011 are summarised in Table 1.2 [14–20]. The complete resection (freezing) rate ranged from 20% to 100%. The results of Study ACOSOG Z1072, a Phase II study of 87 lesions of early-stage breast cancer (including ductal carcinoma in situ), were reported at the meeting of the American Society of Breast Surgeons in 2014. Complete resection (freezing) was confirmed in 60 patients (69.0%). However, it was 100% effective for the treatment of tumours of 1 cm or less in diameter. Therefore, the investigators concluded that cryoablation was a new promising therapeutic option for early-stage breast cancer.

1.4 High-Intensity Focused Ultrasound (HIFU)

Ultrasound ablation is a truly noninvasive ablative technique because it does not require needle insertion or an incision at the tumour site. When an ultrasound beam is focused at a specific point at a certain distance from the transducer, the acoustic energy is converted to heat, leading to tissue coagulation. Frequencies in the range of 0.5–4 MHz can increase the temperature at the focal point to between 60 °C and 90 °C during a single sonication session.

A single ultrasound beam ablates only a small volume of tissue (approximately the size of a grain of rice), so the skin and surrounding tissue experience minimal temperature changes. Therefore, the entire volume of the tumour and margins need to be covered by overlapping multiple beams, which makes the procedure longer

Table 1.3 Studies of focused ultrasound followed by surgical excision

Author (year)	No. of pts.	Tumour size (cm)	Complete ablation (%)
Gianfekice et al. (2003) [21]	17	<3.5	24
Wu et al. (2003) [22]	23	2.0–4.7	100
Zippel and Papa (2005) [23]	10	<3.0	20
Furusawa et al. (2006) [24]	30	0.5–2.5	53.5
Khiat et al. (2006) [25]	26	0.01–11.2	27

than some of the other ablative techniques. Precise targeting for the procedure can be accomplished with MRI guidance.

There have been several studies examining the efficacy of HIFU at ablating breast cancer. As with other forms of ablation, the initial studies consisted of HIFU followed by resection, which have yielded mixed results (Table 1.3) [21–25].

Although the fact that HIFU is noninvasive, as opposed to cryoablation or RFA, which are minimally invasive, and is in some ways advantageous, it also presents some challenges. For example, there is a risk that if the target lesion moves during treatment, complete ablation might not be achieved. The biggest challenge facing the clinical implementation of HIFU for breast cancer is the heterogeneity of results, with histopathology analysis showing complete tumour necrosis in 20–100% of patients treated.

1.5 Studies on Noninvasive Surgical Treatment Without Subsequent Resection

Studies on nonsurgical ablative therapies without resection are summarised in Table 1.4 [26–32]. The number of subjects and duration of observation are both insufficient and the evidence supporting these therapies as new treatment methods is weak.

Another obstacle is that multiple steps are necessary to show equivalency with breast conservation surgery. Most data are from studies of ablation and resection, with strong data for cryoablation, HIFU, and RFA, but there is limited experience with ablation-only trials. The existing data are from small trials with highly selected groups of patients, and in some cases, remain unpublished. Although the completion of the ACOSOG Z1072 trial, a large-scale ablate-and-resect trial of cryoablation, represents a major step forward; a more concerted effort to design and implement multicentre trials is needed for in situ ablation to become a viable alternative to lumpectomy.

For RFA, the results of a large-scale Japanese multicentre clinical study, Radiofrequency Ablation Therapy for Early Breast Cancer as Local Therapy (the RAFAELO study) that began in 2013, are eagerly awaited.

Table 1.4 Studies of in situ ablation without surgical excision

Autor (year)	Type of ablation	No. of pts.	Tumour size (cm)	Posttreatment assessment	Results
Gianfelice et al. (2003) [26]	HIFU	24	0.6–2.5	MRI, CNB	5 (21 %) with residual disease
Wu et al. (2003) [27]	HIFU	22	<5	MRI, CT	5-year recurrence free survival of 89 %
Oura et al. (2007) [28]	RFA	52	<5	FNA, MRI	No local recurrences after median follow/up of 15 months
Furusawa et al. (2007) [29]	HIFU	21	0.5–5	MRI	1 local recurrence (5 %) with a median follow-up of 14 months
Littrup et al. (2009) [30]	Cryo	11	–	MRI	No local recurrences after median follow-up of 18 months
Yamamoto et al. (2011) [31]	RFA	29	Luminal A or DCIS, <1	VAB, MRI	No residual disease in 27/29
					No local recurrences after median follow-up of 17 months
Fukuma et al. (2012) [32]	Cryo	38	Luminal A or DCIS, <1	MRI, CNB	No local recurrences after median follow-up of 43 months

1.6 Conclusion

We expect that nonsurgical ablative therapies including RFA, which are used as minimally invasive local therapies for breast cancer, can achieve outcomes equivalent to surgical resection if the right procedure is carried out for the right indication. We began with evaluating RFA because it has been approved under the Pharmaceutical Affairs Law, thus we believed that it would become prevalent as a therapeutic method of breast cancer in Japan most quickly. In conclusion, we confirmed that cell death can be safely and completely achieved in targeted tumours. However, we identified remaining microscopic intraductal lesions that cannot be detected by diagnostic imaging as a potential problem; this phenomenon also occurs with conservative treatment of breast cancer. The results of long-term observation in prospective studies are awaited to determine whether these microscopic lesions can be controlled in the long term by radiotherapy or medications. Moreover, RFA devices and procedures need continuously to be developed and improved, and medium-to-long term safety, aesthetic outcomes, and capacity for local control need to be evaluated. Although cryoablation, which causes only minor local reactions, and HIFU, which truly does not involve any resection, are promising; given the current state of insufficient evidence, we think they should be used only in clinical studies after obtaining appropriate informed consent under an established monitoring system.

Data on nonsurgical ablative therapies including RFA, cryoablation, and HIFU are steadily accumulating. We believe these therapies can replace lumpectomy, the standard treatment for breast cancer, in the near future. This will trigger further advancement in the field of nonsurgical treatment, because science and technology greatly contribute to the progress of medical technology and diagnostic imaging.

This book was written by experts in nonsurgical ablative therapies for breast cancer and intended for medical professionals whose goal is to treat breast cancer nonsurgically. It is a compilation of their achievements. We hope that the readers will fully utilise this book in order to make future treatment of early-stage breast cancer even less invasive and gentler for patients.

These studies were supported in part by a Grant for Project Promoting Clinical Trials for Developing of New Drugs and Medical Devices from the Japan Agency for Medical Research and Development (AMED).

References

1. Jeffrey SS, et al. Radiofrequency ablation of breast cancer. Arch Surg. 1999;134:1064–8.
2. Izzo F, et al. Radiofrequency ablation in patients with primary breast carcinoma. Cancer. 2001;92:2036–44.
3. Burak WE, et al. Radiofrequency ablation of invasive breast carcinoma followed by delayed surgical resection. Cancer. 2003;98:1369–76.

4. Singletary SE, et al. Radiofrequency ablation for primary breast cancer. Breast Cancer. 2003;10:4–9.
5. Hayashi AH, et al. Treatment of invasive breast carcinoma with ultrasound-guided radiofrequency ablation. Am J Surg. 2003;185:429–35.
6. Fornage BD, et al. Small breast cancer treated with US-guided radiofrequency ablation: feasibility study. Radiology. 2004;231:215–24.
7. Noguchi M, et al. Radiofrequency ablation of small breast cancer followed by surgical resection. J Surg Oncol. 2006;93:120–8.
8. Khatri VP, et al. A phase II trial ogf image-guided radiofrequency ablation of small invasive breast carcinoma: use of saline-cooled tip electrode. Ann Surg Oncol. 2007;14:1644–52.
9. Medina-Franco H, et al. Radiofrequency ablation of invasive breast carcinoma: a phase II trial. Ann Surg Oncol. 2008;15:1689–95.
10. Garbay JR, et al. Radiofrequency thermal ablation of breast cancer local recurrence: a phase II clinical trial. Ann Surg Oncol. 2008;15:3222–6.
11. Imoto S, et al. Feasibility study on radiofrequency ablation followed by partial mastectomy for stage I breast cancer patients. Breast. 2009;18:130–4.
12. Kinoshita T, et al. Radiofrequency ablation as local therapy for early breast carcinomas. Breast Cancer. 2011;18:10–7.
13. Ohtani S, et al. Radiofrequency ablation of early breast cancer followed by delayed surgical resection. – A promising alternative to breast-conserving therapy. Breast. 2011;20(5):431–6.
14. Pfleiderer SO, Freesmeyer MG, Marx C, et al. Cryotherapy of breast cancer under ultrasound guidance: initial results and limitations. Eur Radiol. 2002;12:3009–14.
15. Sabel MS, Kaufman CS, Whitworth P, et al. Cryoablation of early-stage breast cancer: work-in-progress report of a multi-institutional trial. Ann Surg Oncol. 2004;11:542–9.
16. Pfleiderer SO, Marx C, Camara O, et al. Ultrasound-guided, percutaneous cryotherapy of small (<15mm) breast cancers. Invest Radiol. 2005;40(7):472–7.
17. Niu LZ, Xu KC, He WB, et al. Efficacy of percutaneous cryoablation for small solitary breast cancer in termpathologic evidence. Technol Cancer Res Treat. 2007;6:460–1.
18. Morin J, Traore' A, Dionne G, et al. Magnetic resonance-guided percutaneous cryosurgery of breast carcinoma: technique and early clinical results. Can J Surg. 2007;47:347–51.
19. Pusztaszeri M, Vlastos G, Kinkel K, et al. Histopathological study of breast cancer and normal breast tissue after magnetic resonance-guided cryotherapy ablation. Cryobiology. 2007;55 (1):44–51.
20. Manenti G, Perretta T, Gaspari E, et al. Percutaneous local ablation of unifocal subclinical breast cancer: clinical experience and preliminary results of cryotherapy. Eur Radiol. 2011;21:2344–53.
21. Gianfelice D, Khiat A, Amara M, et al. MRI imaging-guided focused ultrasound surgery of breast cancer: correlation of dynamic contrast-enhanced MRI with histopathologic findings. Breast Cancer Res Treat. 2003;12:32–8.
22. Wu F, Wang ZB, Cao YD, et al. A randomized clinical trial of high-intensity focused ultrasound ablation for the treatment of patients with localized breast cancer. Br J Cancer. 2003;89:2227–33.
23. Zippel DB, Papa MZ. The use of MR imaging guided focused ultrasound in breast cancer patients; a preliminary phase one study and review. Breast Cancer. 2005;12:32–8.
24. Furusawa H, Namba K, Thomsen S, et al. Magnetic resonance-guided focused ultrasound surgery of breast cancer: reliability and effectiveness. J Am Coll Surg. 2006;203:54–63.
25. Khiat A, Gianfelice D, Amara M, et al. Influence of post-treatment delay on the evaluation of the response to focused ultrasound surgery by breast cancer by dynamic contrast enhanced MRI. Br J Radiol. 2006;79:308–14.
26. Gianfelice D, Khiat A, Boulanger Y, et al. Feasibility of magnetic resonance imaging-guided focused ultrasound surgery as an adjuvant to tamoxifen therapy in high-risk surgical patients with breast carcinoma. J Vasc Interv Radiol. 2003;14:1275–82.

27. Wu F, Wang ZB, Zhu H, et al. Extracorporeal high intensity focused ultrasound treatment for patients with breast cancer. Breast Cancer Res Treat. 2005;92:51–60.
28. Oura S, Tamaki T, Hirai I, et al. Radiofrequency ablation therapy in patients with breast cancers two centimeters or less in size. Breast Cancer. 2007;14:48–54.
29. Furusawa H, Namba K, Nakahara H, et al. The evolving non-surgical ablation of breast cancer: MR guided focused ultrasound (MRgFUS). Breast Cancer. 2007;14:55–8.
30. Littrup PJ, Jallad B, Chandiwala-Mody P, et al. Cryotherapy for breast cancer: a feasibility study without excision. J Vasc Interv Radiol. 2009;20:1329–41.
31. Yamamoto N, Fujimoto H, Nakamura R, et al. Pilot study of radiofrequency ablation therapy without surgical excision for T1 breast cancer. Breast Cancer. 2011;18:3–9.
32. Fukuma E, Nakashima H, Tozaki M. Nonsurgical cryoablation for small breast cancer (oral presentation). In: American Society of Breast Surgeons 13th Annual Meeting, Edition. Phoenix, April 27–May 1;2012.

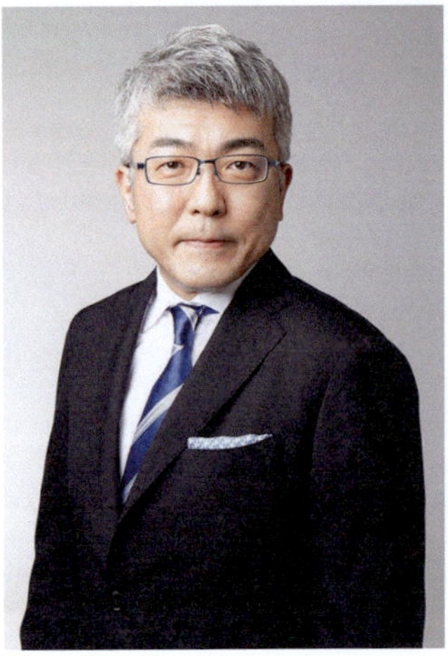

Takayuki Kinoshita

Chapter 2
Evolution of Operative Methods in Japan

Tadashi Ikeda

2.1 Evolution of Operative Methods in Japan

The first operation for a breast cancer patient was performed in the early nineteenth century in Wakayama (1804.11.14), Japan. This operation was performed by Seishu Hanaoka, a Japanese doctor, using general anesthesia [1]. The general anesthetic agent used was called Tsusen-san, which was an extract of Datura metel. This might have been the first breast cancer operation under general anesthesia in the world. After that, no further descriptions of the operative method for breast cancer patients were given in Japan.

The trends in the operative method for breast cancer in the modern era are about the same in Japan as in Western countries, but in Japan, the changes tend to occur more slowly. Notably, however, Shimada et al. reported the 5-year results of total mastectomy with axillary dissection compared to Halsted's mastectomy as early as 1964 [2]. Their comparison showed no difference between the two methods; however, this method did not become popular in Japan at that time.

According to the breast cancer registry of the Japanese Breast Cancer Society (JBCS) (Fig. 2.1) [3], standard radical mastectomy (Halsted's mastectomy), which consisted of total mastectomy with major and minor pectoral muscle resection and axillary dissection, was the most popular operative method until 1980. About 90 % of the cases underwent standard radical mastectomy. Then, modified radical mastectomy, which consisted of total mastectomy with/without minor pectoral muscle resection and axillary dissection, became the most popular operative method during the 1990s. There were several variations of the modified radical mastectomy, including Patey's modified radical mastectomy, Auchincloss' modified radical

T. Ikeda (✉)
Department of Surgery, Teikyo University School of Medicine, 2-11-1 Kaga, Itabashi-ku, Tokyo 160-8582, Japan
e-mail: ikedat@med.teikyo-u.ac.jp

T. Kinoshita (ed.), *Non-surgical Ablation Therapy for Early-stage Breast Cancer*,
DOI 10.1007/978-4-431-54463-0_2

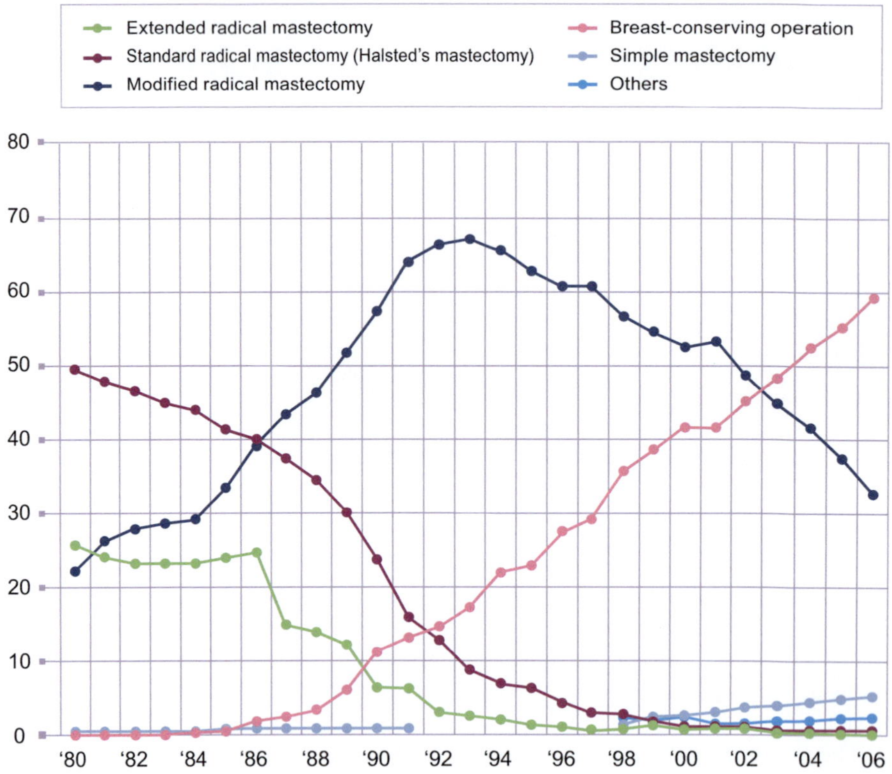

Fig. 2.1 Changing trends in surgical procedures for breast cancer in Japan between 1980 and 2006 (Ref. [3])

mastectomy, and Kodama's method. Patey's modified radical mastectomy was the most popular modified radical mastectomy approach at first, but Auchincloss' method became the most popular during the 1990s. Kodama's method is one type of modified radical mastectomy. High axillary dissection was performed by widening the interpectoral sulcus. With this method, level III axillary lymph nodes could be dissected under direct vision, and the prognosis was comparable to that of radical mastectomy [4].

Breast-conserving operations were initiated around 1986 in Japan. They rapidly increased after the reports of prospective, randomized trials from Western countries [5, 6], and over 60 % of the cases underwent breast-conserving operations in 2006. However, the incidence of breast-conserving operations plateaued at about 70 % in 2011 (Fig. 2.2) [7]. Initially, segmental resection was the most popular breast-conserving operation. At first, the breast-conserving operation was performed without postoperative radiation. With this method, ipsilateral intrabreast tumor recurrence (IBTR) developed in 5.5 % of the 1351 patients treated with breast-conserving operation during a mean follow-up period of 6.5 years [8], which is comparable to the results from Western countries. However, it should be noted that, according to the guideline in Japan for treating breast cancer at that time,

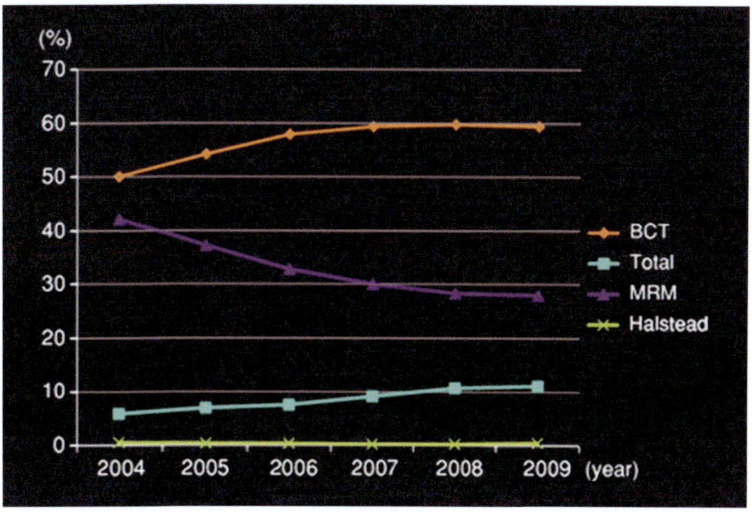

Fig. 2.2 Trends in surgical procedures for breast cancer in Japan from 2004 to 2009 (Ref. [7])

the definition of negative surgical margin was no cancer cells within 5 mm from the cut margin [9], while the definition in Western countries was no cancer cell exposure on the cut surface or within 1 mm [10].

Postoperative radiotherapy is an important component of breast-conserving therapy, and it reduces local recurrence by one-third [11]. Because of this evidence, as well as the operative trend from quadrantectomy (segmental mastectomy) to lumpectomy, lumpectomy with postoperative radiotherapy became the standard procedure for breast-conserving therapy in Japan. The rate of postoperative radiotherapy gradually increased from 60 % in 1992 to 72 % in 2004 and 79 % in 2009 [3, 7].

Because surgical margin status is an important predictive factor for local recurrence, patients with a positive surgical margin for cancer cells are candidates for re-excision. To reduce the reoperation rate, intraoperative frozen section diagnosis and/or print cytology of the surgical margin has been introduced [12]. Since about 27 % of the cases showed pathologically positive surgical margins at the cut end during breast-conserving operations, the evaluation of cut margin status during operation is now commonly performed in Japan.

Preoperative chemotherapy has become more common in Japan, as well as in Western countries, to increase the number of patients eligible for breast-conserving operation. According to the results from the NSABP-B18 trial, the breast-conserving rate increased from 60 % to 68 % after neoadjuvant therapy, while the in-breast recurrence rate increased from 7.6 % to 10.7 % [13]. The surgical margin should be carefully evaluated when performing breast-conserving operations after neoadjuvant chemotherapy, because the intraductal component may be more resistant to chemotherapy and it remains after neoadjuvant chemotherapy. It is important to know the tumor shrinkage pattern, including the concentric, honeycomb pattern, to achieve the appropriate surgical margin. Evaluation of the tumor shrinkage pattern after neoadjuvant chemotherapy by MRI is now commonly performed in Japan [14].

2.2 Surgical Procedures in Axillary Region

With respect to lymph node dissection, axillary dissection was the standard procedure for a lengthy period of time. Parasternal lymph node dissection and/or supraclavicular lymph node sampling were also performed concomitantly with axillary dissection. Level III dissection was also done in the early days, but it was soon abandoned based on the results of a randomized trial. The randomized trial compared level II dissection without minor pectoral muscle resection to level III dissection with minor pectoral muscle resection and showed no difference in terms of both overall and disease-free survival [15]. One other prospective, randomized trial that compared level I dissection to level III dissection also showed no difference in terms of overall survival [16]. Thus, the breast-conserving operation with level I/II dissection became the standard procedure.

However, after the first successful report of sentinel lymph node biopsy (SLNB) [17, 18], this technique was rapidly introduced to clinical settings. As the results of the sentinel node trials revealed no difference in terms of prognosis between SLNB and that of axillary dissection [19], SLNB has been accepted as a standard procedure for early breast cancer with no nodal involvement clinically [20]. According to the breast cancer registry under the auspices of JBCS, SLNB started in 1996, and about 40 % and 60 % of registered institutions began SLNB in 2006 and 2008, respectively. The most used method for SLNB is the blue dye method, followed by a combination method involving the radioisotope (RI) method and the blue dye method. The RI method alone was seldom performed [21]. Only Tc^{99m}-tin colloid and Tc^{99m}-stannous phytate are permitted as radioisotopes, and indocyanine green (ICG) and indigo carmine are permitted as dyes for SLNB by government health insurance. ICG and indigo carmine are proven to be safe, with grade 1 adverse effects occurring in only 0.06 % of patients [22]. Japanese government health insurance approved SLNB for patients with no clinical nodal involvement for reimbursement in 2012. SLNB has not only been accepted as a standard procedure in early breast cancer patients; it has also been accepted in various situations, including large breast cancer, after neoadjuvant chemotherapy, and in-breast cancer recurrence [23].

Given the results of ACOSOG Z-0011 [24], whether backup axillary dissection is needed in patients with 1–2 positive sentinel nodes remains controversial. There is considered to be insufficient evidence to not perform backup dissection, so omitting backup dissection in a patient with macrometastasis is not considered standard procedure in Japan [25]. However, omitting backup dissection has already begun in carefully selected patients at the time of 2013.

In recent years, molecular diagnosis of sentinel nodal metastases has been developed and is currently entering into clinical use [26, 27]. It is now validated to be as accurate as pathological diagnosis for the diagnosis of sentinel node metastasis.

2.3 Reconstruction

Though breast reconstruction after mastectomy has not been commonly performed in Japan, the rate of postmastectomy reconstruction is increasing. According to a questionnaire survey in 2007, about 60 % of the institutions belonging to JBCS did not perform reconstruction [28]. Reconstruction using a latissimus dorsi flap was the most used method, followed by a rectus abdominis flap, and tissue expander immediately after mastectomy. Because government health insurance started to cover breast reconstruction including tissue expander for patients who underwent mastectomy since 2006 and implants this year (2013), the rate of postmastectomy reconstruction is expected to increase. There are no exact statistics concerning secondary reconstruction, but the number of actual cases is considered small [28].

The number of reconstructions after breast-conserving operations is also not large. But among them, many patients who have undergone breast-conserving operations are looking for breast reconstruction due to deformity. Fat grafting is one of the promising methods to reform the deformed breast [29].

Many breast surgeons have noticed the need for oncoplastic surgical procedures during breast-conserving operations. However, there is as yet no established way to perform such procedures, because no method of evaluating the esthetic outcome has been established. One evaluation method that evaluated several issues, including volume, shape, scar, and firmness of the breasts and size, shape, color, and deviation of the nipples, was proposed by a working group of the JBCS [30]. In addition, the Japanese Society of Breast Oncoplastic Surgery was established in 2012.

2.4 Nonsurgical Ablation

The history and procedures for nonsurgical ablation are presented elsewhere in this book, so only the outline of the evolution of these procedures is presented here.

Radiofrequency (RF) ablation for the treatment of hepatocellular carcinoma (HCC) began in the early 1990s. HCC develops with a background of hepatitis B or C infection; therefore, multicentric development occurs. This means that another HCC could develop after resection of one HCC. With this in mind, less invasive methods have been investigated. One less invasive method is RF ablation, which has been covered by government health insurance since 2004. It has become a common treatment for HCC.

In the field of breast cancer treatment, as the concept that breast cancer is a generalized disease from the beginning has been widely accepted, the operative procedure has become less invasive. In addition, core needle biopsy (CNB) has become popular. By performing CNB, one can easily obtain information about hormone receptor status, Her2 overexpression, and other pathological features, which are essential pieces of information needed to plan the treatment of breast cancer patients in the modern era.

Keeping the above in mind, nonsurgical ablation has been tried in Japan. While most patients treated with nonsurgical ablation are treated by the RF method, a few patients are treated by cryoablation or high-intensity focused ultrasonic surgery (HIFU). Details of these methods are described elsewhere in this book. The merit of nonsurgical ablation is obviously a good cosmetic result. On the other hand, the criticisms of nonsurgical ablation include the following: its limited applicability for treating intraductal spreading beyond the main tumor; the completeness of ablation is not guaranteed unless pathological specimens are obtained; the location of the tumor should apart from the skin and/or muscle; and there are no mature data in terms of prognosis. Due to these reasons, nonsurgical ablation has not been presently accepted as a standard procedure to treat breast cancer patients [31] and has mainly been performed in only a clinical trial setting.

References

1. Matsuki A. A study on Seishu Hanaoka's "Nyugan Seimei Roku": a name list of breast cancer patients. (in Japanese). Nippon Ishigaku Zasshi. 2002;1:53–65.
2. Shimada N, Matsuda H, Amaaki T. Carcinoma of the breast. Comparative 5-year survival rates of Halsted's mastectomy and Shimada's mastectomy. Keio J Med. 1964;13:67–75.
3. Sonoo H, Noguchi S. Academic committee of the Japanese Breast Cancer Society: results of questionnaire survey on breast cancer surgery in Japan 2004–2006. Breast Cancer. 2008;15:3–4.
4. Kodama H. Modification of muscle-preserving radical mastectomy. Cancer. 1979;44:1517–22.
5. Veronesi U, Saccozzi R, Del Vecchio M, Banfi A, Clemente C, De Lena M, et al. Comparing radical mastectomy with quadrantectomy, axillary dissection, and radiotherapy in patients with small cancers of the breast. N Engl J Med. 1981;305:6–11.
6. Fisher B, Redmond C, Poisson R, Margolese R, Wolmark N, Wickerham L, et al. Eight-year of a randomized clinical trial comparing total mastectomy and lumpectomy with or without irradiation in the treatment of breast cancer. N Engl J Med. 1989;320:822–8.
7. Saji S, Hiraoka M, Tokuda Y, Fukui N, Ikeda T. Trends in local therapy application for early breast cancer patients in the Japanese Breast Cancer Society breast cancer registry during 2004–2009. Breast Cancer. 2012;19:1–3.
8. Kasumi F, Takahashi K, Nishimura S, Iijima K, Miyagi U, Tada K, et al. CIH-Tokyo experience with breast-conserving surgery without radiotherapy: 6.5 year follow-up results of 1462 patients. Breast J. 2006;12:S181–90.
9. Working group for establishing standardized breast conserving therapy under the auspecies of Japanese Ministry of Health and Welfare. Guideline of breast conserving therapy for the medical staffs (in Japanese). Tokyo: Kanehara Shuppan; 2005. p. 21–25.
10. Grobmyer SR, Cowher MS, Crowe JP. Optimizing clinical management of surgical margins in breast-conserving therapy for breast cancer. In: ASCO educational book. 2013.
11. Early Breast Cancer Trialists' Collaborative Group (EBCTCG), Darby S, McGale P, Correa C, Taylor C, Arriagada R, Clarke M, et al. Effect of radiotherapy after breast-conserving surgery on 10-year recurrence and 15-year breast cancer death: meta-analysis of individual patient data for 10,801 women in 17 randomised trials. Lancet. 2011;378:1707–16.
12. Ikeda T, Enomoto K, Wada K, Takeshima K, Yoneyama K, Furukawa J, et al. Frozen-section-guided breast conserving operation, implications of frozen section diagnosis as a guide to the extent of resection. Surg Today. 1997;27:207–12.

13. Wolmark N, Wang J, Mamounas E, Bryant J, Fisher B. Preoperative chemotherapy in patients with operable breast cancer: nine-year results from national surgical adjuvant breast and bowel project B-18. J Natl Cancer Inst Monogr. 2001;30:96–102.
14. Nakamura S, Kenjo H, Nishio T, Kazama T, Doi O, Suzuki K. Efficacy of 3D-MR mammography for breast conserving surgery after neoadjuvant chemotherapy. Breast Cancer. 2002;9:15–9.
15. Tominaga T, Takashima S, Danno M. Randomized clinical trial comparing level II and level III axillary node dissection in addition to mastectomy for breast cancer. Br J Surg. 2004;91:38–43.
16. Kodama H, Nio Y, Iguchi C, Kan N. Ten-year follow-up results of a randomised controlled study comparing level-I vs level-III axillary lymph node dissection for primary breast cancer. Br J Cancer. 2006;95:811–16.
17. Krag DN, Weaver DL, Alex JC, Fairbank JT. Surgical resection and radiolocalization of the sentinel lymph node in breast cancer using a gamma probe. Surg Oncol. 1993;2:335–9.
18. Giuliano AI, Kirgan DM, Guenther JM, Morton DL. Lymphatic mapping and sentinel lymphadenectomy for breast cancer. Ann Surg. 1994;220:391–8.
19. Krag DN, Anderson SJ, Julian TB, Brown AM, Harlow SP, Costantino JP, et al. Sentinel-lymph-node resection compared with conventional axillary-lymph-node dissection in clinically node-negative patients with breast cancer: overall survival findings from the NSABP B-32 randomised phase 3 trial. Lancet Oncol. 2010;11:927–33.
20. Evidence based guidelines to treat patients with breast cancer (in Japanese), ed by Japanese Breast Cancer Society, 2013. p. 208–11.
21. Tsugawa K, Nakamura S. The results of a questionnaire survey on sentinel lymph node biopsy for breast cancer patients in Japan (in Japanese). Nyu-gan no Rinsho (Jpn J Breast Cancer). 2009;24:265–70.
22. Nakamura S. Current status of sentinel node biopsy for breast cancer in Japan. In: Toi M, Winer EP, editors. Local and systemic management of primary breast cancers. Kyoto: Kyoto University Press; 2010. p. 54–60.
23. Yorozuya K, Ikeda T. Sentinel node biopsy under specific conditions. In: Sonoo H, Fukuda M, Ikeda T, Saeki H, Shikama N, editors. Korekarano Nyuuganshinryou 2013–2014 (breast cancer management in the future) (in Japanese). Tokyo: Kanehara Shuppann; 2013. p. 43–50.
24. Giuliano AE, Hunt KK, Ballman KV, Beitsch PD, Whitworth PW, Blumencranz PW, et al. Axillary dissection vs no axillary dissection in women with invasive breast cancer and sentinel node metastasis. A randomized clinical trial ACOSOGZ0011. JAMA. 2011;305:569–75.
25. Evidence based guidelines to treat patients with breast cancer (in Japanese), ed by Japanese Breast Cancer Society, 2013. p. 216–8.
26. Iinuma H, Tamura J, Omoto D, Kamo N, Ohnaka S, Mitoma Y, et al. Accurate and rapid novel genetic diagnosis for detection of sentinel lymph node metastasis in breast cancer patients. Br J Cancer. 2012;107:724–31.
27. Tamaki Y, Akiyama F, Iwase T, Kaneko T, Tsuda H, Sato K, et al. Molecular detection of lymph node metastases in breast cancer patients: results of a multicenter trial using the one-step nucleic acid amplification assay. Clin Cancer Res. 2009;15:2879–84.
28. Yano K, Tamaki Y. Results of questionnaire survey on the actual medical status of breast reconstruction (in Japanese). Nyuugan-no Rinsho (Clin Breast Cancer). 2007;22:509–14.
29. Asano Y. Cell-assisted lipotransfection to the deformity after breast conserving operation. In: Sonoo H, Fukuda M, Ikeda T, Saeki H, Shikama N, editors. Korekarano Nyuugan Shinryo 2011–2012 (breast cancer management in the future). Tokyo: Kanehara Shuppann; 2011. p. 25–30.
30. Sawai K, Nakajima H, Ishihara S, Yano K, Watanabe O, Kitamura K, et al. Study on the evaluation of deformity after breast conserving operation in relation to resected volume (in Japanese). Proceedings of the 12nd congress of the Japanese Breast Cancer Society; 2004. p. 107.

31. Evidence based guidelines to treat patients with breast cancer (in Japanese), ed by Japanese Breast Cancer Society, 2013 p. 236–7.

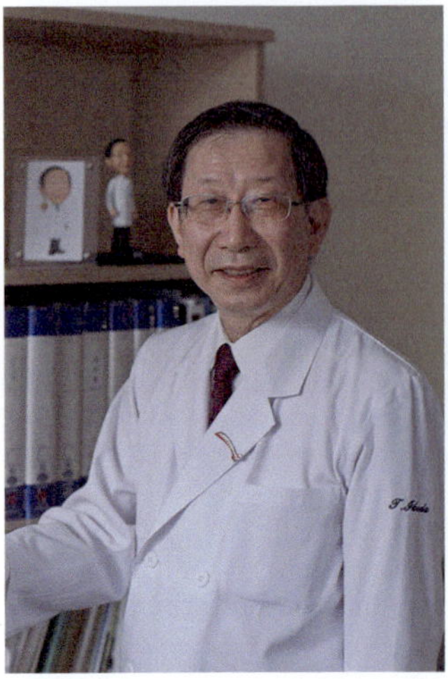

Tadashi Ikeda

Chapter 3
New Trends and Development in Breast Surgery

Takashi Shigekawa and Toshiaki Saeki

3.1 Introduction

Several large, randomized clinical trials have been conducted to define surgical treatment of breast cancer. In this chapter, new trends and developments in breast cancer surgery, including appropriate breast-conserving therapy (BCT), accelerated postoperative irradiation, skin-sparing mastectomy and nipple and areola sparing mastectomy (SSM/NSM) with immediate reconstruction, and sentinel lymph node biopsy (SLNB) for axillary staging, have been described.

3.2 Breast Surgery

BCT comprised the excision of tumors with negative surgical margins, axillary surgery, and postoperative irradiation. In the 1980s, six prospective, randomized clinical trials were conducted worldwide to compare BCT with mastectomy, but none revealed any significant difference in the overall survival (OS) between the two arms for early-stage invasive breast cancer [1–7]. However, in these meta-analyses indicated therapeutic equivalence [8, 9]. BCT has been increasingly accepted as a treatment option for stage I and II and selected stage III breast cancer cases. According to the Japanese Breast Cancer Society Breast Cancer Registry, BCT was performed more frequently compared with mastectomy for early-stage breast cancer patients from 2004 to 2009 in Japan [10].

T. Shigekawa (✉) • T. Saeki
Breast Oncology Service, Saitama Medical University International Medical Center, 1397-1 Yamane, Hidaka, Saitama 350-1298, Japan
e-mail: t.shigekawa@gmail.com

T. Kinoshita (ed.), *Non-surgical Ablation Therapy for Early-stage Breast Cancer*,
DOI 10.1007/978-4-431-54463-0_3

The choice of appropriate patients is important for successful BCT. The absolute contraindications for BCT include the following:

1. Multicentric cancers in different quadrants of the breast
2. Diffuse ductal metastasis (diffuse malignant calcifications on mammography)
3. The cases that cannot receive radiotherapy because of radiation-induced acute and late onset toxicities (history of prior radiotherapy or connective tissue diseases such as active systemic lupus erythematosus or scleroderma)
4. Positive surgical margins after multiple re-excisions

Although tumor size itself is not a contraindication for BCT, both adequate resection with negative margins and acceptable cosmetic results should be accomplished for successful BCT. Previous meta-analyses revealed that neoadjuvant chemotherapy can effectively decrease the tumor size and successfully improve the rate of BCT [11].

Few studies have reported that the rate of local–regional recurrence (LRR) is higher following BCT than mastectomy [1, 4]. Although LRR was thought to not affect OS, a meta-analysis performed by the Early Breast Cancer Trialists' Collaborative Group reported that the higher rate of LRR led to a poorer survival rate [8]; therefore, the risk of LRR should not be overlooked.

One of the most important factors of LRR following BCT is the surgical margin status [12–14]. Although there is no international standard definition of positive surgical margins, in Japan, it has been defined as a positive margin with cancer cells detected at 5 mm or less from the surgical edge. In case of positive margin status (margin exposure $\leq$5 mm), additional re-excision is recommended to achieve a negative margin status. According to the National Comprehensive Cancer Network (NCCN), margins less than 1 mm are considered inadequate [15, 16].

Of the BCT methods discussed so far, only conventional radiotherapy has been evaluated. Conventional radiotherapy delivers 45–50 Gy to the whole breast over 4–5 weeks, which has been considered to effectively decrease the LRR incidence, distant recurrence, and death [17]. Recently, the focus of BCT has increasingly shifted to cosmetic outcome, quality of life, and patient satisfaction; further, accelerated irradiation schedules have increased the convenience of conventional radiation therapy. In a meta-analysis, it was concluded that accelerated irradiation schedules were equivalent to conventional radiation therapy with regard to LRR, OS, breast cosmesis, and early and late onset toxicities [18]. Moreover, because most ipsilateral breast tumor recurrences (IBTRs) occur near the lumpectomy cavity, accelerated partial breast irradiation (APBI) has been developed. APBI delivers higher doses of radiation focused to a limited tissue volume over a shorter period of time to achieve less toxicity, decreased costs, and increased convenience. APBI may enable repeated BCT in case with LRR outside of the previous irradiated cavity. Currently, APBI is being evaluated in a large clinical trial by the National Surgical Adjuvant Breast and Bowel Project (NSABP) and the Radiation Therapy Oncology Group (RTOG) (NSABP B-39/RTOG 0413).

At present, BCT has become a well-established procedure worldwide, and the other modalities that enable noninvasive treatment of primary tumors, including percutaneous ablation, radiofrequency ablation, and cryoablation, have been the focus of several clinical trials that are now ongoing worldwide.

SSM for breast cancer has been widely applied to preserve a majority of the natural skin envelope of the breast. With this procedure, immediate reconstruction is possible to improve the cosmetic outcome [19]. A meta-analysis of such retrospective studies reported no significant difference in the local recurrence rates between patients undergoing SSM with immediate reconstruction and those undergoing conventional mastectomy without reconstruction [20]. More recently, in carefully selected patients, NSM has been performed to preserve the entire natural skin envelope of the breast and allow immediate reconstruction. However, no randomized trials with long-term follow-up periods have been conducted to examine the utility and safety of SSM/NSM; therefore, it is necessary to carefully select patients suitable for SSM/NSM.

3.3 Axillary Staging

Axillary status is one of the most important prognostic factors to predict the outcomes of breast cancer treatment. ALND remains the standard method in clinically node-negative patients and is important for LRR, but its impact on OS is unclear.

The NSABP B-04 trial was performed as two parallel trials, one for clinically node-negative patients and the other for clinically node-positive patients (Fig. 3.1)

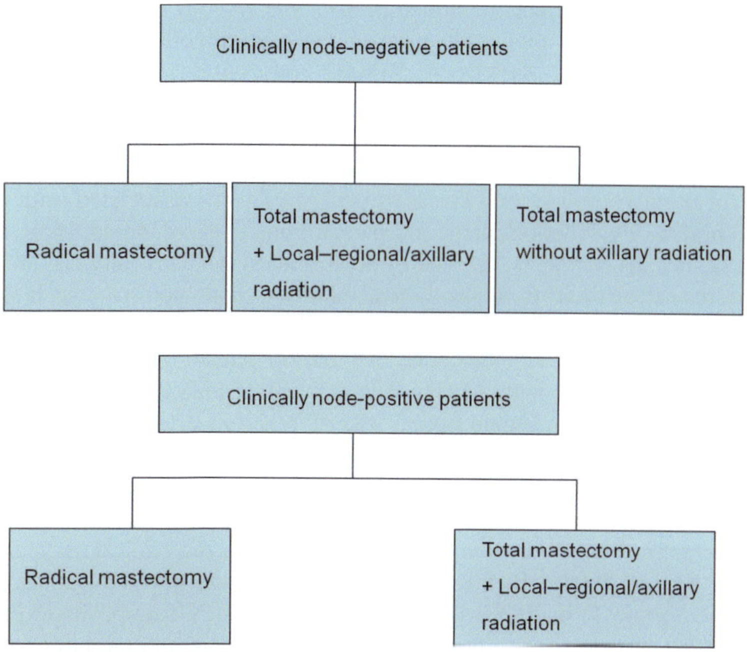

Fig. 3.1 Schema for NSABP B-04 trial

to compare radical mastectomy with less extensive surgical treatments [21]. Between 1971 and 1974, 1079 patients with clinically node-negative disease were randomized to undergo radical mastectomy ($N = 362$), total mastectomy plus local–regional/axillary radiation ($N = 352$), or total mastectomy without axillary radiation ($N = 365$), whereas 586 patients with clinically node-positive disease were randomized to undergo radical mastectomy ($N = 292$) or total mastectomy plus radiation ($N = 294$). None of the patients received systemic treatment [21]. In 2002, 25-year follow-up data were reported, which revealed no significant differences with respect to disease-free survival (DFS), distant disease-free survival (DDFS), and OS among the three groups of patients with clinically node-negative disease or the two groups of patients with clinically node-positive disease [22]. In the clinically node-negative arm, the LRR incidence was lower in the patients who underwent total mastectomy plus radiation (5 %) than in those who underwent radical mastectomy (9 %) or total mastectomy alone (13 %; $P = 0.002$). In the clinically node-positive arm, the LRR incidence revealed no significant difference: 16 % in patients who underwent radical mastectomy and 14 % in those who underwent total mastectomy plus radiation ($P = 0.67$). In this trial, 40 % clinically node-negative patients who underwent radical mastectomy revealed pathological lymph node involvement; therefore, it can be assumed that 40 % clinically node-negative patients who underwent total mastectomy without radiation also had pathological lymph node involvement; however, only 19 % (68/365) patients subsequently experienced nodal recurrence and then underwent ALND. The median time from mastectomy to identification of axillary metastases was 15 months (range, 3–135 months), and most cases were identified within 2 years from the initial surgery. These patients remained in the same arm for survival analyses.

Similarly, in the meta-analysis to compare patients with clinically node-negative disease with or without ALND, ALND did not confer a survival advantage, although the rate of axillary recurrence was decreased [23]. These data suggested that routine ALND for clinically node-negative patients is unnecessary and that ALND after the diagnosis of clinically evident disease in the axilla did not have a significant negative impact on OS. However, ALND was associated with lymphedema, shoulder dysfunction, pain, and paresthesias [24–26]. In addition, in clinically node-negative patients, the rate of nodal metastases was only 20–35 % [27–29]. The results of these trials promoted a shift to more noninvasive breast and axillary surgery.

SLNB was developed as an accurate method to evaluate the axillary status with less morbidity compared with ALND. The concept of SLNB, which was the first method designed to drain lymph nodes, was proposed as a treatment modality for melanoma in the late 1980s and early 1990s [30, 31]. Since Giuliano et al. first reported the results of SLNB for breast cancer treatment [32], larger trials have been conducted to evaluate SLNB as a staging procedure for clinically node-negative breast cancer. The NSABP B-32 trial was a large randomized clinical trial conducted between 1999 and 2004, which randomized 5611 patients into two groups: SLNB plus ALND (group 1) or SLNB plus ALND (only if SLN was positive; group 2) (Fig. 3.2). The primary endpoints were OS, regional control, and morbidity, whereas

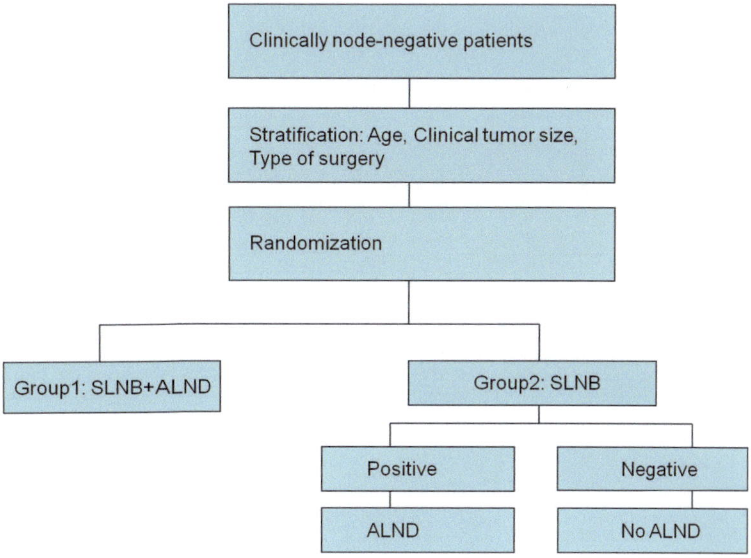

Fig. 3.2 Schema for NSABP B-32 trial

the secondary endpoints were accuracy and technical success [33]. The initial results of technical success and accuracy in 5536 patients were reported in 2007, which revealed that SLN was identified in 5379 patients (97 %) and was positive in 26 % patients in both groups. In group 1, the accuracy of SLNB was 97 %, and the false negative rate was 9.8 %. The OS results were reported in 2010 [33]. A total of 3986 patients with pathologically negative SLN were compared. The two groups were well balanced with regard to age, clinical tumor size, and type of surgery. The use of systemic therapy and radiation was similar between the groups. The 5-year Kaplan–Meier estimates for OS were 97 % and 95 % in groups 1 and 2, respectively, and the 8-year estimates were 92 % and 90 %, respectively ($P=0.12$). Further, the 8-year estimates for DFS were 82 % in both groups, and the rates of regional control were similar as well. Because the OS, DFS, and regional control rates between these treatment groups were equivalent, it was concluded that if SLN is negative, SLNB alone (without ALND) is appropriate for axillary status staging.

Although omission of ALND in patients with a negative SLN has become standard, ALND is recommended for SLN-positive patients [34, 35]. However, the results of the NSABP B-04 trial indicated no survival advantage for patients who received ALND at the time of the initial surgery; further, considering the improvements in systemic treatment, ALND may not be necessary in all SLN-positive patients. To determine whether SLN-positive patients require ALND, the American College of Surgeons Oncology Group (ACOSOG) conducted the Z-0011 trial, which enrolled patients with clinical T1 or T2, N0, M0 breast cancer who underwent BCT and revealed one or two positive SLNs by hematoxylin and eosin staining (Fig. 3.3). These patients were randomized into two arms: those in arm 1 underwent ALND,

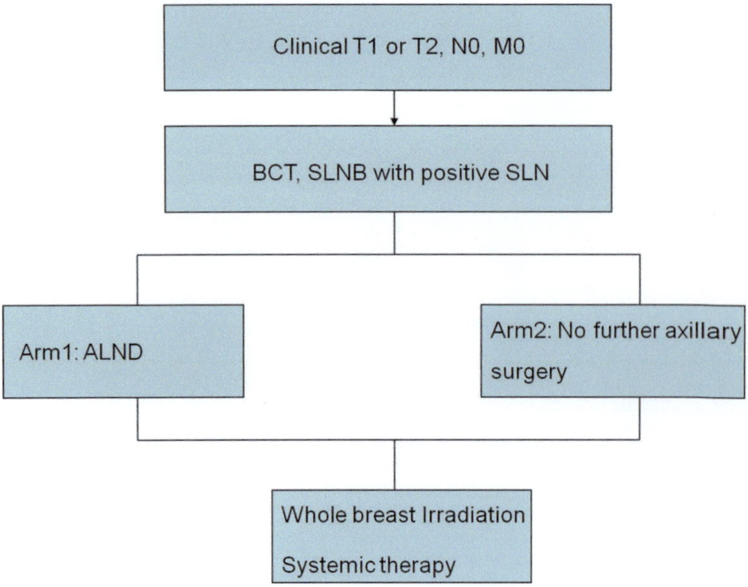

Fig. 3.3 Schema for ACOSOG Z0011 trial

whereas those in arm 2 received no further axillary surgery. All the patients received postoperative whole breast irradiation and were recommended for systemic treatment. The primary endpoint was OS, and the secondary endpoint was DFS. Although this trial was designed for 1900 patients, and enrollment in the trial was initiated in 1999, it was closed in early 2004 after 891 patients were enrolled and randomized (arm 1, 445 patients; arm 2, 446 patients). The reasons for early closure were slow accrual and a lower event rate than anticipated at the time of the study design. Micrometastases were identified in SLNs of 45 % patients in arm 1 and 38 % patients in arm 2. Additional positive lymph nodes were identified in 27 % patients in arm 1. Adjuvant systemic treatment was administered in 96 % patients (chemotherapy, 58 %; hormonal treatment, 46 %) in arm 1 and 97 % patients (chemotherapy, 58 %; hormonal therapy, 47 %) in arm 2. After a median follow-up period of 6.3 years, only 29 incidences of LRR were reported among all patients. The local recurrence rate was 4 % in arm 1 and 2 % in arm 2. Recurrence of the ipsilateral axilla was very rare (0.5 % and 0.9 % in the arms 1 and 2, respectively) [36], and there were no differences in OS or DFS between the two groups. On the basis of these results, the ACOSOG investigators concluded that ALND may be safely omitted in selected patients in line with the eligibility criteria of this trial; however, this trial did not include the following patients: those with T3 tumors, those who underwent mastectomy, those who received neoadjuvant chemotherapy, or those who were administered APBI. Therefore, the ACOSOG investigators cautioned that ALND remains the standard treatment for SLN-positive patients. Further, the International Breast Cancer Study Group (IBCSG) 23-01 trial to investigate the necessity of ALND in SLN-positive patients is currently ongoing. The eligibility criteria were as follows: clinically node negative, breast tumors ≤5 cm, and SLN micrometastasis (≤2 mm). The patients were randomized into two groups: ALND or no further axillary surgery. Unlike the Z-0011 trial, patients who underwent mastectomy were eligible for enrollment. The primary endpoint was DFS, and the secondary endpoints were OS and systemic DFS. Although this trial was designed for 1960 patients, its enrollment began in 2001 and was closed early in 2010 after 934 patients were randomized. The reasons for early closure of the IBCSG 23-01 trial were the same as those for the Z-0011 trial. The initial results were presented in 2011, and after a median follow-up period of 49 months, the 4-year DFS rate was 91 %. The first comparison of outcomes between the two groups will be reported after a median follow-up of 5 years. Considering the low DFS event rate in the IBCSG 23-01 trial, ALND may be omitted in patients undergoing mastectomy with micrometastatic SLNs.

3.4 Summary

Surgical treatments for breast cancer have been developed through randomized clinical trials conducted over the past few decades, ranging from the Halsted radical mastectomy to more noninvasive surgeries. Currently, most patients are able to receive personalized surgical treatment with cosmetically acceptable outcomes as well as favorable oncological outcomes, although other modalities to treat a primary tumor in a more noninvasive way have also attracted attention, including percutaneous ablation, radiofrequency ablation, and cryoablation, which have been assessed in several clinical trials.

References

1. Veronesi U, Cascinelli N, Mariani L, et al. Twenty-year follow-up of a randomized study comparing breast-conserving surgery with radical mastectomy for early breast cancer. N Engl J Med. 2002;347(16):1227–32.
2. Fisher B, Anderson S, Bryant J, et al. Twenty-year follow-up of a randomized trial comparing total mastectomy, lumpectomy, and lumpectomy plus irradiation for the treatment of invasive breast cancer. N Engl J Med. 2002;347(16):1233–41.
3. van Dongen JA, Bartelink H, Fentiman IS, et al. Factors influencing local relapse and survival and results of salvage treatment after breast-conserving therapy in operable breast cancer: EORTC trial 10801, breast conservation compared with mastectomy in TNM stage I and II breast cancer. Eur J Cancer. 1992;28A(4–5):801–5.
4. van Dongen JA, Voogd AC, Fentiman IS, et al. Long-term results of a randomized trial comparing breast-conserving therapy with mastectomy: European organization for research and treatment of cancer 10801 trial. J Natl Cancer Inst. 2000;92(14):1143–50.
5. Poggi MM, Danforth DN, Sciuto LC, et al. Eighteen-year results in the treatment of early breast carcinoma with mastectomy versus breast conservation therapy: the National Cancer Institute randomized trial. Cancer. 2003;98(4):697–702.

6. Blichert-Toft M, Rose C, Andersen JA, et al. Danish randomized trial comparing breast conservation therapy with mastectomy: six years of life-table analysis. Danish Breast Cancer Cooperative Group. J Natl Cancer Inst Monogr. 1992;11:19–25.
7. Arriagada R, Lê MG, Rochard F, et al. Conservative treatment versus mastectomy in early breast cancer: patterns of failure with 15 years of follow-up data. Institut Gustave-Roussy Breast Cancer Group. J Clin Oncol. 1996;14(5):1558–64.
8. Clarke M, Collins R, Darby S, et al. Effects of radiotherapy and of differences in the extent of surgery for early breast cancer on local recurrence and 15-year survival: an overview of the randomised trials. Lancet. 2005;366(9503):2087–106.
9. Morris AD, Morris RD, Wilson JF, et al. Breast-conserving therapy vs mastectomy in early-stage breast cancer: a meta-analysis of 10-year survival. Cancer J Sci Am. 1997;3(1):6–12.
10. Saji S, Hiraoka M, Tokuda Y, et al. Trends in local therapy application for early breast cancer patients in the Japanese Breast Cancer Society breast cancer registry during 2004–2009. Breast Cancer. 2012;19(1):1–3.
11. Gralow JR, Burstein HJ, Wood W. Preoperative therapy in invasive breast cancer: pathologic assessment and systemic therapy issues in operable disease. J Clin Oncol. 2008;26(5):814–19.
12. Park CC, Mitsumori M, Nixon A. Outcome at 8 years after breast-conserving surgery and radiation therapy for invasive breast cancer: influence of margin status and systemic therapy on local recurrence. J Clin Oncol. 2000;18(8):1668–75.
13. Singletary SE. Surgical margins in patients with early-stage breast cancer treated with breast conservation therapy. Am J Surg. 2002;184(5):383–93.
14. Houssami N, Macaskill P, Marinovich ML. Meta-analysis of the impact of surgical margins on local recurrence in women with early-stage invasive breast cancer treated with breast-conserving therapy. Eur J Cancer. 2010;46(18):3219–32.
15. Morrow M. Breast conservation and negative margins: how much is enough? Breast. 2009; Suppl 18(3):S84–86.
16. Blair SL, Thompson K, Rococco J, et al. Attaining negative margins in breast-conservation operations: is there a consensus among breast surgeons? J Am Coll Surg. 2009;209(5):608–13.
17. Darby S, McGale P, Correa C. Effect of radiotherapy after breast-conserving surgery on 10-year recurrence and 15-year breast cancer death: meta-analysis of individual patient data for 10,801 women in 17 randomised trials. Lancet. 2011;378(9804):1707–16.
18. James ML, Lehman M, Hider PN. Fraction size in radiation treatment for breast conservation in early breast cancer. Cochrane Database Syst Rev. 2010;10(11):CD003860.
19. Simmons RM, Adamovich TL. Skin-sparing mastectomy. Surg Clin North Am. 2003;83 (4):885–99.
20. Lanitis S, Tekkis PP, Sgourakis G, et al. Comparison of skin-sparing mastectomy versus non-skin-sparing mastectomy for breast cancer: a meta-analysis of observational studies. Ann Surg. 2010;251(4):632–9.
21. Fisher B, Montague E, Redmond C, et al. Comparison of radical mastectomy with alternative treatments for primary breast cancer. A first report of results from a prospective randomized clinical trial. Cancer. 1977;39:2827–39.
22. Fisher B, Jeong JH, Anderson S, et al. Twenty-five-year follow-up of a randomized trial comparing radical mastectomy, total mastectomy, and total mastectomy followed by irradiation. N Engl J Med. 2002;347(8):567–75.
23. Sanghani M, Balk EM, Cady B. Impact of axillary lymph node dissection on breast cancer outcome in clinically node negative patients: a systematic review and meta-analysis. Cancer. 2009;115(8):1613–20.
24. Fleissig A, Fallowfield LJ, Langridge CI, et al. Post-operative arm morbidity and quality of life. Results of the ALMANAC randomised trial comparing sentinel node biopsy with standard axillary treatment in the management of patients with early breast cancer. Breast Cancer Res Treat. 2006;95(3):279–93.
25. Lucci A, McCall LM, Beitsch PD, et al. Surgical complications associated with sentinel lymph node dissection (SLND) plus axillary lymph node dissection compared with SLND alone in the

American College of surgeons oncology group trial Z0011. J Clin Oncol. 2007;25(24):3657–63.
26. Erickson VS, Pearson ML, Ganz PA, et al. Arm edema in breast cancer patients. J Natl Cancer Inst. 2001;93(2):96–111.
27. Krag DN, Anderson SJ, Julian TB, et al. Technical outcomes of sentinel-lymph-node resection and conventional axillary-lymph-node dissection in patients with clinically node-negative breast cancer: results from the NSABP B-32 randomised phase III trial. Lancet Oncol. 2007;8(10):881–8.
28. Giuliano AE, Hawes D, Ballman KV, et al. Association of occult metastases in sentinel lymph nodes and bone marrow with survival among women with early-stage invasive breast cancer. JAMA. 2011;306(4):385–93.
29. Veronesi U, Paganelli G, Viale G, et al. A randomized comparison of sentinel-node biopsy with routine axillary dissection in breast cancer. N Engl J Med. 2003;349(6):546–53.
30. Cabanas RM. An approach for the treatment of penile carcinoma. Cancer. 1977;39(2):456–66.
31. Morton DL, Wen DR, Wong JH, et al. Technical details of intraoperative lymphatic mapping for early stage melanoma. Arch Surg. 1992;127(4):392–9.
32. Giuliano AE, Kirgan DM, Guenther JM, et al. Lymphatic mapping and sentinel lymphadenectomy for breast cancer. Ann Surg. 1994;220(3):391–8.
33. Krag DN, Anderson SJ, Julian TB, et al. Sentinel-lymph-node resection compared with conventional axillary-lymph-node dissection in clinically node-negative patients with breast cancer: overall survival findings from the NSABP B-32 randomised phase 3 trial. Lancet Oncol. 2010;11(10):927–33.
34. Lyman GH, Giuliano AE, Somerfield MR, et al. American Society of clinical oncology guideline recommendations for sentinel lymph node biopsy in early-stage breast cancer. J Clin Oncol. 2005;23(30):7703–20.
35. National Comprehensive Cancer Network. Clinical practice guidelines in oncology: breast. National Comprehensive Cancer Network; 2008. Version 2.
36. Giuliano AE, McCall L, Beitsch P, et al. Locoregional recurrence after sentinel lymph node dissection with or without axillary dissection in patients with sentinel lymph node metastases: the American College of Surgeons oncology Group Z0011 randomized trial. Ann Surg. 2010;252(3):426–32.

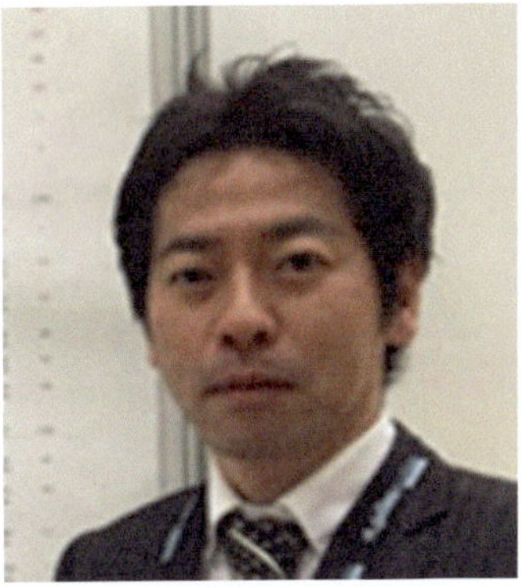

Takashi Shigekawa

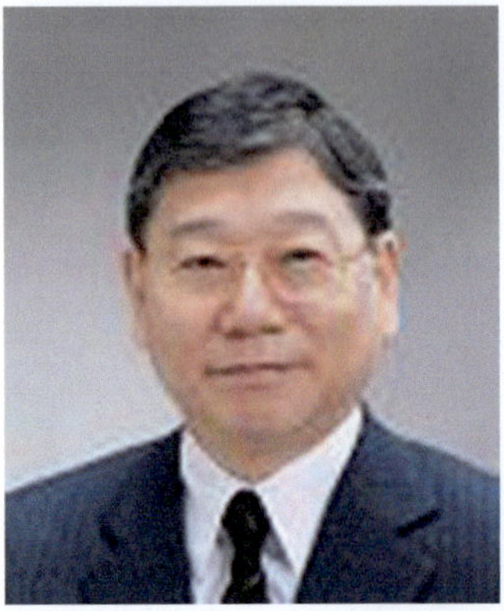

Toshiaki Saeki

Chapter 4
A Theory of Radiofrequency Ablation (RFA)

Kenjiro Jimbo and Takayuki Kinoshita

4.1 Theory of RFA

4.1.1 Electric Field, Magnetic Field, and Electromagnetic Waves

In 1820, the French physicist André Marie Ampere (1775–1836) discovered that a unidirectional, concentric magnetic force (magnetic field) is produced around the electric current flowing in a conducting wire (Ampere's law;Fig. 4.1-a). And in 1831, the English physicist Michael Faraday (1791–1867) demonstrated that a current (an electric field) is induced in a circuit when a magnetic field is produced within the centre of a coil-shaped conducting wire (inside the circuit) and the electric field is induced according to the temporal fluctuations of that magnetic field (Faraday's law of electromagnetic induction;Fig. 4.1-b). Based on these two fundamental principles, the English physicist James Clerk Maxwell (1831–1879) established electromagnetism, and in 1868, showed that an electromagnetic wave is a transverse wave that is generated in a process where electric and magnetic fields are produced alternately. This is a theory whereby the magnetic field generated from an oscillating electric current gives rise to an electric field in a chain-interaction in which a further, subsequent magnetic field is created, and so on, which forms an electromagnetic wave. In other words, an electromagnetic wave was confirmed to be a wave motion due to an oscillation that comprises a fluctuation in the vacuum of the electric and magnetic fields (Fig. 4.1-c).

K. Jimbo (✉) • T. Kinoshita
Surgical Oncology Division, National Cancer Center Hospital, 5-1-1 Tsukiji, Chuo-ku, Tokyo 104-0045, Japan
e-mail: kjimbo@ncc.go.jp

T. Kinoshita (ed.), *Non-surgical Ablation Therapy for Early-stage Breast Cancer*,
DOI 10.1007/978-4-431-54463-0_4

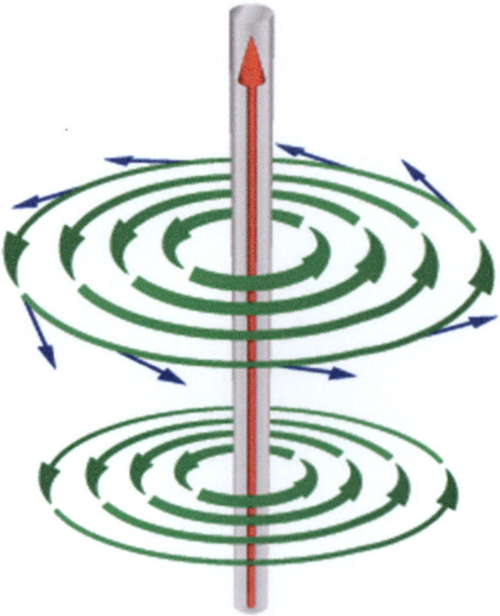

Fig. 4.1-a Ampere's law. A current flowing in a coil generates a magnetic field around it in an anticlockwise sense. The magnetic field is proportional to the strength of the current, and is inversely proportional to the distance from the current

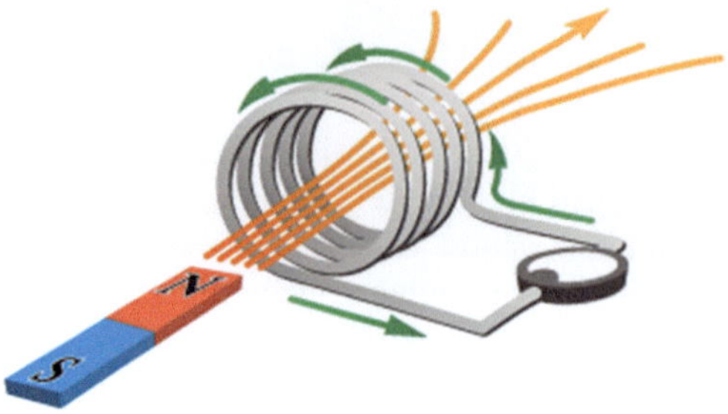

Fig. 4.1-b Faraday's law of electromagnetic induction. The magnetic field which is generated in a closed circuit enclosed by a coil induces a current in that circuit. The current flows in a direction so as to generate an opposing magnetic field which acts to cancel out the magnetic field generated. The current produced depends on the temporal fluctuations of the magnetic field

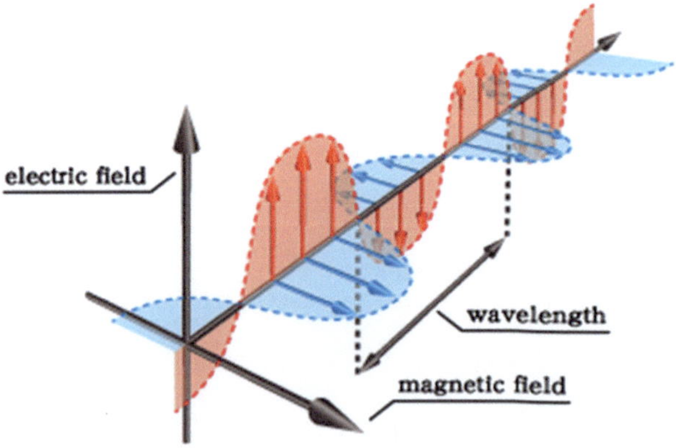

Fig. 4.1-c Maxwell's electromagnetic wave. The electric and magnetic fields are generated alternately to form a wave. It is a chain reaction in which, alternately, the electric field creates a magnetic field, and that magnetic field then creates an electric field, and so on. The wave progresses at the speed of light

4.2 RF (Radio Frequency) and Joule Heat

Electromagnetic waves are classified according to their wavelength, being broadly divided from the short wavelength side into radiation, light, and then radio waves in that order. RF has been defined in electrical engineering as those electromagnetic waves with frequencies in the range (10 kHz–100 GHz). Electromagnetic waves have been applied in various fields in everyday life for each respective frequency (Table 4.1). The RF used in breast cancer therapy is classified as a medium-frequency electromagnetic wave with a frequency range of 460–480 kHz. Due to the RF alternating electromagnetic wave passing into the surrounding tissue from an electrode introduced into a lesion, the molecular ions in the tissue induce molecular vibration. Frictional heating (Joule heat) occurs from the fluctuation of these ionic charges, and thermal coagulation necrosis occurs at the target site. RFA is a medical treatment due to tissue ablation that makes use of this thermal coagulation necrosis. The treatment apparatus requires an RF generator and a puncture electrode to excite the RF within the body, as well as a return electrode to collect the RF current. The electromagnetic wave current that is flowing around inside the body is then recovered by the earthed return electrode.

The Joule heat generated due to the RF is understood from the simple formula given below.

Table 4.1 Type, frequency, and practical application of electromagnetic waves

	Types	Frequency (Hz)	Practical Application
Radiation	γ ray	3×10^{18}	Radiosurgery, sterilisation
	X-ray	3×10^{16}	X-ray examination
Light (sunlight)	Ultraviolet ray	3×10^{15}	Germicidal lamp
	Visible ray	3×10^{13}	Optical instrument
	Infrared light ray	3×10^{12}	Heater, thermography
Electric wave	Terahertz (THz)	3×10^{11}	Optical communication, Radio telescope
	Extremely High Frequency (EHF)	3×10^{10}	Digital convenience radio
	Super High Frequency (SHF)	3×10^{9}	Microwave oven, cell phone
	Ultra High Frequency (UHF)	3×10^{8}	Air route surveillance radar
	Very High Frequency (VHF)	30,000,000	FM broadcasting, terrestrial broadcasting
	High Frequency (HF)	3,000,000	Amateur radio
	Medium Frequency (MF)	300,000	*RFA*, AM broadcasting
	Low Frequency (LF)	30,000	Induction heating
	Very Low Frequency (VLF)	3000	Seabed probe
	Extremely Low Frequency (ELF)	50–60	Power cable

The generated Joule heat Q (J) is found for the ideal state as the output electrical power W (W) × the time the current passes T (s).

$$Q\,(J) = WT$$

Here, because the electrical power W = I (A) · E (V), then

$$Q\,(J) = WT = I \cdot E \cdot T$$

Further, from the fact that E (V) = I (A) · R (Ω) 【Ohm's laws】,

$$Q\,(J) = WT = I^2 \cdot R \cdot T \text{【Joule's laws】}$$

and expressed in this way, we can see that the generated Joule heat Q increases in proportion to the resistance value of the resistor.

In addition, for a constant electrical power supply, the current flowing decreases if the tissue resistance increases, and conversely, a strong current flows if the tissue resistance decreases, and then dielectric heating effects become more significant.

For the Joule heat due to the electromagnetic waves, the higher the frequency (the shorter the wavelength), the force vibrating the molecules gets stronger, and also thermal tissue damage increases the greater this current is (the equation above). Because molecular vibration is even more strongly induced by such as microwaves of ultrashort wavelength with a higher frequency than RF, a strong Joule heat will then be produced. For this reason, although they have been applied extensively in household appliances, and used in microwave ovens, for example, because the frequency is higher than RF, they may possibly cause greater tissue cell damage. When DNA is exposed to microwaves of strong power, they can possibly enter the DNA molecule and cause damage from the ionisation effect. On the other hand, although generally, for low-frequency stimulation with radio waves of less than 100 kHz, the cause of tissue damage is the shock produced in the surrounding tissue, inasmuch as the RF used in medicine is of a relatively high frequency, stimulation of, and shock to, the nerves and muscles is prevented. And because the generated heat is diffused by the impedance drop due to blood flow, danger to surrounding blood vessels is easily avoided. Moreover, the RF used for medical purposes is rapidly attenuated the farther it progresses into deeper regions, which means that the range in which frictional heating occurs is kept in the vicinity of the insertion electrode, implying that localised ablation of the tissue is possible. One of the advantages of thermal ablation treatment using RF is that it is a mild coagulation necrosis effect which is locally limited.

4.3 Thermal Coagulation Necrosis Using RFA and Its Application to Humans

In environment conditions in which there is a gentle temperature rise up to about 40 °C, the cellular homeostatis of human cells can be maintained. However, in environmental conditions of hyperthermia in which it is increased to roughly

42–45 °C, the cells can easily suffer damage from various external invasion [1, 2]. Although it is true that the type of cell comprising the tissue and its cell cycle, for example, as well as the pH of the cell environment and the blood flow in the tissue, all vary greatly in a thermal environment that induces cell death, the time for which the cells are exposed and their temperature are also important factors. In environmental conditions where the temperature is 46 °C, for an exposure of 60 min, the cells suffer irreversible damage leading to cell dysfunction. But for a 60–100 °C environment, the key cytosolic enzyme and mitochondrial enzymes are irreversibly damaged almost instantaneously, and this induces cell protein coagulation [3–5]. And for high-temperature conditions of 105 °C or higher, the cells, or the tissue formed from their aggregates, is subject to boiling and vapouring, and ultimately, for 200 °C or higher, charring of the tissue then begins. As a medical strategy, RFA is the transfer of heat to the target tissue evenly and homogeneously throughout to provoke uniform protein coagulation necrosis in the cell. On the other hand, of equally key importance is that heat has minimal effect on the normal tissue around a tumour. As a technique which can satisfy both of these simultaneously, it was developed as a treatment by applying thermal coagulation using RF to bring on necrosis effectively through protein coagulation with a target tissue temperature of 50–100 °C.

The clinical application of radio-frequency ablation technology has expanded into the area of liver cancer. Under ultrasonic guidance, an electrode is inserted percutaneously into the intended liver lesion, and the coagulation necrosis of the cancer is performed using the dielectric heating which results from the RF released from the electrode. Because the heat generated is seen as a tissue coagulation effect which is confined to the vicinity of the electrode, there is little invasion into the surrounding tissue compared to the modality that uses higher frequencies and shorter wavelengths than RF, such as microwave or laser treatment, and it therefore gained popularity as a localised therapy which could be safely implemented. By making a comparison with the treatment results of PEIT (percutaneous ethanol injection therapy), which was established as a noninvasive, localised therapy, the superiority of RFA in terms of safety and long-term prognosis have also been reported. The inhomogeneity of the coagulation effect on the target tissue that occurred during injection of the ethanol, which was one of the problem points about PEIT, was overcome by using ablation with RF, and RFA was established as a useful localised therapy in the area of liver cancer. Furthermore, RFA has also been applied clinically for both lung tumours and kidney tumours. Up until 1966, every application aimed at human lung tumours involved numerous animal experiments to investigate the possibility and safety of the therapy [6, 7], and for tissue ablation using dielectric heating, the fact was demonstrated that there is little damage to the normal lung tissue surrounding the lung tumour. As energy is concentrated for lung tumours because of the insulation effect from surrounding lung parenchyma, it was suitable as a candidate for RFA. In 1999, Jeffrey et al. [8] were the first to report on ablation results of RFA for the clinical application of RFA to breast cancer in

Table 4.2 Electric and thermal conductivity

Tissue type	Electric conductivity (I/(Ω · m))	Thermal conductivity (W/(m · °C))
Fat	0.057	0.12
Tumour (carcinoma)	0.412	0.28

The tumour tissue has an electrical conductivity which is approximately 7 times that of fat, and the thermal conductivity is approximately double. For the tumour mass, because RF is propagated a long way into it and much heat is transported, it is a suitable environment for performing RFA [10]

relation to five cases of breast cancer. It was a study of advanced breast cancer with tumour sizes of 4–7 cm as its subject matter, but reported a high ablation rate of four cases (80%). Many feasibility studies also followed after that up until 2003, and further progress in the clinical application of RFA was made which showed a high complete ablation rate in relation to early-stage breast cancer of comparatively small invasive size [9].

In RFA, for the safe and complete ablation of the target site, it is important that a necessary and sufficient amount of heat is transferred to the target site homogeneously and evenly to cause cell degeneration. Because the current density varies according to the distance from the electrode, the amount of heat generation at individual points may also show a certain difference in their distributions. Additionally, the strength of the current at each site is dependent on that tissue resistance, in that, if the resistance of an individual site is increased, the total resistance (impedance) increases as well, and for constant voltage driving, it is difficult for the current to flow at sites where the impedance is high, and the heat cannot be conducted very easily. For tissue sites with low resistance, there is greater heat generation because a greater current starts to flow, and tissue coagulation is achieved at a relatively earlier stage. Of these, the sections with a high resistance start to coagulate, which may also be the reason for uneven tissue coagulation. For example, because the value of the tissue resistance for fat is higher than that for a tumour, the electronic and thermal conductivity is lower compared with the tumour tissue [10] (Table 4.2). Mammary glands are often surrounded by fatty tissue, and it is not uncommon for fat to be mixed in with the tumour itself. Therefore, from the differences in the tissue resistance, differences arise in the ablation speed between tissues. Additionally, when tumours make contact with a blood vessel, as it takes a lot of current, the surrounding tissue is hardly ablated at all. On the other hand, although great heat is generated in the vicinity of the electrode for RF heat conduction when using a monopolar electrode, the tissue temperature tends to drop further away from the electrode [11] (Fig. 4.2-a). Furthermore, when the ablation effectiveness intensifies for sites in contact with the electrode, boiling and vapouring are induced in the tissue there, and the gas which is generated then cuts off conduction of the heat in the area. The gas that is generated increases the impedance to conduction of the RF, which further inhibits the dispersion of the heat. In order to avoid excessive heating in the vicinity of this electrode, a device is used during ablation which uses cooling water to cool the electrode itself. This is the Cool-tip method that we are using ourselves in the area of the breast cancer. By

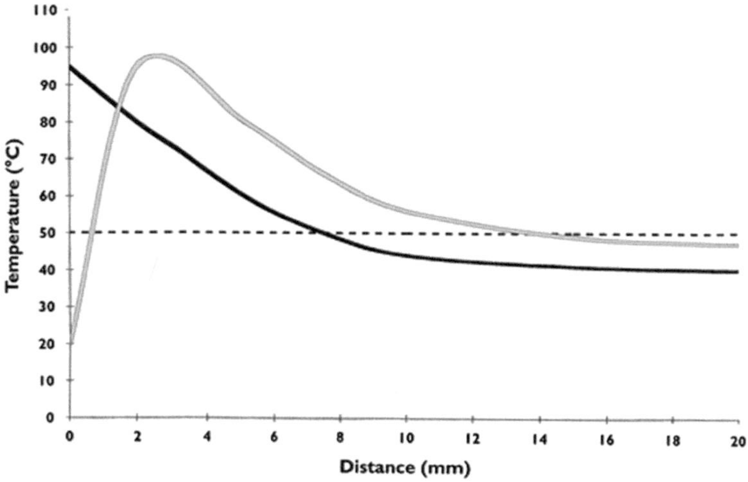

Fig. 4.2-a Graph showing tissue temperature profile for thermal ablation with and without cooling of energy applicator. Temperatures were generated by applying RF for 12 min at maximum tissue temperature of 95 °C to in vivo swine muscle. Internal cooling permits greater energy deposition in tissues resulting in greater heating at distance from electrode. Solid black line represents conventional RF, solid gray line is cooling, and broken line is coagulation threshold [11]

circulating cooling water within the electrode, the tissue in immediate contact with the electrode is cooled and excessive heat coagulation, boiling, and vapouring are prevented. The resistance of the tissue which is in contact with the electrode needle does not rise excessively, and the RF heat conduction is propagated into the tissue effectively (Fig. 4.2-b). In practice, because the generated heat is propagated to the surrounding tissue, after a constant period of time has elapsed, we can expect that the heat is produced uniformly and also that the tissue near the electrode undergoes heat coagulation to bring about the required amount of cell damage.

In the treatment of breast cancer with RFA, the centre of the target cancer is penetrated with the needle electrode. Adequate tissue coagulation is achieved in a range up to 5 mm from the tip of the needle electrode, and thus the ablation is started with the tip protruding from the tumour by about 5 mm. The measurement of the initial resistance value of the tissue before ablation is taken as that value measured when 1 W of electrical power is passed through the tip of the needle electrode from the generator. If the initial resistance value just before passing the RFA current is greater than or equal to 250 Ω, there may not be sufficient current passing through the tissue with this high initial resistance; it is then necessary to alter the route for the needle, and measure the resistance value again. When the value for the initial resistance exceeds 300 Ω, we ourselves would have serious misgivings about ablation using RFA being adequate, and it is assumed that this line of treatment in such a case should be properly justified. We start by passing an initial 5 W of electrical power through the tissue, and then increase it in steps of

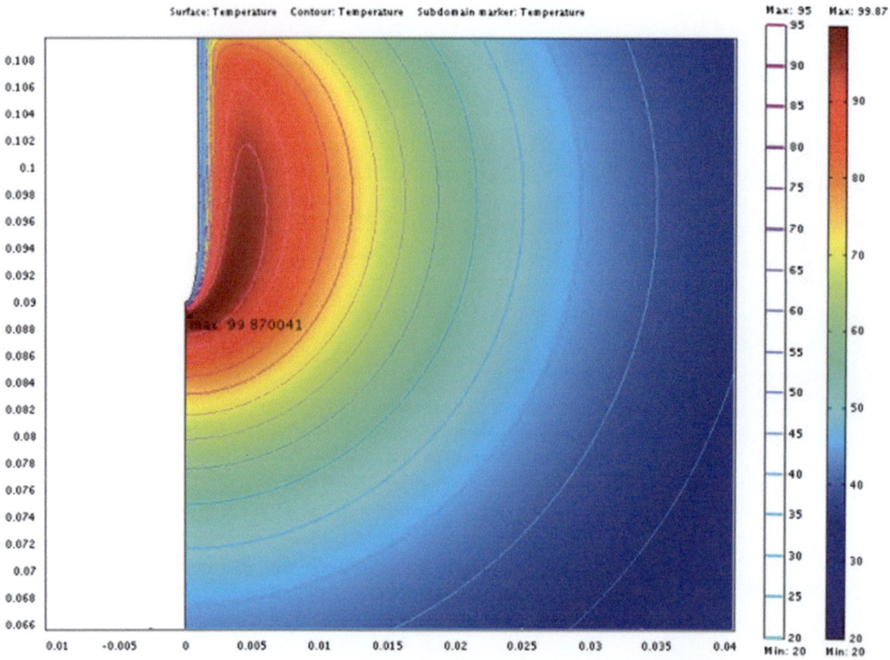

Fig. 4.2-b Distribution of the heat transmitted into the fatty tissue from the needle electrode. Contours are at 5 °C intervals, and colour coding at 10 °C intervals. The heat is concentrated in the vicinity of the needle electrode, and the amount of heat drops drastically with distance [10]

10 W every minute. We think that it is important to avoid an increase in the tissue resistance due to a sudden, high electrical power. Tissue ablation progresses as the supplied power is gradually increased, but if it progresses sufficiently, the value of the tissue resistance will, at some point, start to go up rapidly. If the continued measured value for the resistance increases very suddenly (this is expressed as either 'break' or 'roll-off') for an increase from the initial resistance within a width of 30 Ω (or a resistance value corresponding to 130% of the initial resistance), the power supply from the generator is cut off, as it is then determined that the target tissue has been ablated sufficiently. In the United States ultrasonography, the tumour is confirmed to be ill-defined, included within a 'cocoon'-shaped ablation region with a 'high'-ish echo, and the tip temperature of the needle electrode is measured with a built-in sensor. If the tissue temperature is 60 °C or more, it is judged that sufficient tissue ablation has been achieved. And to check whether the tissue interior is also similarly 60 °C or more, the needle electrode is withdrawn about 1 cm. The needle electrode is drawn out on determining that sufficient ablation has been achieved. The tissue temperature achieved is almost always around 80–100 °C.

References

1. Seegenschmiedt MH, Brady LW, Sauer R. Interstitial thermoradiotherapy: review on technical and clinical aspects. Am J Clin Oncol. 1990;13:352–63.
2. Overgaard J. Hyperthermia as an adjuvant to radiotherapy: review of the randomized multicenter studies of the European society for hyperthermic oncology. Strahlenther Onkol. 1987;163:453–7.
3. Larson TR, Bostwick DG, Corica A. Temperature-correlated histopathologic changes following microwave thermoablation of obstructive tissue in patients with benign prostatic hyperplasia. Urology. 1996;47:463–9.
4. Goldberg SN, Solbiati L, Gazelle GS, Tanabe KK, Compton CC, Mueller PR. Treatment of intrahepatic malignancy with radio-frequency ablation: radiologic–pathologic correlation in 16 patients (abstr). AJR 1997;168 [American Roentgen Ray Society 97th Annual Meeting Program Book suppl]:121.
5. Thomsen S. Pathologic analysis of photothermal and photomechanical effects of laser-tissue interactions. Photochem Photobiol. 1991;53:825–35.
6. Goldberg SN, et al. Radiofrequency tissue ablation in the rabbit lung: efficacy and complications. Acad Radiol. 1995;2:776–84.
7. Goldberg SN, et al. Radiofrequency tissue ablation of VX2 tumor nodules in the rabbit lung. Acad Radiol. 1996;3:929–35.
8. Jeffery SS, Birdwell PL, Ikeda DM, et al. Radiofrequency ablation of breast cancer: first report of an emerging technology. Arch Surg. 1999;134:1064–8.
9. Noguchi M. Minimally invasive surgery for small breast cancer. J Surg Oncol. 2003;84:94–101.
10. Ekstrand V, Wiksell H, Schultz I, Sandstedt B, Rotstein S. Influence of electrical and thermal properties on RF ablation of breast cancer: is the tumour preferentially heated? Biomed Eng Online. 2005;4:41.
11. Goldberg SN, Gazelle GS, Mueller PR. Thermal ablation therapy for focal malignancy: a unified approach to underlying principles, techniques, and diagnostic imaging guidance. Am J Roentgenol. 2000;174(2):323–31.

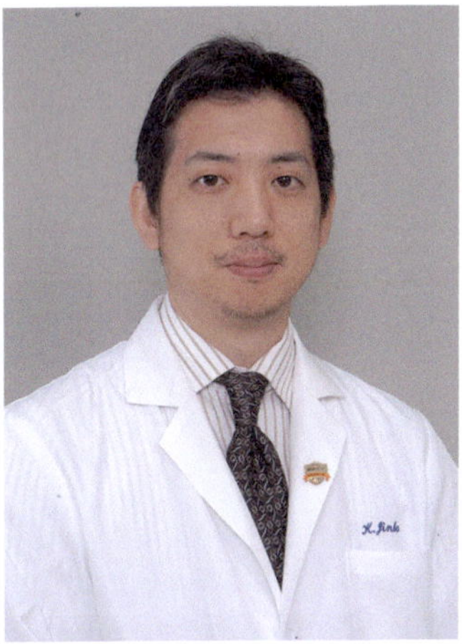

Kenjiro Jimbo

Chapter 5
RFA of Breast Cancer: Criteria and Procedure

Noriaki Wada

5.1 Introduction

Image-guided tumor ablation is currently the most promising treatment alternative to surgery for breast cancer. Continued advances in therapeutic energy devices, application techniques, and therapeutic efficacy have accompanied increasing interest.

In this chapter, the criteria and procedures for RFA in clinical percutaneous tumor ablation technologies are described. Other methods such as chemical ablation, cryoablation, microwave ablation, and focused ultrasound surgery will not be discussed. The RFA technique uses thermal energy in the form of a high-frequency alternating current, which flows from an uninsulated electrode into the surrounding tissue [1].

Minimally invasive tumor ablation therapy for focal malignancies encompasses several specific objectives. Most importantly, the primary goal of most ablation procedures is to eradicate all viable malignant cells within a designated target volume. Furthermore, excellent cosmetic results can be achieved without the appearance of surgical scars.

Therefore, the objective of RFA is to achieve a curative effect for the small volume of breast tumors. Because studies of patients with large tumors, tumors that infiltrate the skin or muscle, or tumors treated by postprimary systemic or palliative therapy are relatively few, such cases will not be addressed in this chapter.

N. Wada (✉)
Department of General and Breast Surgery, Tokyo Dental College Ichikawa General Hospital, 5-11-13 Sugano, 272-8513 Ichikawa, Chiba, Japan
e-mail: nowada@tdc.ac.jp

T. Kinoshita (ed.), *Non-surgical Ablation Therapy for Early-stage Breast Cancer*,
DOI 10.1007/978-4-431-54463-0_5

5.2 Pre-radio-frequency Ablation Procedures

5.2.1 *Pretreatment Imaging*

Pretreatment imaging with mammography, ultrasound, and magnetic resonance imaging (MRI) to accurately define the tumor extent and volume is important for appropriate patient selection. The selection of ablation is largely based on tumor size and extent of disease. It is advisable to exclude patients carrying tumors with undefined borders and definite signs of wide-ranging intraductal components. Accurate assessment of the extent of disease prior to RFA is essential for treatment success.

Although the diagnostic accuracy of MRI in the detection and measurement of tumor size remains somewhat controversial, MRI should still be considered for appropriate patient selection [2], particularly to exclude those with extensive intraductal components [3], as well as a modality to assess therapeutic effects [4] because it is reported to reliably predict histological findings [5].

Patients with multifocal or multicentric breast lesions diagnosed by MRI are unsuitable candidates for curative RFA. Also, patients with tumors that cannot be detected using dynamic contrast-enhanced MRI should be excluded because a follow-up with MRI is not possible [6].

5.2.2 *Essential Histological Diagnosis*

Ultrasound (US) is a well-established imaging modality for the detection and monitoring of both malignant and benign breast disease. Furthermore, US-guided techniques, including percutaneous core needle biopsy (CNB), have proven to be indispensable for the diagnosis of breast cancer. Prior to an ablative procedure, CNB is necessary to establish a histopathological diagnosis, histological grade, and receptor status or subtypes (estrogen receptor, progesterone receptor, Her2/neu, Ki67, etc.). Disease characteristics to determine additional treatment for breast cancer cannot be obtained after RFA because ablation induces thermal denaturation effects in the primary breast tumor [7–9]. Patients diagnosed by only aspiration cytology are required to undergo CNB before RFA.

5.2.3 *Suitable Histological Types*

The ideal candidate will have a single, small, biopsy-proven, invasive ductal carcinoma (IDC). The presence of an extensive intraductal component is a contra-indication to RFA. However, a small ductal carcinoma in situ (DCIS) having a clear margin and appearing localized on imaging should be considered as a candidate for

RFA. RFA can act preferentially on breast cancer tumors because tumor strands absorb heat to a relatively greater extent compared with adjacent normal tissue [10].

RFA should be discouraged in patients with invasive lobular carcinoma because exact determination of the extent of lobular carcinoma in the breast can be difficult. Palussière et al. [11] reported that two-thirds of patients with lobular carcinoma treated with RFA experienced local recurrence. There are no reports in the literature regarding the success and failure of RFA by histological subtypes (i.e., luminal, non-luminal, HER2-enriched, and triple-negative breast carcinoma). The subtype is not typically considered as an indication for RFA.

5.2.4 *Tumor Location*

Tumor location is an important factor to consider in ablation. Also, the effect of heat transmission during ablation to the surrounding normal tissue should be considered. Patients with skin or nipple infiltration cannot be treated by RFA because of technical factors; RFA cannot treat the entire tumor without burning the skin.

Similarly, tumor ablation may allow the delivery of high temperature to a position adjacent to the greater pectoral muscle or rib. In general, a minimum distance of 1 cm between the tumor margin and the skin, nipple, pectoral muscle, and chest wall is advised [12].

5.2.5 *Suitable Tumor Size*

A suitable tumor size is a major concern for RFA. Complete tumor eradication is dependent on both tumor size and performance of the needle device. Considering potential complications, currently available needle devices have limitations. Although a smaller tumor size is desirable for RFA, tumor size limitations remain unclear in currently available treatments.

The 2014 NCCN guidelines do not address RFA in the management of breast cancer [13]. Although there are currently no guidelines for the inclusion of patients on the basis of tumor size, a previous study reported consistent complete destruction of breast tumors measuring up to 2 cm in diameter [14].

Zhao et al. [15] conducted a systematic review of breast cancer patients who underwent minimally invasive RFA from 1999 to 2009. The majority of tumors analyzed in this study were in the early stage, and the breast lesions ranged from 0.5 to 2.0 cm in size with demarcated margins. Nine investigators reported the feasibility and safety of RFA for small breast tumors. The ablated tumor was removed immediately or 1–4 weeks after RFA, and tumor viability was evaluated by histopathological examinations. Complete coagulation necrosis rates of 76–100 % have been reported. Similarly, Soukup et al. [16] conducted a literature review of

17 studies published from 2003 to 2010 and found that some groups reported 100 % success rates [12, 17, 18].

Results from several studies have suggested that complete tumor ablation may be dependent on tumor size. For example, Kinoshita et al. [19] reported that of 49 patients who completed treatment using the single cooled needle method, complete ablation was achieved in 30 patients (61 %) by hematoxylin and eosin staining and/or nicotinamide adenine dinucleotide diaphorase staining. In an evaluation of ablation efficacy in 20 patients with tumors measuring >2 cm in diameter and 29 with tumors measuring ≤2 cm in diameter, complete tumor ablation rates were 30 % and 86 %, respectively. They concluded that RFA is a safe and promising minimally invasive treatment for small breast carcinomas with a pathological tumor size of ≤2 cm in diameter and without an extended intraductal component.

Similar results were obtained in another study [20] of 25 patients with a mean tumor size of 2.08 cm (range, 0.9–3.8 cm). There was a significant difference ($p < 0.05$) between tumors measuring ≤2 cm (complete necrosis in 13 of 14 cases, 93 %) and those measuring >2 cm (complete necrosis in 6 of 11 cases, 55 %; $p < 0.05$).

These results are in agreement with those of several other studies where tumors measuring <2 cm achieved ablation rates of 90–100 % [5, 12, 18, 21]. The strong agreement between the good success rates in the ≤2-cm groups suggested that RFA may be more appropriate for the treatment of smaller tumors [16].

5.2.6 Larger Tumors

Our ideal goal for curative treatment is complete ablation at one time with puncture in one direction. Percutaneous RFA using the US-guided technique in patients with difficult anatomical access because of tumor size and location of the breast presents some limitations. For larger tumors (generally defined as those measuring >3 cm in diameter), a single ablation treatment may be insufficient to eradicate all target lesions. In such patients, multiple overlapping puncture of the tumor from different directions or simultaneous use of multiple needles may be required for successful ablation. It is, however, difficult to define an ablative margin and penetrate the unablated target lesion repeatedly using a needle under US-guided techniques [22]. If possible, multiple needle placements should be avoided to achieve a curative effect.

5.2.7 Other General Conditions

The general physical condition of the patient needs to be sufficient to withstand general anesthesia and radiation therapy. However, no special conditions are required. Because of the localized nature of RFA, there are no systemic side effects.

Most RFA procedures in Japan are performed under general anesthesia. However, it is possible to perform RFA under local anesthesia and, occasionally, light sedation. Percutaneous ablation for focal malignancies is suitable for the treatment of both elderly patients and those who are intolerant to general anesthesia. A small pilot study concluded that RFA treatment of early-stage breast cancer in inoperable elderly patients (age >75 years) was both feasible and safe under local anesthesia with satisfactory outcomes [23]. A recent study reported that US-guided RFA for the treatment of small breast carcinomas under local anesthesia was feasible and resulted in only mild pain and no adverse events [2].

Relative contraindications to US-guided ablation include active local inflammation and infection, implanted cardiac pacemaker, implantable cardioverter–defibrillator, pregnancy, sepsis, and coagulopathy. Whenever possible, the use of anticoagulants or antiplatelet drugs should be discontinued before ablation. RFA for radical cure is contraindicated in patients with distant metastasis. Moreover, patients with definitive regional lymph node metastases should undergo simultaneous axillary lymph node dissection if the surgery is switched to a procedure other than minimally invasive surgery. Ablation only offers a cosmetic benefit in the breast.

With regard to primary systemic therapy, Fornage et al. [12] reported that patients treated with neoadjuvant chemotherapy were poor candidates for ablation because viable tumor cells that are undetectable on preprocedural imaging may remain in the peripheral tissue after chemotherapy-induced shrinkage of a larger primary tumor compromising accurate image-guided targeting. Indications of previous therapy (chemotherapy, hormone therapy, and radiation therapy) for the tumor remain challenges.

Before RFA, all patients and their relatives are informed of the procedural characteristics, including the risk of incomplete ablation, technical failure of appropriate needle placement, and device malfunction. Consequently, a new surgical treatment may be required. Written informed consent is obtained from all patients before treatment.

Table 5.1 lists the criteria of the RAFAELO study using the Cool-tip™ RFA system in Japan.

5.3 Electrode Selection

5.3.1 Two Types of Electrode Designs

RF energy from an electrode causes cell death by coagulative necrosis. The ideal electrode would supply uniform heating to all areas of the tumor. It has long been established that a tissue temperature of approximately 45 °C is required before necrotic cell death [24].

Table 5.1 Criteria in the RAFAELO study using the Cool-tip RF ablation system in Japan for reference

Inclusion criteria
1. Pathological confirmation of DCIS or IDC using CNB
2. Tumor size ≥1.5 cm in diameter [largest size measured by required scans (mammogram, ultrasound, and MRI) will be used to determine eligibility]
3. No previous therapy (chemotherapy, hormone therapy, and radiation therapy) for this tumor
4. Female sex, age of 20–79 years
5. Good general health and the ability to tolerate radiation therapy
6. No past history of cerebral infarction, cardiac infarction, or thromboembolic event and the ability to tolerate general anesthesia
7. No suspicious axillary lymph node metastasis with palpation and diagnostic imaging
8. Current written informed consent
Exclusion criteria
1. Pregnancy or suspicion of pregnancy
2. Previous malignancy other than breast cancer, except for those listed below. In case of a prior history of non-breast malignancy, the patient must have survived disease-free for 5 years after curative treatment, with a very low risk of recurrence
3. Implanted cardiac pacemaker or implantable cardioverter–defibrillator
4. Active local inflammation or infection
5. Serious heart disease or brain disease
6. Inability to place the return electrode in the patient
7. Hemostatic problems because of antiplatelet or anticoagulant therapy
8. Wide range with intraductal component or multicentric disease
9. Diffuse microcalcification on mammography
10. Simultaneous bilateral breast malignancy
11. Metachronous breast malignancy, including ipsilateral breast tumor recurrence
12. Distant metastasis
13. Impropriety for this study as determined by the investigator

The shape of the ablated volume is dependent on the shape, size, and design of the RF electrode [25]. Currently, there are two different types of electrode designs in RFA systems operating in a monopolar mode. One deploys multi-arrays to enable more tissue contact and equal heat generation within the tumor. The multi-array electrode contains secondary electrodes that are deployed to form a star or umbrellalike array around the primary electrode. The second design employs a straight needle with continuous infusion of cold saline to prevent charring at the contact point and decreases tissue impedance, thereby increasing heat deposition and ablation volume [26].

There are three major monopolar RFA devices currently available in the market: a multi-array electrode system (StarBurst™ system, AngioDynamics, Queensbury, NY, USA, and LeVeen CoAccess™ electrode system, Boston Scientific, Natick, MA, USA) and a straight needle system (Cool-tip™ RF ablation system, Covidien, Boulder, CO, USA).

5.3.2 *Electrode Selection*

Each device manufacturer provides various sizes of the active length of the electrode. The ablation zone is dependent on tissue vascularization, type, temperature, and impedance. Proper needle selection differs according to tumor size, location, and use of a familiar device. Therefore, it is important to refer to the manufacturer's guidelines.

An ex vivo model suggested that the single cooled needle system is more efficacious for tumor ablation [27]. However, Hung et al. [26] reported a comparative study of two needle designs. The results of ten patients with breast cancer who underwent RFA with a multi-array LeVeen electrode were compared with those of ten patients who were treated with a saline-infused Cool-tip electrode. Both needles had the same efficacy for breast cancer ablation, but the Cool-tip electrode was easier to insert and had a shorter ablation time [28]. It has been established that the efficacy of RFA is mainly dependent on operator experience and tumor size. (Please see other chapters.)

The generators manufactured by the three major RFA companies provide a maximum output of 150–200 W and deliver a high-frequency (450–500 kHz) alternating current via RF electrodes with a gauge range of 14–17. These RF generators have different ablation protocols. The main protocols of monopolar systems include impedance control, time, and temperature feedback.

5.3.3 *Manufactured Devices (Figs. 5.1 and 5.2)*

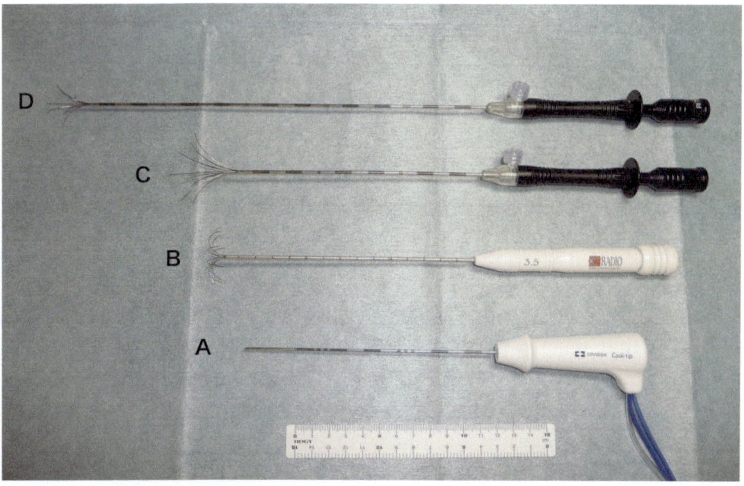

Fig. 5.1 (**a**) Cool-tip RF ablation system (Covidien, Boulder, CO, USA), (**b**) LeVeen CoAccess electrode system (Boston Scientific, Natick, MA, USA), (**c**, **d**) StarBurst XL RFA device (AngioDynamics, Queensbury, NY, USA)

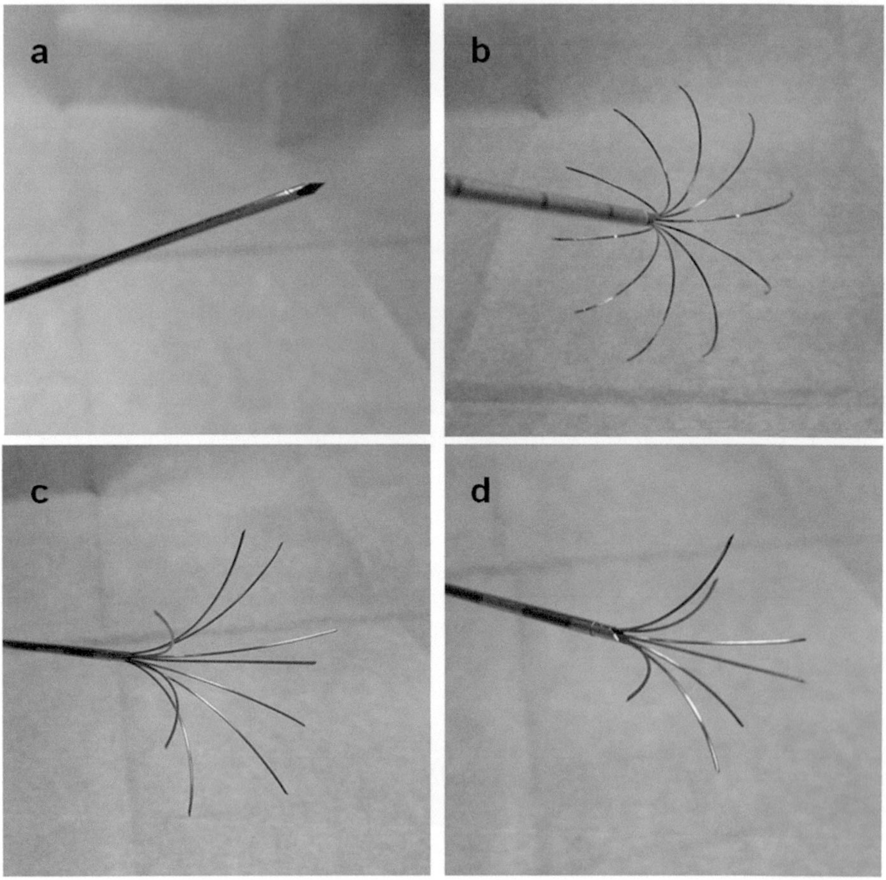

Fig. 5.2 (**a**) Cool-tip™ RF ablation system (Covidien, Boulder, CO, USA) is a straight needle design with trocar-style tips and internally circulates chilled water, cooling the tissue adjacent to the exposed electrode to maximize energy deposition and eliminate tissue charring. (**b**) LeVeen CoAccess™ electrode system (Boston Scientific, Natick, MA, USA) is a coaxial system with an umbrella-shaped array-type electrode. (**c**, **d**) StarBurst™ XL RFA device (AngioDynamics, Queensbury, NY, USA) is a multi-array needle electrode system with nine arrays plus active trocar tips and five thermocouples

5.3.3.1 Cool-tip RF Ablation System

The Cool-tip RF ablation system consists of a 17-gauge straight needle design with trocar-style tips that insert and position like biopsy needles. The Cool-tip is now available with both 2.0- and 3.0-cm active electrode probe tips for breast cancer. This design circulates water internally to cool the tissue adjacent to the electrode to limit tissue charring and permits increased energy deposition for potentially larger ablation volumes. The Cool-tip temperatures are intended to prevent excessive heating and carbonization of tissue immediately adjacent to the electrode, which can pose high impedance to current flow and prevent optimal penetration of energy.

5.3.3.2 LeVeen CoAccess Electrode System

The LeVeen CoAccess electrode system is a coaxial system with an array-type electrode. On deployment, the tines of the array splay radially outward and arch backward, each in a semicircular fashion, to form an umbrellalike pattern. The coaxial RFA device is available with array diameters of 3.0, 3.5, and 4.0 cm and is designed to provide full coverage and volumetric feedback to deliver a more consistent heat pattern throughout the lesion. An electrode algorithm compensates for tissue variability and has been developed to facilitate complete, homogeneous thermal lesion creation.

5.3.3.3 StarBurst XL RFA System

The StarBurst XL RFA device is a multi-array needle electrode system. It consists of a primary electrode—that is, a stainless-steel cannula with a noninsulated distal tip that acts as an electrode—and secondary electrodes, which are curved, flexible stainless-steel prongs that are contained within and can be deployed outside of the primary electrode. A single device can offer the capability to produce scalable, spherical ablations (3–5 cm) and to deliver precise amounts of normal saline to the ablation zone via ports in the electrode. Its real-time, multipoint temperature feedback system ensures sustained target temperatures during the procedure.

5.4 Procedural Steps

Table 5.2 shows the standard procedure for using the Cool-tip RF ablation system.

RFA is delivered in the operating room with patients under general anesthesia. Prior to RFA, a sentinel lymph node biopsy is performed using an established method (e.g., combination of blue dye and a radioisotope), if needed.

5.4.1 Needle Placement

Accurate tumor puncture is crucial for successful RFA. Under real-time US guidance, the electrode is inserted using a free-hand technique, choosing the best pathway to cross the center of the tumor while remaining parallel to the chest wall. The electrode tip should be placed beyond the distal edge of the tumor to allow appropriate ablative margins, according to the manufacturer's

Table 5.2 Ablation procedure

1. RFA is delivered in the operating room with the patient under general anesthesia
2. Use ultrasound guidance to identify the safest access site and determine patient positioning
3. Select a proper active length of Cool-tip (2 or 3 cm) according to the tumor size
4. Place one ground pad on the patient's thigh. If using two ground pads on the patient's thighs (one per leg), place them with both pairs equidistant from the ablation site
5. Hook up all lines and, prior to needle insertion, confirm that the tip of the needle is cold because the tip circulates water internally to cool the tissue adjacent to the electrode
6. Make a small skin incision with a number 11 surgical blade or 18-gauge injection needle at the puncture site
7. Place the electrode in the center of the lesion under US-guided imaging and create the axis parallel to the chest wall
8. Verify the position of the electrode on three-dimensional imaging. Optimally, the tip site will only slightly penetrate the lesion
9. Subcutaneously inject approximately 20–40 mL of 5 % glucose into the retromammary space to avoid burning of the skin and muscle by RFA-induced heat
10. RFA is started at 5 W and increased to an output of 10 W after 1 min. Then, the output is continuously increased in increments of 10 W at 1-min intervals until a major increase in impedance occurs (roll-off). The generator will shut off automatically, thereby stopping the flow of current
11. Place sterile ice packs on the skin above the tumor to prevent burning of the skin until the end of ablation
12. Measure the core temperature of the tumor using a thermometer at the tip of the needle after the roll-off, stopping the pump to circulate cold saline
13. If the temperature is below 70 °C, start the second phase until a second roll-off occurs
14. Remove the electrode and close the wound using a Steri-Strip
15. If necessary, in principle, perform sentinel lymph node biopsy prior to RFA

This table explains a standard procedure using the Cool-tip RF ablation system. In reference to the above table, modify the settings according to the patient's condition in practice

recommendation for the specific RFA system. US imaging with at least two orthogonal views to confirm appropriate positioning of the electrode is essential.

An ideal ablated zone includes an additional 0.5–1.0-cm ablative margin of normal-appearing parenchyma, while limiting damage to large areas of normal tissue. However, there are inherent problems with this technique. For example, it is difficult to accurately determine the three-dimensional proportions of the tumor using US. In addition, matching of the RFA zone to the tumor shape is difficult because of the inability to accurately visualize the ablation zone [16].

5.4.2 Output Setting and Power Distribution

Thermal ablation therapy such as RFA exploits energy–tissue interactions. The electrode attached to the RF generator induces a current in the tissue adjacent to the electrode, and heating of the tissue is due to resistive (Joule) heating. As the tissue is heated, conductivity is reduced, thereby limiting the extent of ablation. Such an occurrence of rapid reduction in conductivity (or increase in impedance) is known as "roll-off."

Adequate heat induces irreversible injury to the target cells. Minimal ablation temperatures are 50–54 °C for 4–6 min [25, 29], which has become the standard surrogate end point for thermal ablation therapies in both experimental studies and current clinical paradigms [25].

If the temperature rapidly increases to above 100 °C, then boiling, vaporization, and carbonization occur, all of which decrease energy transmission and limit the ablation effect. The ideal objective is to heat the surrounding tissues to 50–100 °C for more than 9 min, without causing charring or vaporization. The generator output can be gradually increased. Power and impedance are monitored continuously during treatment with a generator. When impedance roll-off is reached, the generator will shut off automatically.

Output setting of RF energy can differ slightly among devices [30]. Most studies begin at an initial power setting that is 5–20 W and is subsequently increased by 5 or 10 W every 1–5 min, until a rapid increase in impedance occurs or until the power reaches 60 W [11, 12, 19, 21, 31, 32].

Many commercially available devices are designed to directly monitor either tissue temperature (StarBurst™ system, AngioDynamics, Queensbury, NY, USA) or impedance (LeVeen CoAccess™ electrode system, Boston Scientific, Natick, MA, USA; Cool-tip™ RF ablation system, Covidien, Boulder, CO, USA) to prevent excessive heating. Algorithms and protocols used for each RFA device may vary (ramped energy deposition or impedance regulation). In a practical sense, we need to check the specific algorithm, set the manufacturer-recommended starting power, and increase the wattage every minute.

For example, for the Cool-tip RF ablation system, the initial ablation setting is 5 W, and after 1 min, the power is increased to 10 W. Thereafter, the power is increased in intervals of 10 W every minute until a roll-off occurs. Immediately thereafter, the pump is turned off, and after 30 s, the maximum temperature of the tumor is measured with a thermometer at the tip of the needle, which is usually 60–90 °C. If the maximum temperature is <70 °C, treatment (second phase) is repeated.

Kinoshita et al. [19] reported that the duration of RFA with the Cool-tip was 3–18 min (mean, 8.7 min). The mean tumor impedance was 195.1 Ω, with a mean reduction of 53.4 Ω during treatment. A median of one cycle and a mean power of 48.5 W (range, 5–118 W) were used to achieve tumor ablation.

Real-time US should be used to guide and monitor the treatment procedure. Unfortunately, US is technically limited by hyperechogenicity of the heated breast tissue (the so-called "fog effect") coupled with reflection of the US beams by gas formed during ablation, which hampers the differentiation between ablated and viable residual tumor [21, 31].

5.4.3 Prevention of Complications

To prevent burns to the skin and muscle, in cases with a close distance to the skin or muscle, approximately 20–40 mL of 5 % glucose solution can be injected under the skin over the tumor and/or in the retromammary space to increase the distance (hydrodissection). A sterile ice pack may also be placed on the skin directly over the area to be ablated to avoid an increase in skin temperature during the ablation procedure and for 1–2 h after the procedure. This precaution is particularly important if the tumor is located only 1 cm below the skin surface. Gentle lateral compression and elevation of the breast throughout the entire ablation procedure can prevent burns in addition to increasing the distance between the target lesion and chest wall [5, 30].

5.4.4 Procedure Completion

At the completion of the procedure, the electrode is withdrawn. Bleeding from the hole is rarely observed. Sterile skin closure strips (3M Company, St. Paul, MN, USA) may be used to close the skin. Following ablation, patients are monitored for 4–5 h in a dedicated recovery room. Overnight hospitalization for up to 24 h may be necessary if the principal physician prefers to monitor the patient for immediate adverse events. Many patients do not require analgesic agents.

If it is difficult to assess the margin of the ablated lesions, then radiotherapy for the breast is essential to prevent local recurrence, similar to that in conventional conservative breast surgery.

Apparently, RFA without surgical resection is a promising minimally invasive technique for the management of primary small breast tumors, which offers several advantages over conventional treatments. Although preceding studies have reported encouraging results, further research and observation are necessary to establish optimal indications and techniques based on careful evaluations of the long-term prognosis and cosmetic effects of RFA.

References

1. Van Esser S, van den Bosch MA, van Diest PJ, et al. Minimally invasive ablative therapies for invasive breast carcinomas: an overview of current literature. World J Surg. 2007;31:2284–92.
2. Schässburger K-U, Löfgren L, Lagerstedt U, et al. Minimally-invasive treatment of early stage breast cancer: a feasibility study using radiofrequency ablation under local anesthesia. Breast. 2014;23:152–8.
3. Wiksell H, Löfgren L, Schässburger K-U, et al. Feasibility study on the treatment of small breast carcinoma using percutaneous US-guided preferential radiofrequency ablation (PRFA). Breast. 2010;19(3):219–25.

4. Nagashima T, Sakakibara M, Sangai T, et al. Surrounding rim formation and reduction in size after radiofrequency ablation for primary breast cancer. Jpn J Radiol. 2009;27:197–204.
5. Manenti G, Bolacchi F, Perretta T, et al. Small breast cancers: in vivo percutaneous US-guided radiofrequency ablation with dedicated cool-tip radiofrequency system. Radiology. 2009;251:339–46.
6. Hayashi AH, Silver SF, van der Westhuizen NG, et al. Treatment of invasive breast carcinoma with ultrasound-guided radiofrequency ablation. Am J Surg. 2003;185:429–35.
7. Imoto S, Wada N, Sakemura N, et al. Feasibility study on radiofrequency ablation followed by partial mastectomy for stage I breast cancer patients. Breast. 2009;18:130–4.
8. Khatri VP, McGahan JP, Ramsamooj R, et al. A phase II trial of image-guided radiofrequency ablation of small invasive breast carcinomas: use of saline-cooled tip electrode. Ann Surg Oncol. 2007;14:1644–52.
9. Noguchi M. Is radiofrequency ablation treatment for small breast cancer ready for "prime time"? Breast Cancer Res Treat. 2007;106:307–14.
10. Ekstrand V, Wiksell H, Schultz I, et al. Influence of electrical and thermal properties on RF ablation of breast cancer: is the tumour preferentially heated? Biomed Eng Online. 2005;4:41.
11. Palussière J, Henriques C, Mauriac L, et al. Radiofrequency ablation as a substitute for surgery in elderly patients with nonresected breast cancer: pilot study with long-term outcomes. Radiology. 2012;264:597–605.
12. Fornage BD, Sneige N, Ross MI, et al. Small (< or = 2-cm) breast cancer treated with US-guided radiofrequency ablation: feasibility study. Radiology. 2004;231:215–24.
13. NCCN. NCCN Clinical Practice Guidelines 2014 in Oncology (NCCN Guidelines) Breast Cancer. NCCN.org 2014. http://www.nccn.org/professionals/physician_gls/f_guidelines.asp
14. Van der Ploeg IMC, van Esser S, van den Bosch MJ, et al. Radiofrequency ablation for breast cancer: a review of the literature. Eur J Surg Oncol. 2007;33:673–7.
15. Zhao Z, Wu F. Minimally-invasive thermal ablation of early-stage breast cancer: a systemic review. Eur J Surg Oncol. 2010;36:1149–55.
16. Soukup B, Bismohun S, Reefy S, Mokbel K. The evolving role of radiofrequency ablation therapy of breast lesions. Anticancer Res. 2010;30:3693–7.
17. Earashi M, Noguchi M, Motoyoshi A, Fujii H. Radiofrequency ablation therapy for small breast cancer followed by immediate surgical resection or delayed mammotome excision. Breast Cancer. 2007;14:39–47.
18. Noguchi M, Earashi M, Fujii H, et al. Radiofrequency ablation of small breast cancer followed by surgical resection. J Surg Oncol. 2006;93:120–8.
19. Kinoshita T, Iwamoto E, Tsuda H, Seki K. Radiofrequency ablation as local therapy for early breast carcinomas. Breast Cancer. 2011;18:10–7.
20. Medina-Franco H, Soto-Germes S, Ulloa-Gómez JL, et al. Radiofrequency ablation of invasive breast carcinomas: a phase II trial. Ann Surg Oncol. 2008;15:1689–95.
21. Burak WE, Agnese DM, Povoski SP, et al. Radiofrequency ablation of invasive breast carcinoma followed by delayed surgical excision. Cancer. 2003;98:1369–76.
22. Dodd GD, Frank MS, Aribandi M, et al. Radiofrequency thermal ablation: computer analysis of the size of the thermal injury created by overlapping ablations. AJR Am J Roentgenol. 2001;177:777–82.
23. Susini T, Nori J, Olivieri S, et al. Radiofrequency ablation for minimally invasive treatment of breast carcinoma. A pilot study in elderly inoperable patients. Gynecol Oncol. 2007;104:304–10.
24. Dickson JA, Calderwood SK. Temperature range and selective sensitivity of tumors to hyperthermia: a critical review. Ann N Y Acad Sci. 1980;335:180–205.
25. Goldberg SN, Gazelle GS, Halpern EF, et al. Radiofrequency tissue ablation: importance of local temperature along the electrode tip exposure in determining lesion shape and size. Acad Radiol. 1996;3:212–8.
26. Hung WK, Mak KL, Ying M, Chan M. Radiofrequency ablation of breast cancer: a comparative study of two needle designs. Breast Cancer. 2011;18:124–8.
27. Quaranta V, Manenti G, Bolacchi F, et al. FEM analysis of RF breast ablation: multiprobe versus cool-tip electrode. Anticancer Res. 2007;27:775–84.

28. Grotenhuis BA, Vrijland WW, Klem TMAL. Radiofrequency ablation for early-stage breast cancer: treatment outcomes and practical considerations. Eur J Surg Oncol. 2013;39:1317–24.
29. Ahmed M, Brace CL, Lee FT, Goldberg SN. Principles of and advances in percutaneous ablation. Radiology. 2011;258:351–69.
30. Leylek AM, Whitman GJ, Vilar VS, et al. Radiofrequency ablation for breast cancer. Tech Vasc Interv Radiol. 2013;16:269–76.
31. Izzo F, Thomas R, Delrio P, et al. Radiofrequency ablation in patients with primary breast carcinoma: a pilot study in 26 patients. Cancer. 2001;92:2036–44.
32. Vilar VS, Goldman SM, Ricci MD, et al. Analysis by MRI of residual tumor after radiofrequency ablation for early stage breast cancer. AJR Am J Roentgenol. 2012;198: W285–91.

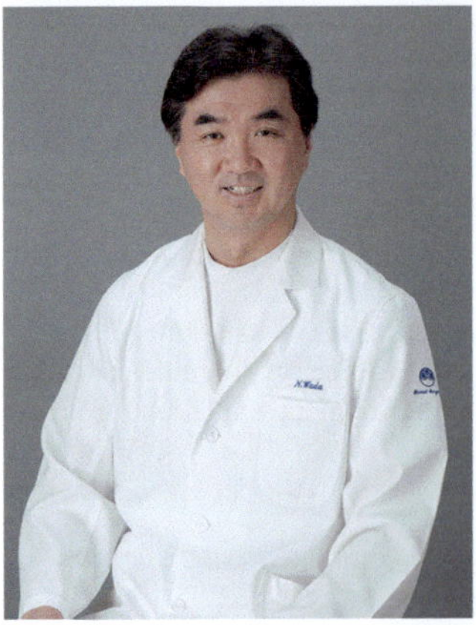

Noriaki Wada

Chapter 6
RFA of Breast Cancer: Technique 1, Requisite Skills and Pitfalls to Avoid

Tomomi Fujisawa

6.1 Materials and Methods

6.1.1 Eligibility Criteria

The main inclusion criterion was the presence of an invasive breast cancer of 1.5 cm or less at the greatest diameter measurable by sonography or by MRI/CT. The tumor had to be clearly identified and unequivocally measurable using US. To avoid the risk of injury to the skin and the membrane of pectoral muscle, a distance of at least 1 cm was required between the tumor and the overlying skin and between the tumor and the chest wall [1].

A histopathological diagnosis of invasive or noninvasive breast cancer had to have been established before RFA by the evaluation of biological study of a tumor specimen obtained by US-guided core needle biopsy or by vacuum-assisted biopsy. In addition, histopathological study including evaluation of ER,PgR,HER2,Ki67 status should be finished before the ablation procedure. Other inclusion criteria included the absence of any axillary lymph node metastasis on palpation or by an imaging examination and the absence of any distant metastases using an imaging examination, eligible for general anesthesia and without serious complications of their breast cancer. Exclusion criteria were previous treatment for breast cancer, previous history of other cancer, pregnancy, presence of an active infection, bleeding tendency, spreading ductal component, and bilateral breast cancer. All

T. Fujisawa (✉)
Department of Breast Oncology Gunma Prefectural Cancer Center, Takabayashi-nishi cho, 617-1, Ota-shi, Gunma 373-8550, Japan
e-mail: fujisawa@gunma-cc.jp

T. Kinoshita (ed.), *Non-surgical Ablation Therapy for Early-stage Breast Cancer*,
DOI 10.1007/978-4-431-54463-0_6

patients signed an informed consent form before being registered for the study and undergoing any study-related procedures.

6.2 Protocol Schedule

6.2.1 Pretreatment Imaging Examinations

Before the operation, the shape and location of the cancer in the breast were recorded by palpation. Mammography and sonography were performed in order to visualize the tumor's shape and size. The tumor's measurements were obtained in three dimensions; the maximum diameter and the transverse and longitudinal lengths of the tumor were calculated. All margins of tumor should be visualized under sonographical study before operation. The distances between the anterior wall of the lesion and the skin and between the posterior margin of the tumor and the membrane of pectoral muscle should be measured. Moderate lateral compression of the breast was allowed, if necessary, to increase these distances. If such compression was used, it was applied to the breast during the entire RFA procedure. CT and MRI scans were performed to visualize the tumor using a 5-mm slice range.

6.2.2 Pretreatment Pathological Study

Core needle or vacuum-assisted biopsies were performed, and the presence of invasive or noninvasive breast cancer was confirmed. The tumors should be undergone routine histopathological evaluation (i.e., assessment of histopathological grade, Ki67 expression, expression of estrogen receptor, progesterone receptor, exist of overexpression of HER2/neu) because after RFA has been performed, viable tumors are not always available for these analyses.

To compare the viability after ablation, H-E staining is not effective, so Nicotinamide Adenine Dinucleotide diaphorase (NADH-diaphorase) viability studies were performed [2]. NADH-diaphorase activity stop after irreversible cellular injury, and this test can therefore be used after RFA to discriminate between viable and nonviable cells in the ablated tissue.

For this analysis, 8-mm unfixed frozen sections were placed on glass slides. Incubation media consisted of 1 mL of reduced α-NADH (Sigma-Aldrich Corp., St Louis, MO) at a concentration of 2.5-mg/mL distilled water, 1 mL of phosphate-buffered saline (pH 7.4) at a concentration of 2 mg/mL, and 0.5 mL of Lactated Ringer's solution. Each tissue section slide was covered with 100 μL of incubation media for 15 min under aerobic conditions at room temperature. Then, each slide was washed in distilled water for 2 min and mounted with glass cover slips using an aqueous medium. Slides were evaluated for characterization of staining within 24 h of processing. A section of normal breast tissue was used as a positive control, and a section of normal breast tissue placed in phosphate-buffered saline and heated to 100 °C was used as a negative control [3, 4].

6.3 The Radio-Frequency Ablation Procedure

6.3.1 Anesthesia

General anesthesia is recommended when carrying out the ablation procedure; local anesthesia is not permitted.

6.3.2 Sentinel Lymph Node Biopsy

After general anesthesia was induced, a sentinel lymph node biopsy (SLNB) was performed. Tracers and dye for SLNB should be injected into the subareolar parenchyma to prevent the interference of fluid with intraoperative US imaging.

6.3.3 Intraoperative US Imaging

After the SLNB was completed, the tumor was visualized by US using the Toshiba Aplio XG SSA-790A (Toshiba Medical Systems Corporation, Otawara, Japan) with a PLT-1204AT (12 MHz) probe. The probe was wrapped with a sterile cover. Under sonographical guidance, the 17-gauge Cool-tip RFA system E series™ (Covidien, Energy-Based Devices, Interventional Oncology, Boulder, CO) pierced the center of the tumor [5] (Figs. 6.1 and 6.2).

The needle penetrated the widest point of the tumor at a right angle. The needle pierced the skin at the margin of the subareolar, to reduce conspicuousness of any later scarring (Fig. 6.3).

From the point at which the needle pierced the tumor, estimated to be its center, the range over which the heat from the ablation spread was measured. The horizontal range was taken as 5 × 30 mm and the vertical range as 5 × 10 mm. An image was taken of the spread of the ablation's heat from the needle to the skin and from the needle to membrane of pectoral muscle (Fig. 6.4).

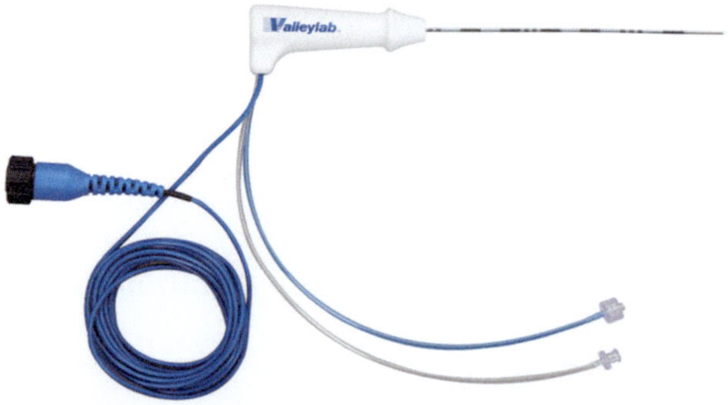

Fig. 6.1 Needle of RFA system

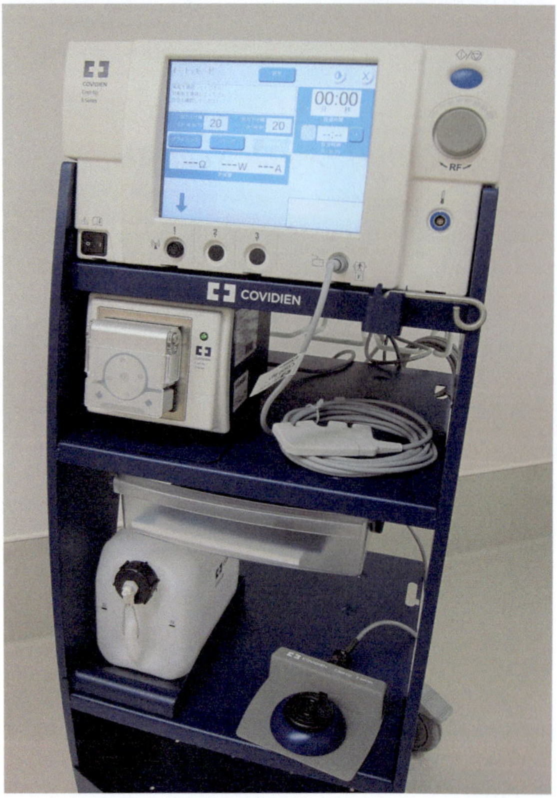

Fig. 6.2 Generator of RFA system

6.3.4 Five Percent Glucose Injection

Assuming that the distance from the needle to skin and to the membrane of pectoral muscle was within 1.5 cm, 5 % glucose was injected between the needle and skin and membrane of pectoral muscle to avoid burning by ablation heat. The glucose injection disturbs the position of the tumor, and therefore in order not to lose the location of the tumor, the needle must not be moved (Fig. 6.5).

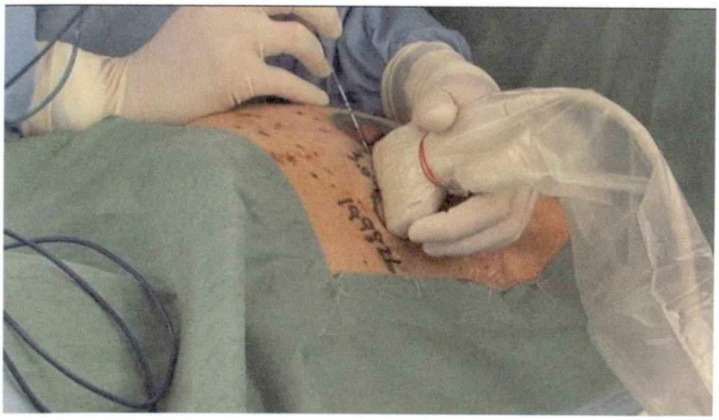

Fig. 6.3 Stick a RFA needle under sonographical finding

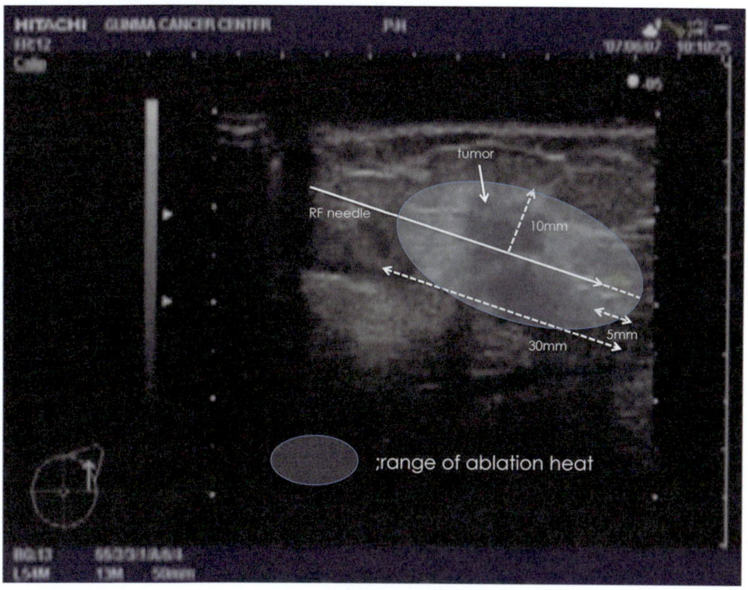

Fig. 6.4 Measurement of tumor under sonographical finding

6.3.5 Ablation

Following the expansion of the distance between the needle and skin and needle and membrane of pectoral muscle by the injection of 5 % glucose, ablation was started. The needle electrode was attached to a 500-kHz monopolar RF generator capable of producing 200-W power. Tissue impedance was monitored continuously using circuitry incorporated into the generator. A peristaltic pump (Watson-Marlow, Medford, MA) was used to infuse 0 °C normal saline solution into the lumen of

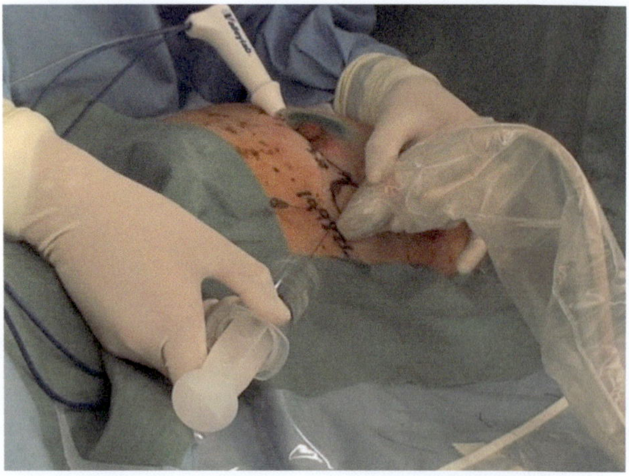

Fig. 6.5 Injection of 5 % glucose

the electrode at a rate sufficient to maintain a tip temperature of 15–25 °C. RF energy was applied to tissue with an initial power setting of 5 W and gradually increased by 10 W per minute to a maximum power of 55 W. Saline circulating internally within the electrode cools the adjacent tissue, maximizing energy deposition and reducing tissue charring. Tissue impedance was continuously monitored. The power setting was left at this point until power "roll-off" occurred. Power roll-off implies that there is an increase in the tissue impedance caused by loss of sodium chloride, which occurs with tissue coagulation around the monopolar electrode. When this occurs, the power generator will shut off, stopping the flow of current and further tissue coagulation. The appearance and progression of hyperechogenicity on the US, referred to as "microbubbles," was used to guide the therapy [7] (Fig. 6.6). Radio frequency was applied until the tumor was completely hyperechoic. A rise in internal temperature of more than 70 °C is required to achieve cell death by ablation. Thus, in cases where the temperature did not rise to 70 °C, the RF energy was reapplied until the internal temperature rose by at least 70 °C. In cases where the ablation had caused coagulation in the tissue surrounding the needle, impedance was elevated, and the power roll-off was induced, causing the generator to shut off too soon with the result that the internal temperature was not raised enough. To avoid this happening, the RF energy supply was increased gradually by 5 W per minute.

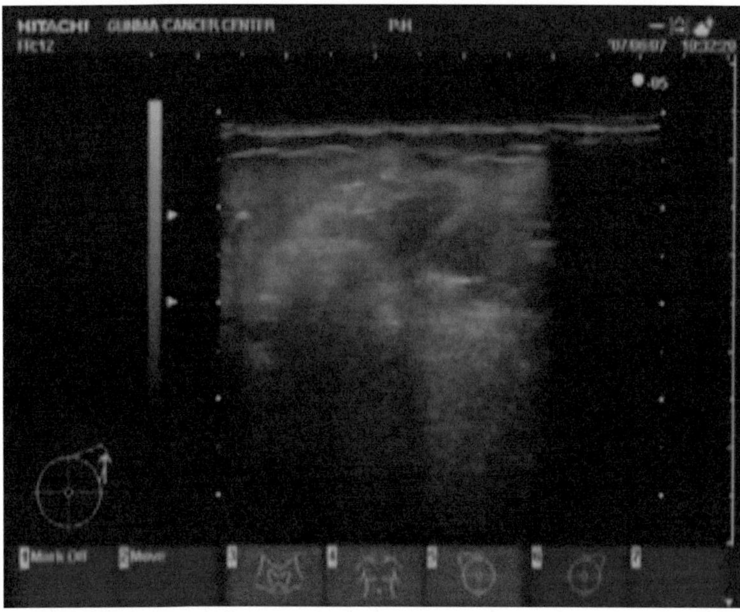

Fig. 6.6 Observation of microbubble under sonographical finding

6.4 After the RFA Procedure

6.4.1 Adjuvant Radiotherapy

In our clinical trial, the protocol prescribed adjuvant radiotherapy (50 Gy/25 Fr) to the whole breast after ablation. The decision on whether to increase the ablation of the lesion by an additional 10 Gy was left to the judgment of the individual facility.

6.4.2 Breast Imaging and Biopsy After Operation

After the RFA procedure, patients were evaluated by US examination every 3 months for the first 2 years after the operation and then every 6 months up to 5 years. After ablation, while the ablated area could be visualized on the US scan by an unclear margin and no vascular flow, contrast-enhanced ultrasonography was sometimes used to detect new vessel flow produced by the residual tumor.

Post-RFA, MRI scans were examined every 6 months for the first 3 years and then every 12 months up to 5 years post-RFA. These scans could detect residual enhancement surrounding the ablated area, for those tumors that had pre-RFA enhancement in the scan.

Mammography was carried out as usual, every 12 months for 5 years.

Vacuum-assisted biopsy was performed post-RFA, as per protocol: at 3 months after the radiation therapy, when the ablated tissue was examined pathologically to determine the residual viability of cancer cells.

6.4.3 *Adjuvant Therapy*

Post-RFA, patients received adjuvant systemic therapy with hormone therapy (when hormone receptor positive) and/or chemotherapy, as recommended by the guidelines for adjuvant therapy [8], based on the intrinsic subtype and histological examination of the needle biopsy before RFA and the results of the SLNB.

6.5 Complications and How to Limit Their Occurrence

6.5.1 *Inadequate Ablation*

The needle electrode was attached to a 500-kHz, monopolar RF generator capable of producing 200-W power. However, sometimes the internal temperature does not reach a high enough temperature for ablation. In such situations, it is likely that the inadequate thermal effect in the cancerous cells will not induce cell apoptosis. One cause of this was thought to be the direct effect of bleeding as a result of the needle puncturing the tumor, as excessive bleeding can negatively influence the thermal effect. In addition, excessive 5 % glucose injection, to expand the distance from ablated tumor to skin and from tumor to membrane of pectoral muscle, might also prevent the temperature reaching an adequate level for ablation.

To avoid bleeding from tumor vessels, US was used to observe the spread of vessels supplying the tumor, before puncturing it with the needle. For the same reason, the 5 % glucose solution was not to be injected too close to the tumor.

In other situations, the 5 % glucose increased the impedance and caused the "roll-off," which stopped the electrical supply. In many Japanese patients, the volume of breast tissue is not so large and the ablation heat has a tendency to reach the skin and membrane of pectoral muscle, resulting in burns. To avoid this happening, over-injection of 5 % glucose can occur and this can cause the "roll-off." When this happens, and with the needle already in place, the ablation is stopped to allow the 5 % glucose to be absorbed by the surrounding breast tissue. The volume of injected 5 % glucose is reduced, until equilibrium is achieved and normal impedance levels return.

6.5.2 *Skin Burn*

With adequate ablation introduced from an electric supply, the temperature at the tip of the needle can be elevated to 80–90 °C leading to apoptosis of the cancer

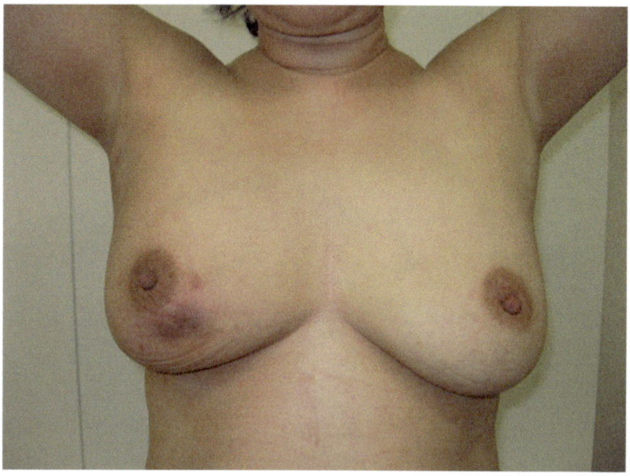

Fig. 6.7 Burn of skin due to RFA heat

cells. However, if the tip of needle comes too close to the skin, it can cause burning (Fig. 6.7). To avoid this, a sterile ice pack was placed on the skin above the tumor [1]. One or two ice packs are usually sufficient to maintain a good surface temperature and avoid skin burns.

Generally, a 2-cm or 3-cm diameter electrode provides a range sufficient to reach the ablation heat. Therefore, it is important to measure the range carefully from needle to skin and to deep muscle to confirm the relative position of the needle's tip.

Skin burn-induced RFA is a direct result of the heat of ablation, and an indirect result of the lack of blood supply induced by damage of vessels by the ablation. Thus, it is hard to heal such a complicated injury.

6.5.3 Bleeding

Bleeding from tumor vessels supplying the tumor, or from the tumors themselves, is not considered as a severe adverse event because of the ease of stopping the bleeding (Fig. 6.8). Nevertheless, because of its direct effect of decreasing the thermal effect, and the indirect effect of a bleeding-induced hematoma, bleeding is also regarded as a side effect that is best avoided. To avoid such problems, the Doppler mode in the sonography function should be used to visualize the vessels.

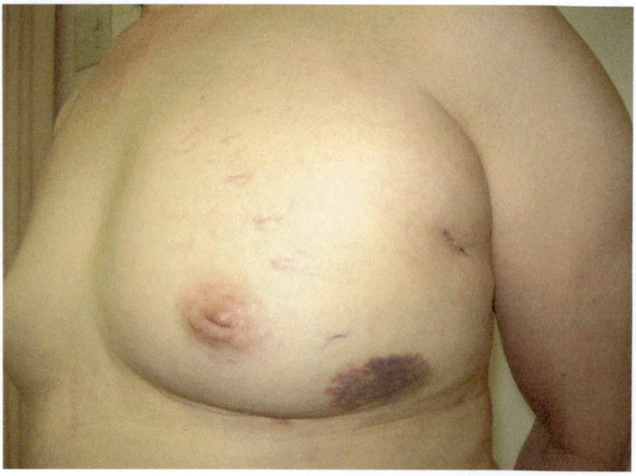

Fig. 6.8 Subcutaneous bleeding after RFA

References

1. Kinoshita T, Iwamoto E, Tsuda H, Seki K. Radiofrequency ablation as local therapy for early breast carcinomas. Breast Cancer. 2011;18(1):10–7.
2. Khatri VP, McGahan JP, Ramsamooj R, Griffey S, Brock J, Cronan M, Wilkendorf S. A phase II trial of image-guided radiofrequency ablation of small invasive breast carcinomas: use of saline-cooled tip electrode. Ann Surg Oncol. 2007;14(5):1644–52.
3. Tsuda H. Radiofrequency ablation therapy for primary breast cancer: expectations and problems as a novel breast conservation therapy. Breast Cancer. 2011;18(1):1–2.
4. Tsuda H, Seki K, Hasebe T, Sasajima Y, Shibata T, Iwamoto E, Kinoshita T. A histopathological study for evaluation of therapeutic effects of radiofrequency ablation in patients with breast cancer. Breast Cancer. 2011;18(1):24–32.
5. Yoshinaga Y, Enomoto Y, Fujimitsu R, Shimakura M, Nabeshima K, Iwasaki A. Image and pathological changes after radiofrequency ablation of invasive breast cancer: a pilot study of nonsurgical therapy of early breast cancer. World J Surg. 2013;37(2):356–63.
6. Oura S, Tamaki T, Hirai I, Yoshimasu T, Ohta F, Nakamura R, Okamura Y. Radiofrequency ablation therapy in patients with breast cancers two centimeters or less in size. Breast Cancer. 2007;14(1):48–54.
7. Hung WK, Mak KL, Ying M, Chan M. Radiofrequency ablation of breast cancer: a comparative study of two needle designs. Breast Cancer. 2011;18(2):124–8.
8. Goldhirsch A, Winer EP, Coates AS, Gelber RD, Piccart-Gebhart M, Thurlimann B, Senn HJ. Personalizing the treatment of women with early breast cancer: highlights of the St Gallen International Expert Consensus on the Primary Therapy of Early Breast Cancer. Ann Oncol. 2013 Sep;24(9):2206–23.

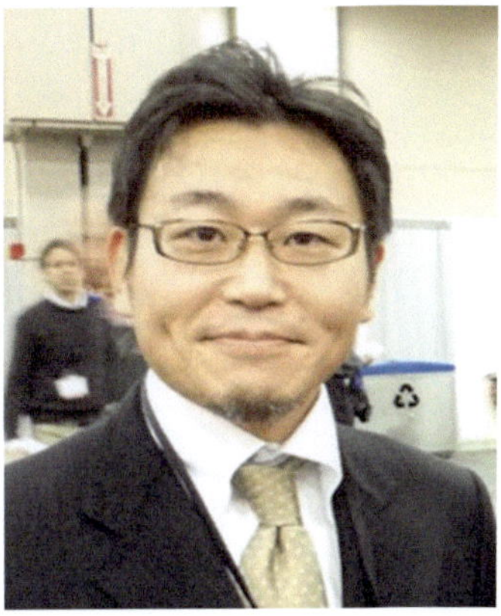

Tomomi Fujisawa

Chapter 7
RFA of Breast Cancer: Technique2, Knack and Pitfall

Toshikazu Ito

7.1 Introduction

This study was done with the approval of the institutions' ethics committees. The primary end points of the study were technical success, safety, and complete necrosis of the target tumors.

Secondary end points were recurrence free survival and cosmetic appearance. Technical success of radio-frequency (RF) ablation was defined as correct placement of the ablation device into the target tumor with completion of the planned ablation protocol—i.e., the target temperature of 70 °C or more [1–10]. The safety assessment included identification of treatment- related complications.

7.2 Patients and Methods

Inclusion criteria were age greater than 18 years; biopsy-proven invasive or non-invasive ductal carcinoma, tumor diameter of 2 cm or smaller in greatest diameter, is detected by ultrasound (US) and contrast-enhanced MRI. Exclusion criteria were patients with a wide extensive intraductal component in invasive cancer, diffuse calcification suggestive of extensive or multifocal ductal carcinoma in situ, and patients who were pregnant or breastfeeding.

Accurate biological tumor characteristics such as estrogen and progesterone receptors, nuclear grade, Ki-67, and human epidermal growth factor receptor

T. Ito (✉)
Department of Surgery, Rinku General Medical Center, 2-23 Rinku Orai-kita, Izumisano, Osaka, Japan
e-mail: t-ito@rgmc.izumisano.osaka.jp

T. Kinoshita (ed.), *Non-surgical Ablation Therapy for Early-stage Breast Cancer*,
DOI 10.1007/978-4-431-54463-0_7

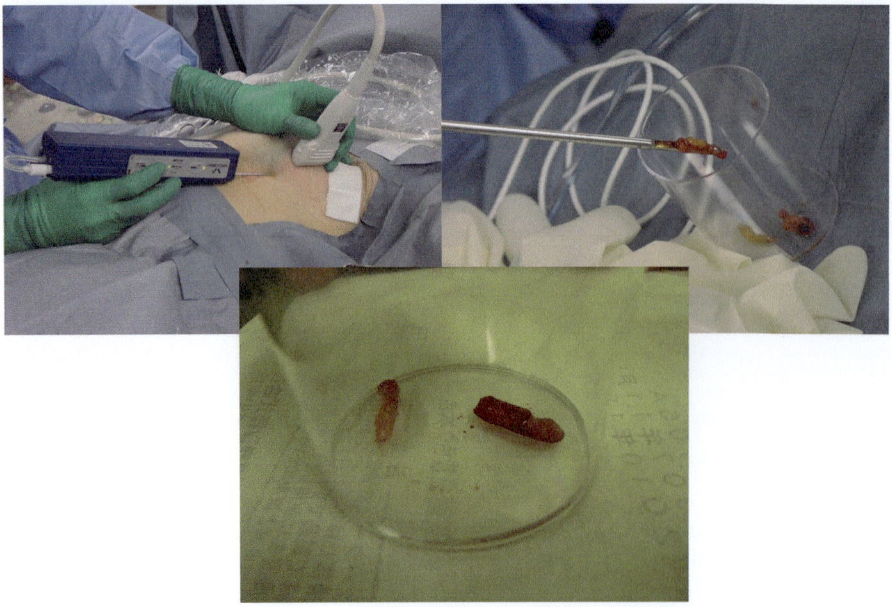

Fig. 7.1 Ten-gauge vacuum-assisted biopsy before RF ablation. Vacuum-assisted biopsy and/or core biopsy had to be adequate for routine pathologic evaluation because after RF ablation has been performed, a viable tumor may not be available

2 (HER-2/neu) status were estimated from tumor tissue taken with core needle biopsy and/or vacuum-assisted biopsy (Fig. 7.1).

7.3 Pretreatment Assessments

Approval for this study was obtained from our institutional ethics committee, and written informed consent was obtained from each patient prior to the procedure. All patients were admitted to the hospital the day before RF ablation. Preablation imaging workup included mammography, an unenhanced and a contrast-enhanced US [11, 12], and MRI of the breast.

A 0.015-mL/kg body weight bolus of a perflubutane microbubble contrast agent Sonazoid® (Daiichi Sankyo Co., Ltd., Tokyo, Japan) with a median diameter of 2–3 μm was injected into an antecubital vein via a 20-gauge cannula and followed by a 10-mL normal saline flush. Contrast-enhanced US was performed with a low mechanical index for up to 5–10 min after the administration of contrast material. Ultrasound systems included APLIO 500, XG (Toshiba Medical Systems, Tokyo, Japan), and a LOGIQ E9 (GE Medical systems, Milwaukee, WI, USA) with a 6–12-MHz linear arrayed transducer. All breast carcinomas were recognized and recorded with tumor location, size, and color flow by unenhanced US. And then

Table 7.1 Contrast-enhanced US in differentiation of malignant and benign lesions

	Accuracy	Sensitivity	Specificity
Contrast-enhanced US (CEUS)	**86.7 %**	**92.9 %**	**84.0 %**
Unenhanced US (UEUS)	66.9 %	86.5 %	58.5 %
Contrast-enhanced MRI (CE-MRI)	69.5 %	86.5 %	62.2 %
CEUS vs UEUS (GEE)	3.215	2.028	3.728
	($P<0.001$)	($P=0.177$)	($P<0.001$)
CEUS vs CE-MRI (GEE)	2.849	2.028	3.188
	($P<0.001$)	($P<0.001$)	($P<0.001$)

The diagnostic accuracy of CEUS was about 20 % higher than the accuracy of unenhanced US and MRI
CEUS was superior in specificity
The sensitivity of contrast-enhanced US was the highest of all at 90 % or more

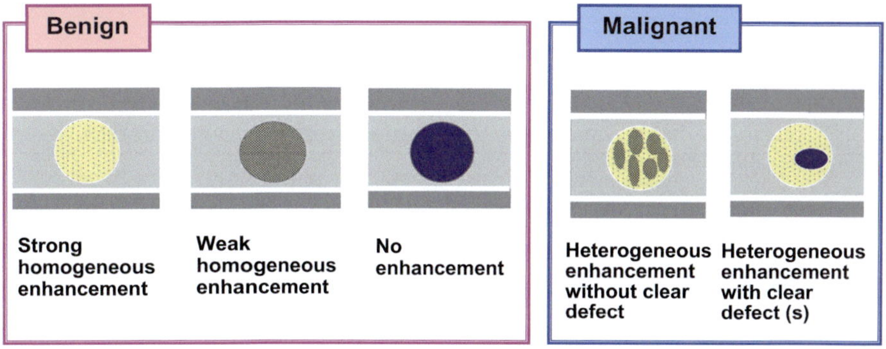

Fig. 7.2 Enhancement patterns of contrast-enhanced US

contrast-enhanced US using Sonazoid® was done for detection of breast tumor lesion and extensive intraductal component.

It had been reported that contrast-enhanced US significantly improved the differential diagnosis of breast lesions compared to unenhanced US and contrast-enhanced MRI (Table 7.1) [11, 12].

The blinded reviewers in DD723 (Sonazoid®) study assessed the lesions of interest for differential diagnoses according to the following enhancement pattern, with the detection of one or a few patterns being enough to make the diagnosis. For benign lesions, these patterns included strong homogeneous enhancement of the entire lesion, weak homogeneous enhancement of the entire lesion, or no enhancement of the entire lesion. For malignant lesions, these patterns included heterogeneous enhancement with or without clear defect, rapid washout from the lesion compared with washout from the surrounding mammary tissues, and enhancement extending outward beyond the expected borders of the lesion (Fig. 7.2) [11, 12].

Additional workup for patients with metastatic disease included contrast-enhanced CT of the chest and abdomen, whole body bone scintigraphy, and MRI of the brain if focal neurologic deficits were defected.

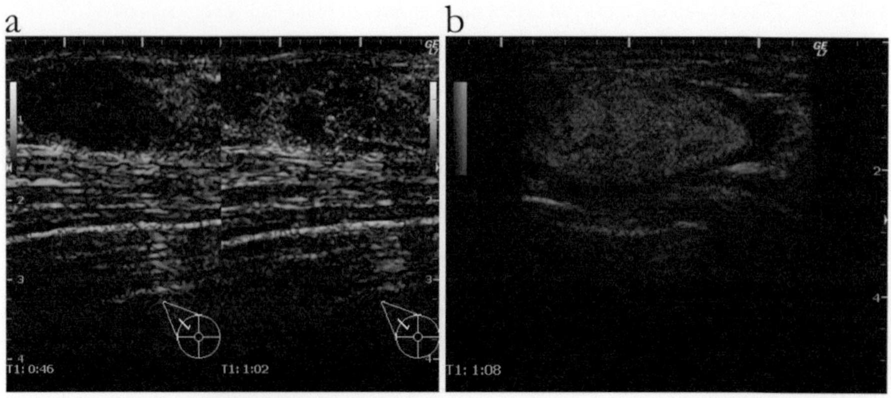

Fig. 7.3 Contrast-enhanced US before and after RF ablation. (**a**) Before RF ablation, the tumor shows a heterogeneous enhancement with clear defect. (**b**) After RF ablation, ablation zone shows a lack of contrast enhancement

It was reported a clinical application about using the ultrasonography contrast agent Sonazoid® before and after RF ablation treatment with primary breast carcinomas (Fig. 7.3).

7.4 Treatment

All RF ablation procedures were performed in an operation room by surgeon. The patient was placed in the dorsal decubitus position. Under general anesthesia, a sentinel lymph node biopsy was performed initially with an indocyaningreen (Daiichi Sankyo, Tokyo, Japan) for axillary staging. In the case of positive sentinel node with histological diagnosis in frozen section, axillary lymph node dissection was performed.

All patients underwent breast ultrasound preoperatively to determine if the invasive tumor and intraductal component were visible, as it would facilitate ultrasound-guided RF ablation.

A single-needle 17-gauge electrode 15 or 10 cm in length with a 3-cm or 2-cm active tip (Cool-tip RF system, Valleylab, Boulder, CO, USA) was used for RF ablation [2–4]. The skin entry site that allowed path of maximum tumor diameter plane was chosen. The needle was placed into the target tumor, and its correct placement was checked by the use of two-dimensional ultrasound and multiplanar image reconstructions (Fig. 7.4). It was then connected to the generator and the heating procedure began.

The device induces an ablation sphere of 3–4 cm in diameter. Because the maximum size of the target tumors was 2.0 cm in diameter, the ablation protocol was planned with the aim to destroy the visible tumor mass plus at least a 0.5-cm safety margin around the tumor. Needle penetration at the center of the tumor was confirmed by US, and the head of the Cool-tip needle was placed outside the tumor

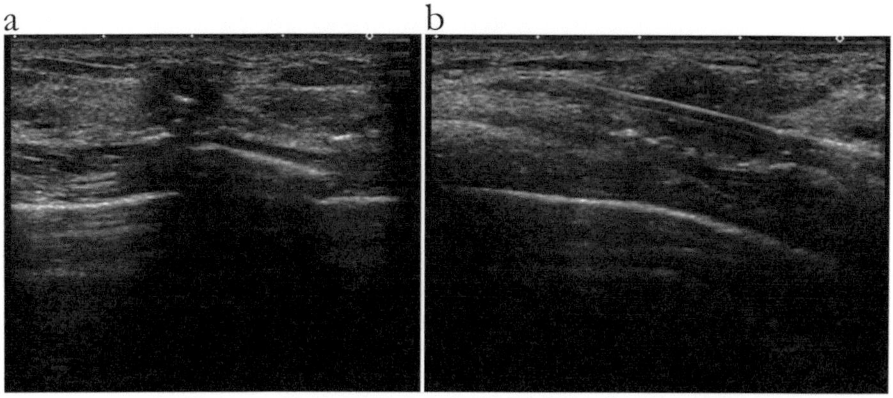

Fig. 7.4 Intraoperative breast ultrasound. (**a**) Cool-Tip™ RF needle electrode is seen traversing the breast tumor. (**b**) Needle is seen "end-on" and noted to be in the center of the lesion

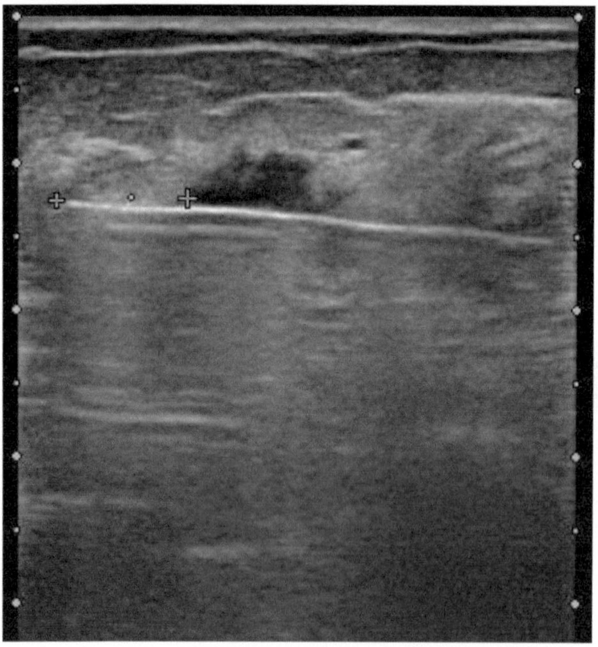

Fig. 7.5 A margin of surround breast tissue. The tip of the needle was placed outside of the tumor approximately 8 mm from the edge of the tumor

approximately 5–10 mm from the edge of the tumor (Fig. 7.5). The shaft of the needle electrode kept aligned with the scanning plane and as parallel to the chest.

Thermal ablation was performed using a generator with two large dispersive electrodes (ground pads) placed on patient's thighs. RF ablation was started at 5-W output. Output was raised to 10 W 1 min later and thereafter increased by 10 W every 1 min until the generator automatically stopped delivering RF energy [1, 2].

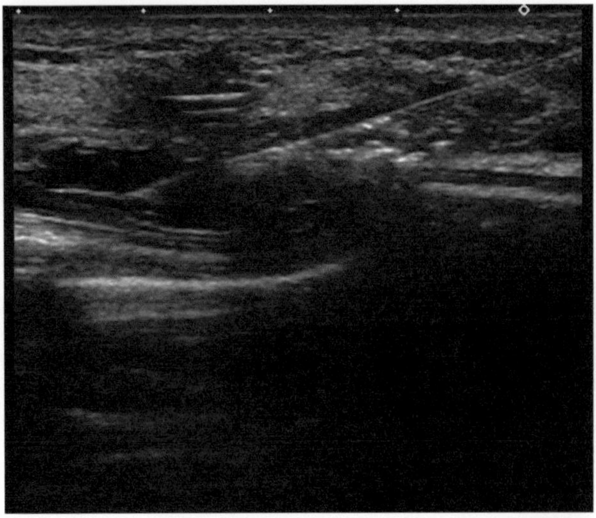

Fig. 7.6 Five percent glucose injection. To minimize thermal injury to the muscle fascia, 5 % glucose was injected into the retromammary space

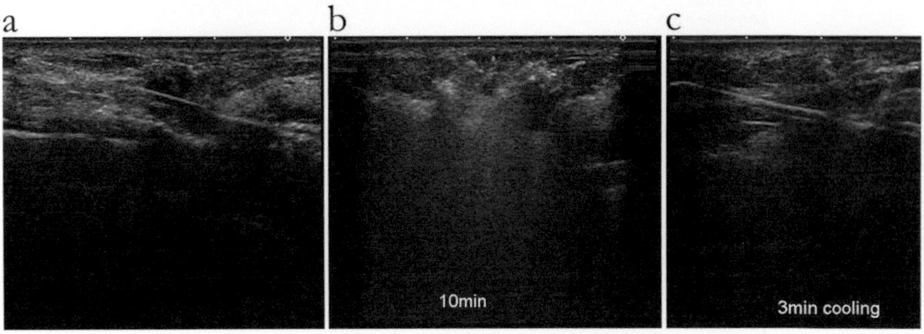

Fig. 7.7 Intraoperative breast ultrasound. (a) Before RF ablation. (b, c) 3-min cooling after RF ablation

About 20 mL or more of 5 % glucose solution was injected into the retromammary space to avoid burns of the major pectoral muscle from ablation induced heat (Fig. 7.6). The skin just above the tumor was cooled with an ice pack after the start of RF ablation until 3–4 h later from end of the operation. If necessary, multiple overlapping ablations were performed in different sections of the tumor when the safety margin was not wide enough around the tumor, and repositioning of the electrode was possible after the first heating session. After the beginning of RF ablation, the amount of gas has increased over time. However several minutes cooling, the amount of gas has decreased (Fig. 7.7). After completion of the procedure, US imaging was obtained to assess technical success zone of ablation and to detect any complications.

7.5 Posttreatment Follow-Up and Evaluation of Efficacy

Posttreatment MRI, contrast-enhanced US assessment, and histological examination were performed 1 month after RF ablation and before radiotherapy. MRI and contrast-enhanced US are valuable for clinical follow-up of breast cancer patients undergoing RF ablation [10]. We considered ablations complete and technical success achieved if the ablation zone completely covered the tumor, and there was no irregular enhancement at the treatment margin (Fig. 7.8). Ablated tumor tissues were obtained using a 10- or 8-gauge needle of vacuum-assisted biopsy under US guidance. When enhancement of the tumor was seen in the center of the ablation zone or when a nodular aspect associated with a tumor-type enhancement was observed in any nodule inside or outside the ablation zone.

Other new technology of ultrasound such as 3D/4D ultrasonography, elastography (Fig. 7.9), and virtual sonography (RVS or Volume navigation) will be valuable for evaluation of RF ablation (Fig. 7.10).

Virtual MRI or CT sonography using magnetic navigation and volume navigation provides cross-sectional images of MRI or CT volume data corresponding to the angle of the transducer in the magnetic field in real time.

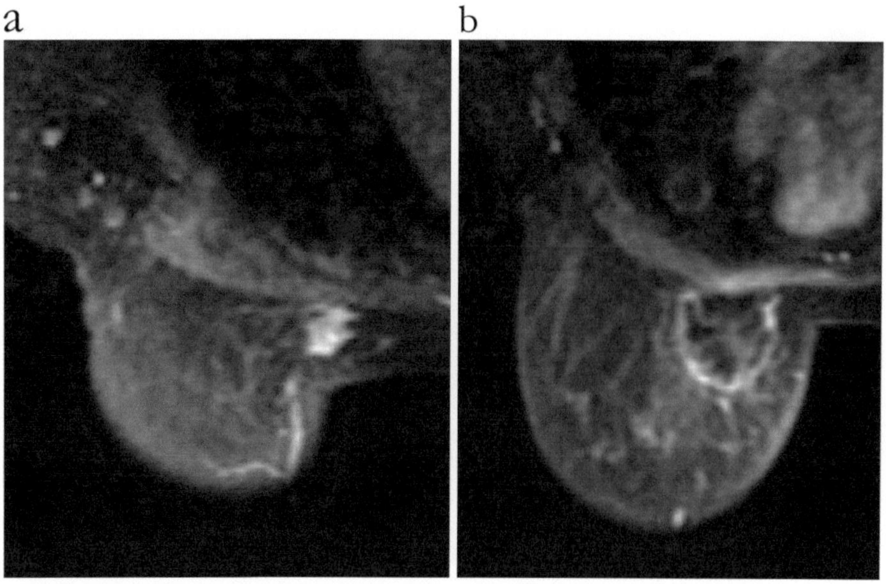

Fig. 7.8 Contrast-enhanced MRI before and after RF ablation. (**a**) Before RF ablation. (**b**) After RF ablation

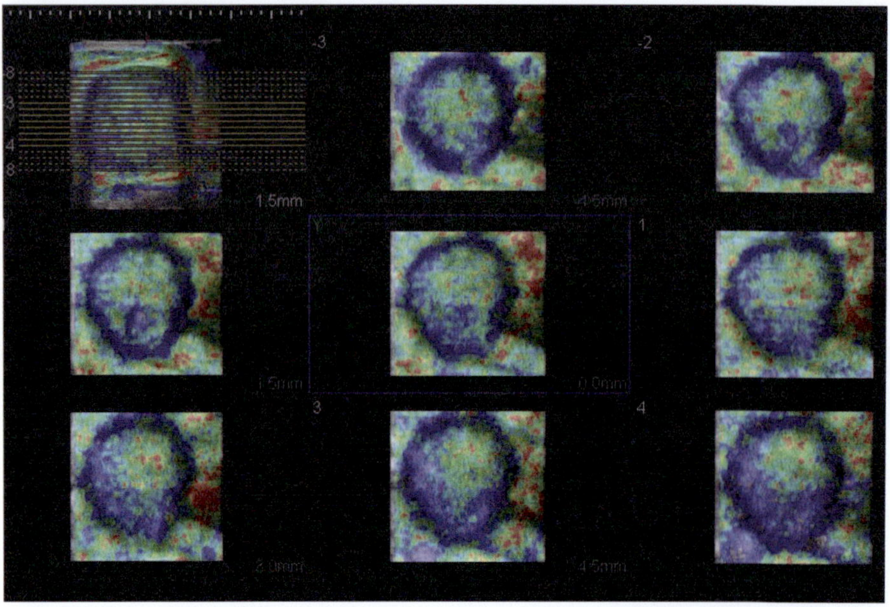

Fig. 7.9 4D elastography of ablation zone

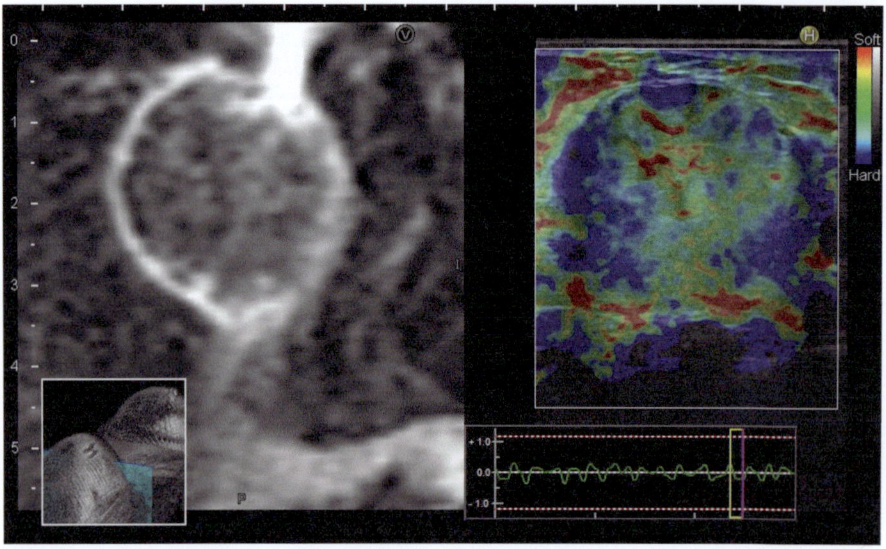

Fig. 7.10 Virtual elastography of ablation zone

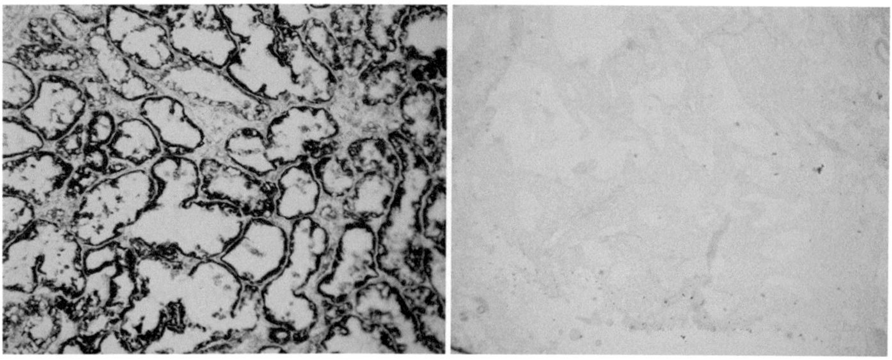

Fig. 7.11 Pathologic evaluation using NADH diaphorase. (**a**) Before RF ablation. (**b**) After RF ablation

7.6 Pathologic Evaluation

Pathologists were informed of the study and looked specifically at the ablation zone, which was identified as an area wherein epithelial and stromal structures were replaced by necrotic cells and inflammatory cells. The ablation zone was defined as an area of coagulative necrosis and fatty tissue necrosis. To evaluate the effects of RF ablation, in addition to routine hematoxylin-eosin (H&E) staining, single-stranded DNA staining and cryosection of 5–6-μm thick were made for cell viability staining with a nicotinamide dinucleotide, reduced NADH diaphorase (Fig. 7.11).

7.7 Adjuvant Treatment

Following RF ablation treatment, patient underwent standard whole-breast radiation therapy (50 Gy ± boost 10 Gy) as part of breast conservation therapy. Decisions regarding adjuvant therapy were based on the status of the lymph node, prognostic factors such as estrogen and progesterone receptor unclear grade, Ki-67, and HER-2/neu status as determined by the pretreatment core biopsy or vacuum-assisted biopsy.

7.8 Long-Term Follow-Up

If successful RF ablation treatment was confirmed, patients received adjuvant radiotherapy and, if needed, adjuvant systemic therapy. Follow-up visits were scheduled 1 and 6 months after treatment and then at 6-month intervals for up to

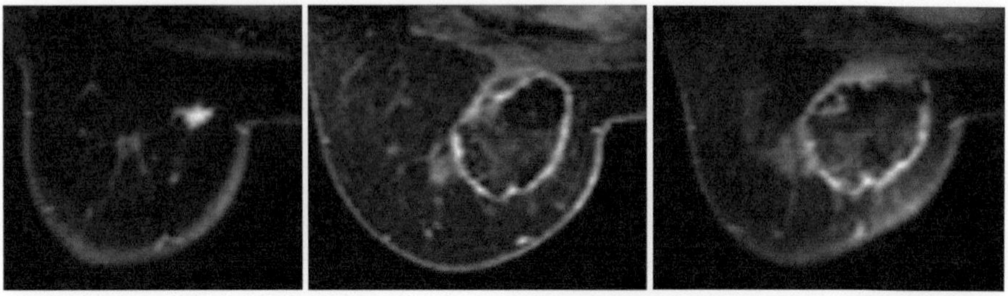

Fig. 7.12 Contrast-enhanced MRI before and after. (**a**) Before RF ablation. (**b**) 6 months after RF ablation. (**c**) 12 months after RF ablation

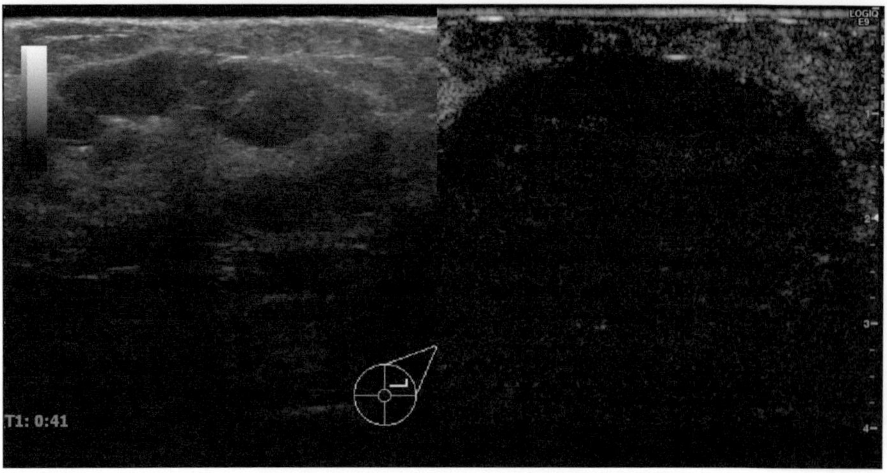

Fig. 7.13 Contrast-enhanced US after RF ablation (Photo caption: Toshikazu Ito)

5 years or more. The following were done at each follow-up visit: physical examination, US, MR imaging (Fig. 7.12), and/or contrast enhancement US (Fig. 7.13) for tumor assessment. Lack of focal enhancement within or at the periphery of a tumor at follow-up contrast-enhanced imaging was considered radiographic evidence of complete necrosis.

7.9 Complications

- Skin burn

Two types of skin burn are possible; one is at the electrode puncture site and the other is at the grounding pad attachment site.

Skin burn at the site of ground pad attachment site is possible, but has not yet been in our institution.

Application of an ice pack to the skin just above the tumor can prevent skin burn.

- Muscle burn and local pain

About 20 mL or more of 5 % glucose solution was injected into the retromammary space to avoid burns of the major pectoral muscle.

Pain is the most common symptom associated with the procedure. Oral or drip infusion painkiller is helpful in reducing pain. But the day after RF ablation, almost all patients have no pain.

- Nipple retraction
- Bleeding

At the end of the procedure, after the automatic cool down of the RF ablation system, the generator was reactivated to ablate the track from the tumor to the subcutaneous tissue to prevent bleeding or tumor cell dissemination.

References

1. Singletary S,E. Minimally invasive surgery in breast cancer treatment. Biomed Pharmacother. 2001;55:510–4.
2. Oura S, Tamaki T, Hirai I, et al. Radiofrequency ablation therapy in patients with breast cancers two centimeters or less in size. Breast Cancer. 2007;14(1):48–54.
3. Yamamoto N, Fujimoto H, Nakamura R, et al. Pilot study of radiofrequency ablation therapy without surgical excision for T1 breast cancer: evaluation with MRI and vacuum-assisted core needle biopsy and safety management. Breast Cancer. 2011;18(1):3–9.
4. Khatri VP, McGahan JP, Ramsamooj R, et al. A phase II trial of image-guided radiofrequency ablation of small invasive breast carcinomas: use of saline-cooled tip electrode. Ann Surg Oncol. 2007;14(5):1644–52.
5. Medina-Franco H, Sato-Germes S, Ulloa-Gomez JL, et al. Radiofrequency ablation of invasive breast carcinomas: a phase II trial. Ann Surg Oncol. 2008;15:1689–95.
6. Manenti G, Bolacchi F, Perretta T, et al. Small breast cancers: in vivo percutaneous US-guided radiofrequency ablation with dedicated cool-tip radiofrequency system. Radiology. 2009;251:339–46.
7. Garbay J-R, Mathieu M-C, Lamuraglia M, et al. Radiofrequency thermal ablation of breast cancer local recurrence: a phase II clinical trial. Ann Surg Oncol. 2008;15:3222–6.
8. Fornage BD, Sneige N, Ross MI. Small (<2-cm) breast cancer treated with US-guided radiofrequency ablation: feasibility study. Radiology. 2004;231:215–24.
9. Earashi M, Noguchi M, Motoyoshi A, et al. Radiofrequency ablation therapy for small breast cancer followed by immediate surgical resection or delayed mammotome excision. Breast Cancer. 2007;14:39–47.
10. Nagashima T, Sakakibara M, Sangai T, et al. Surrounding rim formation and reduction in size after radiofrequency ablation for primary breast cancer. Jpn J Radiol. 2009;27:197–204.
11. Miyamoto Y, Ito T, Takada E, Omoto K, et al. PhaseIIclinical study of DD-723 (perflubutane): dose-response study in patients with breast tumors. J Med Ultrasonics. 2012;39:79–86.
12. Miyamoto Y, Ito T, Takada E, Omoto K et al. Efficacy of SONAZOID® (perflubutane) contrast-enhanced ultrasound in the differentiation of focal breast lesions: phase 3 multicenter clinical trial. AJR. 2014;202(4):W400–7.

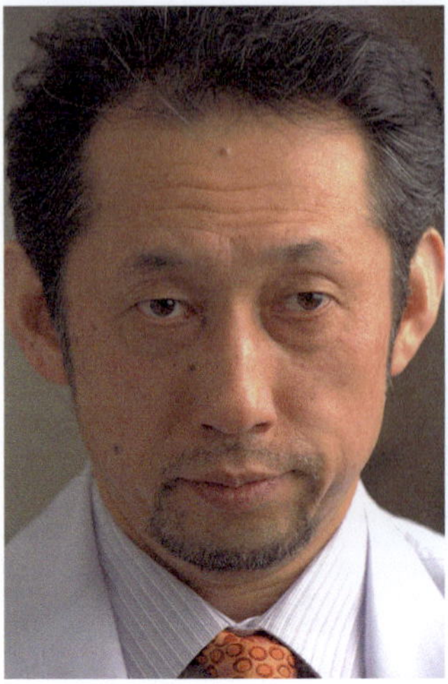

Toshikazu Ito

Chapter 8
Histopathological Evaluation of the Therapeutic Effect of RFA for Early Breast Cancer

Hitoshi Tsuda, Masayuki Yoshida, Kunihiko Seki, Eriko Iwamoto, Kenjiro Jimbo, Sota Asaga, and Takayuki Kinoshita

8.1 Introduction

Between 2006 and 2011, we performed a pilot study to evaluate the efficacy and safety of radiofrequency ablation (RFA) for primary breast cancer at the National Cancer Center Hospital [1]. Patients had the RFA procedure and subsequent surgical resection, mastectomy, or partial resection, with sentinel lymph node biopsy of the primary breast cancer. The study was approved by the internal review board for ethical issues in the National Cancer Center, Tokyo, Japan. All patients provided written informed consent.

An additional goal of the study was to establish reliable criteria for evaluating the RFA effect. RFA has been used for the treatment of hepatocellular carcinoma

H. Tsuda (✉)
Department of Basic Pathology, National Defense Medical College, 3-2 Namiki, Tokorozawa, 359-8513, Saitama, Japan

Department of Pathology and Clinical Laboratories, National Cancer Center Hospital, 5-1-1 Tsukiji, Chuo-ku, Tokyo, 104-0045, Japan
e-mail: hstsuda@gmail.com

M. Yoshida
Department of Pathology and Clinical Laboratories, National Cancer Center Hospital, 5-1-1 Tsukiji, Chuo-ku, Tokyo, 104-0045, Japan

K. Seki
Department of Pathology and Clinical Laboratories, National Cancer Center Hospital, 5-1-1 Tsukiji, Chuo-ku, Tokyo, 104-0045, Japan

Clinical Laboratory Division, JR Tokyo General Hospital, 2-1-3 Yoyogi, Shibuya-ku, 151-8528, Tokyo, Japan

E. Iwamoto • K. Jimbo • S. Asaga • T. Kinoshita
Department of Breast Surgery, National Cancer Center Hospital, 5-1-1 Tsukiji, Chuo-ku, 104-0045, Tokyo, Japan

T. Kinoshita (ed.), *Non-surgical Ablation Therapy for Early-stage Breast Cancer*,
DOI 10.1007/978-4-431-54463-0_8

and early breast cancer, and nicotinamide adenine dinucleotide (NADH) diaphorase staining methods have been used for the evaluation of the therapeutic effect [2–5]. In our pilot study, we assessed hematoxylin and eosin (H&E) staining findings as well as NADH diaphorase staining findings in order to try to propose histopathological criteria for the therapeutic effect of RFA [6].

In this article, we review the method, utility, and limitations of histopathological criteria to evaluate the RFA effect in early breast cancer.

8.1.1 NADH Diaphorase Staining Method

Evaluation of NADH diaphorase activity is the standard method for assaying cell viability in tissues receiving RFA [6]. NADH diaphorase is an enzyme that can transfer hydrogens (and electrons) and reduce substrates, for example, various dyes. NADH plays a central role as a coenzyme in various major redox systems, especially oxidative phosphorylation in mitochondria. The reaction of NADH is briefly expressed with the following formula:

$$\mathrm{NAD}^{+} + \mathrm{Substrate}(2\mathrm{H}^{+} + 2\mathrm{e}^{-}) \Leftrightarrow \mathrm{NADH} + \mathrm{H}^{+} + \mathrm{Substrate},$$

where the oxidized form of NADH is expressed as NAD^{+}, and its reduced form is expressed as NADH. Tetrazolium salts (e.g., nitro blue tetrazolium (NBT)) are substrates that can be reduced by NADH diaphorase and converted to formazans as follows:

$$\mathrm{NADH} + \mathrm{H}^{+} + \mathrm{NBT} \overset{\text{NADH diaphorase}}{\longrightarrow} \text{Formazan dye} + \mathrm{NAD}^{+}$$

The evaluation of NADH diaphorase activity, based on the reduction of NBT to formazan via oxidation of NADH, is a reliable marker of cell viability [6]. With this enzyme histochemical method, sites of enzymatic activity on fresh frozen tissue sections are stained purple blue (water-insoluble formazan pigment). In contrast, enzymatically inactive sites on the tissue are not stained.

From the surgically resected fresh tissue specimen obtained after RFA, representative sections including the entire cut surface of the tumor and surrounding noncancerous tissue were prepared, mounted in OCT compound (Sakura Finetek, Tokyo, Japan), immediately frozen, cut into 4- to 8-μm-thick sections with a cryostat (Leica), and lay a section on a glass slide (Matsunami Glass Co., Kishiwada, Japan). After immediate dry of the slides in order to adhere the section to the glass, the slide was either stained with hematoxylin and eosin (H&E) or stored in a deep freezer until NADH diaphorase staining. The remaining tissues were fixed in 10 % buffered formalin and processed for routine histopathological examination.

For the histochemical assay, frozen tissue slides were incubated in 0.8 mg/mL β-NADH (Sigma), 0.5 mg/mL NBT (Sigma), and 0.05 M Tris-buffered saline (pH 7.4) for 1 h at 37 °C. The slides were then fixed in 10 % buffered formalin, washed in distilled water, and included with cover slips [6].

8.1.2 Evaluation of the RFA Effect

Grossly, the cut surface of the ablated area in the resected specimen shows grayish white to tan discoloration around the needle track (Fig. 8.1) [6]. A red congestive limbic zone surrounds the ablated area.

The therapeutic effect of RFA as the gold standard was evaluated based on NADH diaphorase staining. Non-ablated breast tissue was the positive control. When purple-blue staining was absent throughout the tumor tissue, we concluded that the RFA was completely (100 %) effective. If there were areas of purple-blue staining in the tumor tissue, we concluded that the RFA was incomplete. Representative viable and nonviable areas in a tissue cut surface, as detected by NADH diaphorase staining, are shown in Fig. 8.2.

Fornage et al. described the effect of RFA on breast cancer tissue [7]. A thermal effect was evident in all target lesions, with characteristics of cellular damage that included hemostasis, cytoskeleton denaturation, increased cytoplasmic eosinophilia, pyknotic nuclei, spindling, and cell shrinkage. The authors attempted to classify the extent of the histological therapeutic effect into mild, moderate, and high, but the NADH diaphorase staining was always negative [7].

Based on the results from the previous studies, we evaluated RFA damage to epithelial and stromal cells and fibrous stroma in permanent H&E-stained sections

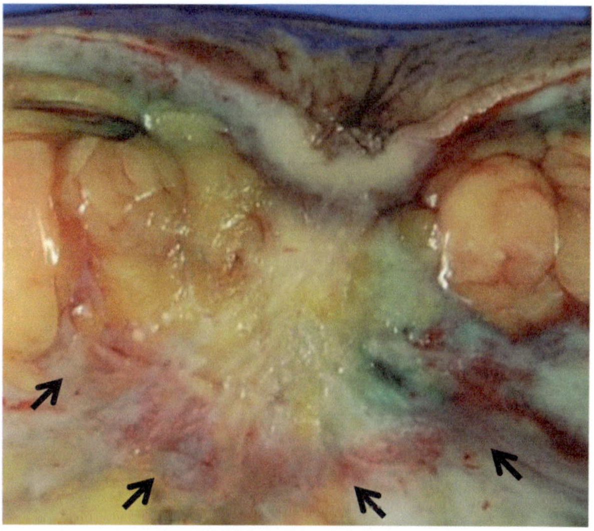

Fig.8.1 Gross appearance of an ablated breast tissue from a resected specimen. The cut surface of the ablated area including the tumor shows *grayish white* to *tan* discoloration. A *reddish* congestive limbic zone surrounding the ablated area is indicated with *arrows* (Figure partially reproduced from Seki et al. [6])

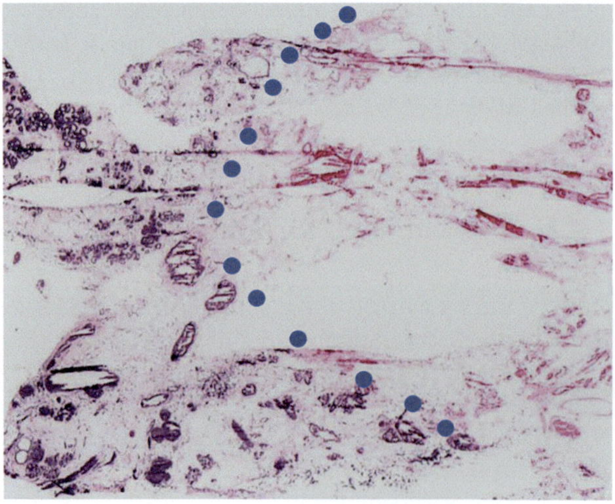

Fig. 8.2 Frozen section of a surgically resected tissue specimen immediately after RFA, with NADH diaphorase staining. The boundary between the ablated area (*right*) and non-ablated area (*left*) is indicated. In the non-ablated area, NADH diaphorase staining labels viable cells *purple blue*, whereas the ablated area is not stained because of non-viability of the constituent cells (Figure partially reproduced from Seki et al. [6])

[6]. Epithelial cells, both cancerous and noncancerous, were characterized by elongated eosinophilic cytoplasm with pyknotic "streaming" nuclei. The intercellular boundaries and details of the nuclear and cytoplasmic morphology were unclear. Collagen matrix in fibrous connective tissue also showed degenerative changes with dense, homogeneous, and highly eosinophilic features. The original delicate, wavy appearance entirely disappeared. Fibroblasts in the area also showed thermal degenerative changes identical to those seen in epithelial cells [6].

We assessed the therapeutic effect of RFA for the 28 cases according to these criteria. If these findings were seen in the entire tumor area examined, the histopathological therapeutic effect was considered complete. Representative H&E-stained frozen sections are shown in Fig. 8.3.

8.1.3 Correlation Between H&E and NADH Diaphorase Stain

The RFA procedure was successful in 26 cases, but the elevation of the voltage during the procedure was suboptimal in the other two cases. In these 28 cases, the RFA effect was considered to be complete in 22 cases (79 %), whereas in the other six, the RFA effect was determined to be incomplete since NADH diaphorase staining was positive in 5–100 % of the tumor area. Of the 22 cases showing completely negative NADH diaphorase staining, 16 (73 %) were determined to be a complete RFA effect by H&E. In contrast, in all of the six cases showing partial or completely positive NADH diaphorase staining, the therapeutic effect was also incomplete by H&E.

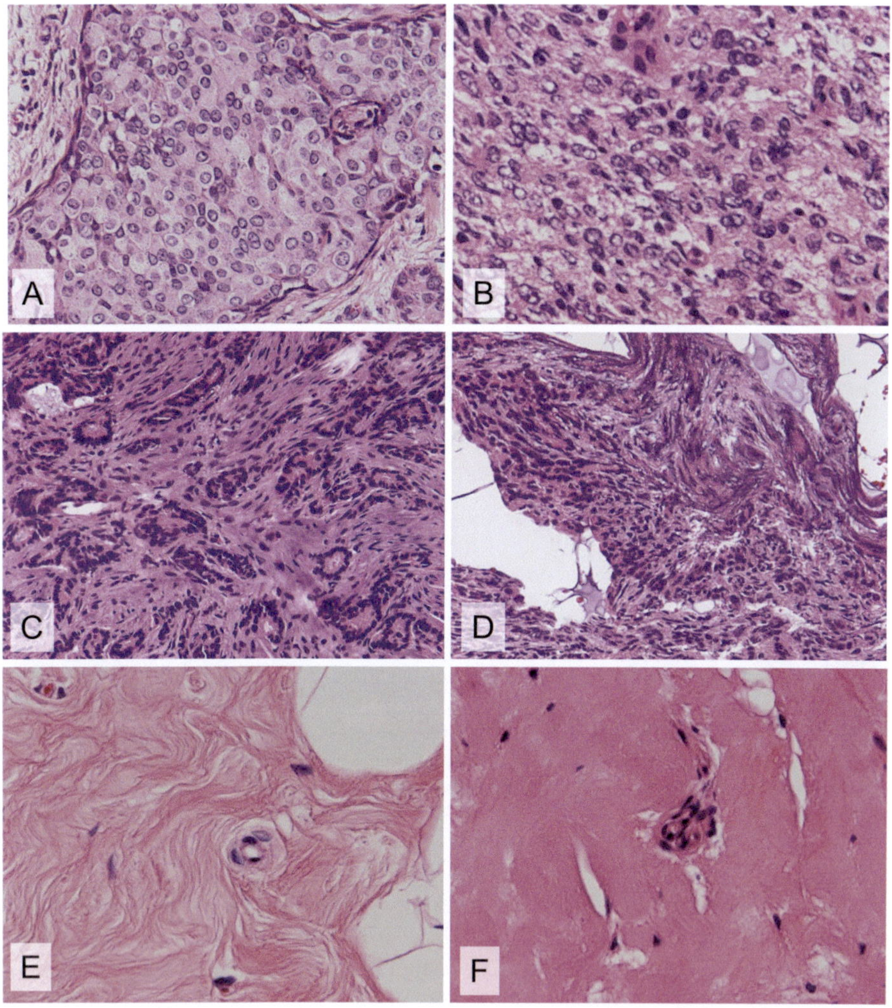

Fig. 8.3 Permanent H&E-stained sections of breast cancer tissues after RFA. (**a**) Non-ablated breast cancer tissue. (**b–d**). Ablated breast cancer tissues. (**b**) Mild cytoplasmic eosinophilia, unclear intercellular boundaries, pyknosis, and unclear chromatin structure in nuclei are seen. (**c**) Moderate to marked heat degeneration in both cancer cells and stromal matrix. Marked pyknosis, nuclear streaming in cancer cells, and degenerative changes of collagen matrix are seen. (**d**) Marked heat degeneration with unclear structure of cells. (**e**) Non-ablated collagenous stroma. (**f**) Collagenous stromal tissue of the mammary gland that was highly degenerated by RFA

If the two cases in which RFA procedure was not optimal were excluded from calculation, the RFA effect was considered to be complete in 85 % (22 of 26) with NADH diaphorase staining. Other four cases (15 %) that showed positive NADH diaphorase staining were considered to be incomplete therapeutic effect.

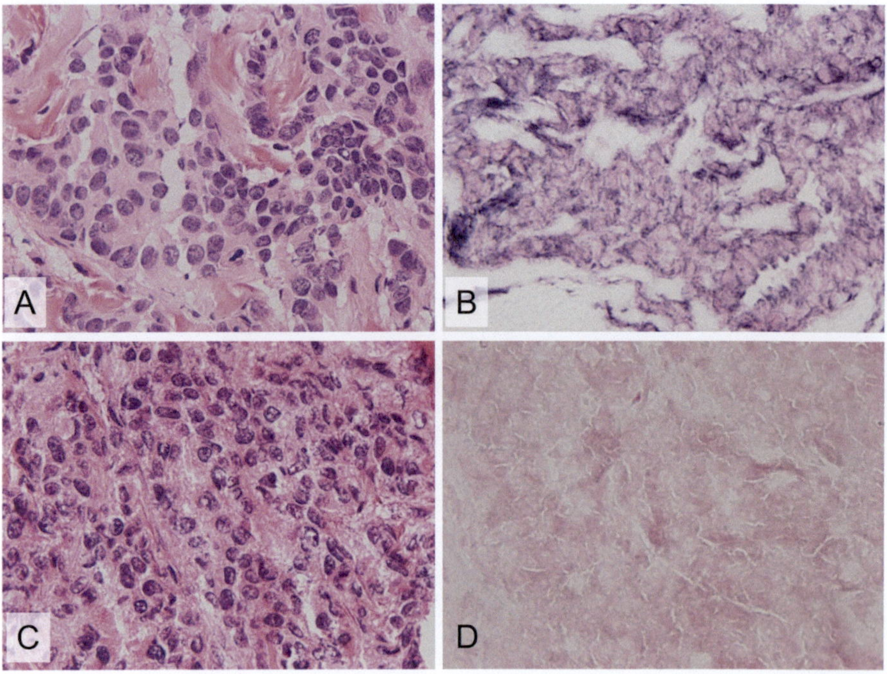

Fig. 8.4 Comparison between H&E-stained and NADH diaphorase-stained frozen sections from breast cancer tissues. (**a**, **b**) Frozen sections of a non-ablated breast cancer. (**a**) H&E-stained section. (**b**) NADH diaphorase-stained section. (**c**, **d**) Frozen sections of an ablated breast cancer. (**c**) H&E-stained section. The extent of degeneration is not very strong, and cytoplasmic eosinophilia and pyknosis can be detected. (**d**) NADH diaphorase-stained section. No staining is observed (Figure partially reproduced from Seki et al. [6])

When the RFA effect was compared between NADH diaphorase and H&E staining in all the 28 cases, most cases had similar results, but there were some discrepancies (Fig. 8.4). All of the 16 cases of complete RFA effects by H&E were also complete RFA effects by NADH diaphorase staining. In the 12 cases of incomplete RFA effects by H&E, six showed a complete effect, whereas the other six showed an incomplete effect by NADH diaphorase staining. Therefore, the therapeutic effect evaluated by H&E staining was significantly correlated with the effect evaluated by NADH diaphorase staining ($P = 0.0088$) (Table 8.1). Nonetheless, the correlation was not perfect: when negative NADH diaphorase staining was defined as the true therapeutic effect, the sensitivity by H&E evaluation was 73 % (16 of 22), whereas the specificity of H&E evaluation was 100 % (6 of 6). The positive predictive value, the negative predictive value, and the accuracy of H&E evaluations were 100 % (16 of 16), 50 % (6 of 12), and 79 % (22 of 28), respectively.

Table 8.1 Correlation of the therapeutic effects by NADH diaphorase staining and by H&E staining in the 28 primary breast carcinomas

	Number of cases		
	Therapeutic effect by NADH		
Therapeutic effect by H&E	Complete (100 %)	Incomplete (≤100 %)	*P*
Complete (100 %)	16	0	0.0088
Incomplete (≤100 %)	6	6[a]	
Total	22	6	

H&E hematoxylin and eosin, *NADH* nicotinamide adenine dinucleotide
[a]Two cases in which RFA procedure was suboptimal are included

8.1.4 Correlation of RFA Efficacy and Tumor Size

The mean tumor size and the mean diameter of invasive carcinoma component of the 28 primary tumors were 2.2 cm (ranging from 0.6 to 5.0 cm) and 1.4 cm (ranging from 0 to 5.0 cm), respectively. The complete RFA effect on breast cancer tissue by NADH diaphorase staining was overwhelmingly correlated with tumor size evaluated by histopathological examination of the resected specimen: all of the 11 tumors ≤1.5 cm in diameter showed a complete effect, whereas 11 (65 %) of the 17 tumors >1.5 cm in diameter showed a complete effect; these percentages differ significantly ($P=0.033$). For the 21 tumors ≤3.0 cm in diameter, 20 (95 %) showed a complete therapeutic effect by NADH diaphorase staining. In contrast, for the seven tumors >3.0 cm in diameter, only two (29 %) showed a complete effect. These rates differ significantly ($P=0.0012$).

In the 26 cases in which RFA procedure was optimal, the complete RFA effect detected with NADH diaphorase staining was observed in all of 20 tumors ≤3.0 cm in diameter, whereas such a complete effect was observed only in two (33 %) of six tumors >3.0 cm in diameter ($P=0.001$) (Table 8.2).

From the measurements of the whole resected specimens, the largest diameters of RFA effect including tumor and non-tumor areas ranged from 1.7 to 6.6 cm (mean = 3.71 cm, standard deviation = 1.33 cm). Twenty-five cases had an RFA effect of 2.5 cm or longer, and the diameters for the remaining three cases were 1.7 cm, 1.7 cm, and 1.9 cm. A primary tumor 1.5 cm or smaller in diameter is therefore expected to be completely ablated by the RFA method.

The therapeutic effect by NADH diaphorase staining was not correlated with histological type or nuclear grade (Table 8.2). In the 26 cases in which RFA procedure was successful, a complete RFA effect was achieved in 82 % (18 of 22) of invasive ductal carcinomas, and differences in histological subtypes (papillotubular, solid-tubular, and scirrhous carcinoma) were not correlated with the RFA effect. Two mucinous carcinomas, one ductal carcinoma in situ (DCIS), and one invasive ductal carcinoma with a predominantly intraductal component

Table 8.2 Correlation of the therapeutic effect by NADH diaphorase staining and histopathological parameters in the 26 tumors

Parameter	Total	Number of cases (%) Therapeutic effect by NADH Complete (100%)	Incomplete (<100%)	*P*
A. Tumor size				
≤1.0 cm	5	5 (100)	0 (0)	0.001
>1.0 cm, ≤1.5 cm	6	6 (100)	0 (0)	
>1.5 cm, ≤2.0 cm	4	4 (100)	0 (0)	
>2.0 cm, ≤3.0 cm	5	5 (100)	0 (0)	
>3.0 cm	6	2 (33)	4 (67)	
B. Histological type of carcinoma				
Invasive ductal	22	18 (82)	4 (18)	N.S.
Papillotubular	8	8 (100)	0 (0)	
Solid-tubular	6	4 (67)	2 (33)	
Scirrhous	8	6 (75)	2 (25)	
Mucinous	2	2 (100)	0 (0)	
DCIS/Predom. DCIS	2	2 (100)	0 (0)	
C. Nuclear grade				
Grade 1	16	14 (87)	2 (13)	N.S.
Grade 2	5	4 (80)	1 (20)	
Grade 3	4	3 (75)	1 (25)	
Not evaluated	1	1 (100)	0 (0)	
Total	26	22	4	

NADH nicotinamide adenine dinucleotide, *N.S.* not significant, *Predom DCIS* Invasive ductal carcinoma with a predominantly intraductal component

showed a complete RFA effect, but the number of cases of these histological types is too small to draw any conclusions.

Likewise, in all 28 cases, based on histopathological criteria by H&E staining, a complete therapeutic effect was obtained in the tumors ≤1.0 cm in diameter (5 of 5), but 9 % of tumors ≤1.5 cm in diameter showed an incomplete RFA effect by H&E (1 of 11) [5]. For tumors ≤2.0 cm in diameter, 19 % showed an incomplete RFA effect by H&E (3 of 16). In the 26 cases in which RFA procedure was optimal, the complete RFA effect detected with H&E staining was observed in 13 (87 %) of 15 tumors ≤2.0 cm in diameter, whereas such a complete effect was observed only in 3 (27 %) of 11 tumors >2.0 cm in diameter ($P = 0.0048$) (Table 8.3). Histological type/subtype and nuclear grade were not correlated with therapeutic effect evaluate from H&E staining results.

Table 8.3 Correlation of the therapeutic effect by H&E staining and histopathological parameters in the 26 tumors

Parameter	Number of cases (%)			P
		Therapeutic effect by H&E		
	Total	Complete (100%)	Incomplete (<100%)	
D. Tumor size				
≤1.0 cm	5	5 (100)	0 (0)	0.0048
>1.0 cm, ≤1.5 cm	6	5 (83)	1 (17)	
>1.5 cm, ≤2.0 cm	4	3 (75)	1 (25)	
>2.0 cm, ≤3.0 cm	5	3 (60)	2 (40)	
>3.0 cm	6	0 (0)	6 (100)	
E. Histological type of carcinoma				
Invasive ductal	22	13 (59)	9 (41)	N.S.
Papillotubular	8	6 (75)	2 (25)	
Solid-tubular	6	3 (50)	3 (50)	
Scirrhous	8	4 (50)	4 (50)	
Mucinous	2	1 (50)	1 (50)	
DCIS/Predom. DCIS	2	2 (100)	0 (0)	
F. Nuclear grade				
Grade 1	16	8 (50)	8 (50)	N.S.
Grade 2	5	4 (80)	1 (20)	
Grade 3	4	3 (75)	1 (25)	
Not evaluated	1	1 (100)	0 (0)	
Total	26	16	10	

H&E hematoxylin and eosin, *N.S.* not significant, *Predom DCIS* Invasive ductal carcinoma with a predominantly intraductal component

NADH diaphorase staining is currently the gold standard method for the evaluation of an RFA effect. H&E staining could be a surrogate marker for an RFA effect if the criteria for evaluation are applied appropriately, although the sensitivity of H&E staining is imperfect.

8.1.5 Evaluation of the Therapeutic Effect in the RAFAELO Study

A multi-institutional phase II study to evaluate the efficacy of radiofrequency ablation therapy for early breast cancer as local therapy (the RAFAELO study), and standardize the method, was launched in 2012. That study also aimed at standardizing the technology of RFA procedure and the methods of histological

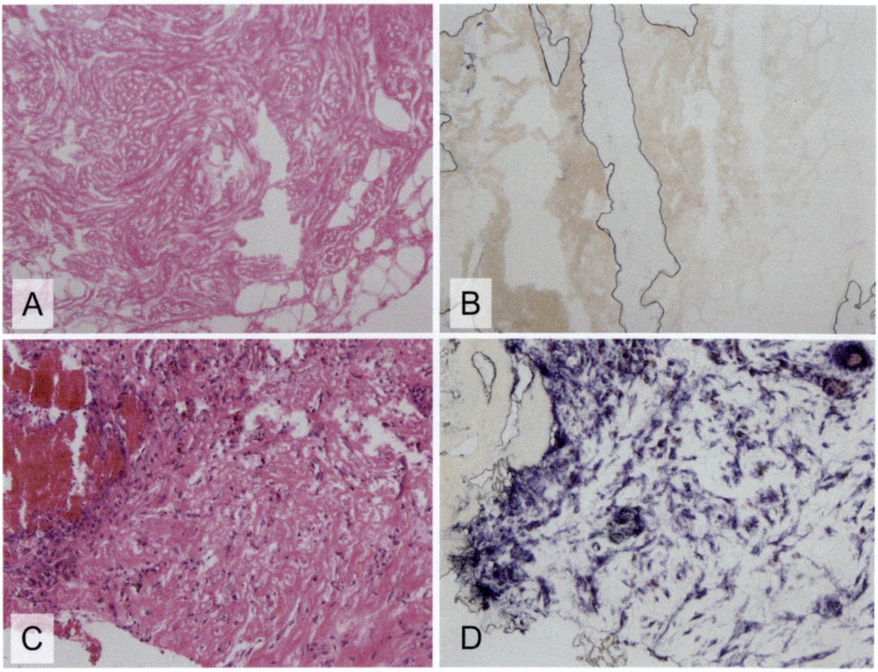

Fig. 8.5 A core needle biopsy specimen of breast cancer tissue 3 months after RFA and whole breast irradiation. (**a**, **b**) Necrotic cancer tissue without organization. (**a**) H&E staining. (**b**) NADH diaphorase staining. (**c**, **d**) Granulation tissue and fibrosis surrounding the necrotic tissue. (**c**) H&E staining. (**d**) NADH diaphorase staining

and histochemical evaluation of RFA effect on the tumor. In that study, patients receive RFA therapy and subsequent whole breast irradiation to the primary breast cancer (no surgery) and are followed up for 5 years. Only patients with a single early breast cancer $\leq$1.5 cm in diameter and without clinical regional lymph node metastasis (cN0) are eligible to enroll in the study [8]. The primary end point is local recurrence-free survival 5 years after RFA.

In the RAFAELO study, core needle or vacuum-associated biopsies will be evaluated for the RFA effect, using both NADH diaphorase and H&E staining, at 3 and 12 months after whole breast irradiation.

From a histopathological standpoint, highly heat-degenerated tumor tissue may change into necrotic tissue, granulation tissue, or fibrosis during follow-up (Fig. 8.5). Heat-degenerated tissue may be replaced by coagulative necrosis and then be absorbed and replaced by granulation tissue and fibrosis. Otherwise, the necrotic area may form a cyst.

If DCIS components extended significantly from the main invasive cancer tissue, the evaluation of the extent of the DCIS component would be difficult using core needle/vacuum-assisted biopsy specimens. In the RAFAELO protocol, the biopsies 3 months after irradiation may include specimens not only from the area where the main tumor existed but also from the mammary gland tissue that surrounds the tumor. Evaluating the viability of noninvasive carcinoma components is sometimes difficult because of cellular atypia caused by irradiation of noncancerous mammary glandular epithelial cells.

8.2 Conclusions

NADH diaphorase staining is currently the best method to evaluate the RFA effect. When evaluation of tumor extent and RFA method are conducted well, most of early ($\leq$1.5 cm in diameter) breast cancer would be the indication of the RFA therapy. Limitations of H&E staining include lower sensitivity and lower negative predictive value despite specificity, and positive predictive value of H&E method is sufficient. Uncertain interobserver reproducibility also needs to be addressed.

Acknowledgments These studies were supported in part by a grant for Project Promoting Clinical Trials for Development of New Drugs and Medical Devices from the Japan Agency for Medical Research and Development (AMED).

Disclosure of Conflict of Interest The authors have no conflict of interest to declare.

References

1. Kinoshita T, Iwamoto E, Tsuda H, Seki K. Radiofrequency ablation as local therapy for early breast carcinomas. Breast Cancer. 2011;18(1):10–7.
2. Mutsaerts EL, Van Coevorden F, Krause R, Borel Rinkes IH, Strobbe LJ, Prevoo W, Tollenaar RA, van Gulik TM. Initial experience with radiofrequency ablation for hepatic tumours in the Netherlands. Eur J Surg Oncol. 2003;29(9):731–4.
3. Imoto S, Wada N, Sakemura N, Hasebe T, Murata Y. Feasibility study on radiofrequency ablation followed by partial mastectomy for stage I breast cancer patients. Breast. 2009;18 (2):130–4.
4. Yamamoto N, Fujimoto H, Nakamura R, Arai M, Yoshii A, Kaji S, Itami M. Pilot study of radiofrequency ablation therapy without surgical excision for T1 breast cancer: evaluation with MRI and vacuum-assisted core needle biopsy and safety management. Breast Cancer. 2011;18 (1):3–9.
5. Noguchi M, Motoyoshi A, Earashi M, Fujii H. Long-term outcome of breast cancer patients treated with radiofrequency ablation. Eur J Surg Oncol. 2012;38(11):1036–42.
6. Seki K, Tsuda H, Iwamoto E, Kinoshita T. Histopathological therapeutic effect of radiofrequency ablation to primary breast cancer: with special reference to changes in cancer cells and stromal structure and comparison with enzyme histochemistry. Breast Cancer. 2011;18(1):18–23.
7. Fornage BD, Sneige N, Ross MI, Mirza AN, Kuerer HM, Edeiken BS, Ames FC, Newman LA, Babiera GV. Singletary SE Small (< or = 2-cm) breast cancer treated with US-guided radiofrequency ablation: feasibility study. Radiology. 2004;231(1):215–24.

8. Tsuda H, Seki K, Hasebe T, Sasajima Y, Shibata T, Iwamoto E, Kinoshita TA. Histopathological study for evaluation of therapeutic effects of radiofrequency ablation in patients with breast cancer. Breast Cancer. 2011;18(1):24–32.
9. Kinoshita T. RAFAELO study. A multicenter prospective study of image-guided radiofrequency ablation for small breast carcinomas. https://upload.umin.ac.jp/cgi-open-bin/ctr/ctr.cgi?function=brows&action=brows&recptno=R000010016&type=summary&language=E.

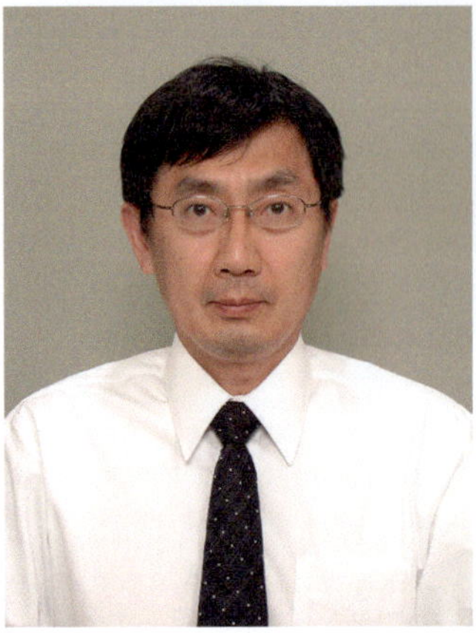

Hitoshi Tsuda

Chapter 9
Importance of Breast Imaging Before and After RFA Therapy

Rikiya Nakamura and Naohito Yamamoto

9.1 Evidence of the Utility of Follow-Up Imaging for Standard Breast-Conserving Therapy

The local recurrence rate after breast-conserving surgery is reported to be 5–20 % [1, 2]. Although one previous randomized controlled trial comparing breast-conserving surgery and total mastectomy for early breast cancer shows no significant differences in the overall survival of the patients, the Early Breast Cancer Trialists' Collaborative Group (EBCTCG) meta-analysis found that the higher rate of local recurrence after breast-conserving surgery negatively affects the overall survival of patients [9].

Follow-up imaging after breast-conserving surgery aims to discover any potential remnant tumor. Currently, mammography (MMG) is the only evidenced method used for breast cancer screening in healthy people [3]. However, there has been no randomized controlled trial examining the clinical efficacy of MMG as a follow-up imaging modality for patients undergoing breast-conserving surgery; therefore, it is currently unknown whether follow-up MMG after breast-conserving surgery contributes to overall survival. On the other hand, the use of follow-up breast magnetic resonance imaging (MRI) for the evaluation of recurrence after breast-conserving surgery has been reported to be both sensitive and specific and thus highly useful [4]. However, Coulthard et al. [5] conversely reported that the utility of MRI as a routine test in the posttreatment follow-up of breast cancer patients was limited and that the posttreatment MRI findings were poor predictors of local recurrence.

R. Nakamura (✉) • N. Yamamoto
Division of Brest Surgery, Chiba Cancer Center Hospital, 666-2 Nitona-chou, chuo-ku, Chiba-shi, Chiba 260-8717, Japan
e-mail: rnakamura@chiba-cc.jp

T. Kinoshita (ed.), *Non-surgical Ablation Therapy for Early-stage Breast Cancer*, DOI 10.1007/978-4-431-54463-0_9

It is needless to say that there are no data on the follow-up breast imaging after the RFA procedure. In this chapter, we will explain the breast imaging after RFA procedure.

9.2 Clinical Criteria of Radiofrequency Ablation (RFA) in Our Hospital

One of the most important risk factors for local recurrence after breast-conserving surgery is a positive surgical margin [6]. Therefore, in addition to good cosmetic results, the main goal of breast-conserving surgery is negative surgical margins [7]. However, pathological evaluation of the surgical margins during breast-conserving surgery is difficult to achieve after RFA therapy, and this represents a major disadvantage of RFA therapy. Accordingly, in order to ensure successful RFA therapy, it is key to accurately evaluate both the preoperative and postoperative diagnostic imaging findings. By performing careful preoperative diagnostic imaging, cases eligible for RFA can be selected, and by performing early postoperative imaging, ablation zone assessment (corresponding to surgical margin evaluation after breast-conserving surgery) can be performed accurately.

In the recent reports, the risk factors for local recurrence after breast-conserving surgery were found to be the surgical margin status, tumor diameter, tumor grade, number of involved nodes, molecular marker (estrogen receptor [ER] and human epidermal growth factor receptor 2 [HER2]) status, and patient age [9, 8]. Moreover, several groups have reported that, in cases of standard breast-conserving surgery, the proportion of invasive cancer cells in the surgical margin, as determined by histopathological examination, is 13–51 % [10–12]. Thus, it is of utmost importance to evaluate the presence or absence of intraductal spread during preoperative diagnosis to judge the indication for breast-conserving surgery, and the eligibility criteria for RFA rather than standard breast-conserving surgery need to be strict. Specifically, familiarity with MMG, breast ultrasonography (US), and breast MRI as means for pre-RFA imaging is essential.

MMG is the most superior imaging technique in terms of visualization of potential calcification. When MMG shows extensive calcification, further intraductal spread should be considered. Furthermore, there are numerous reports of the usefulness of contrast MRI in the expanse diagnosis of breast cancer, whereas evidence of the usefulness of breast US for the preoperative diagnosis of intraductal spread is limited [13].

On the other hand, during RFA, the breast tumor is punctured under ultrasound guidance; therefore, the ablation zone after RFA depends greatly on the US image and puncture technique used. In other words, during preoperative diagnosis, it is important to precisely evaluate the presence of intraductal spread from breast tumors by using MMG and MRI, whereas the main purpose of US is to visualize the tumor identified on MRI during RFA.

Accordingly, the eligibility criteria for RFA therapy in our hospital were as follows:

1. Invasive carcinoma without any other specific carcinoma, as established by core-needle biopsy; tumor diameter of 2 cm or less, as measured by US; no diffuse microcalcification revealed on MMG; no evidence of extensive ductal spread of cancer or multiple tumors on MRI or MMG; and no swelling of axillary lymph nodes, as demonstrated by US and contrast-enhanced multidetector computed tomography with 1.3 mm thin slices.
2. Availability of accurate data on biological tumor characteristics such as ER, progesterone receptor, and HER2 expression estimated from the tumor tissue obtained with core needle biopsy.
3. Possibility of performing pre- and postoperative MRI and follow-up MMG.
4. Patients treated with preoperative chemotherapy were also excluded.

Thus, the eligibility criteria for RFA therapy are based on the long-term results of the standard treatment, such as breast-conserving surgery. As a result, in addition to factors such as no or limited recurrences after breast-conserving surgery, it is also essential to perform a postoperative imaging study to evaluate the success of the RFA procedure.

9.3 Post-RFA Effect Assessment by Imaging Studies

As mentioned, a major disadvantage of RFA is that the pathological surgical margin cannot be easily evaluated, unlike during standard treatment, and the disappearance rate of cancer cells in the ablation zone after RFA therapy is reported to be approximately 64–100 % [14–16. Kinoshita et al. [17] reported that 24 of 29 patients (83 %) with breast carcinomas 2 cm in size or smaller treated by RFA showed complete ablation of the tumor on the basis of histopathology and enzyme histochemistry, suggesting the possibility of remnant cancer cells both within and beyond the ablation zone.

The comparison of the extent of disease spread as determined during preoperative diagnosis and the ablation zone of RFA is a critical aspect of postoperative diagnostic imaging. In other words, it is important to confirm that the extent of disease spread as identified by preoperative imaging was sufficiently targeted by RFA, by postoperative imaging. In cases of insufficient ablation zones, surgical resection needs to be performed or RFA therapy needs to be administered again. In our hospital, US and MRI are performed 4 weeks after RFA therapy and before irradiation. In addition, ablated tumors are evaluated with hematoxylin and eosin and nicotinamide adenine dinucleotide diaphorase staining. Based on the postoperative findings, if needed, adjuvant chemotherapy and/or endocrine therapy is subsequently administered.

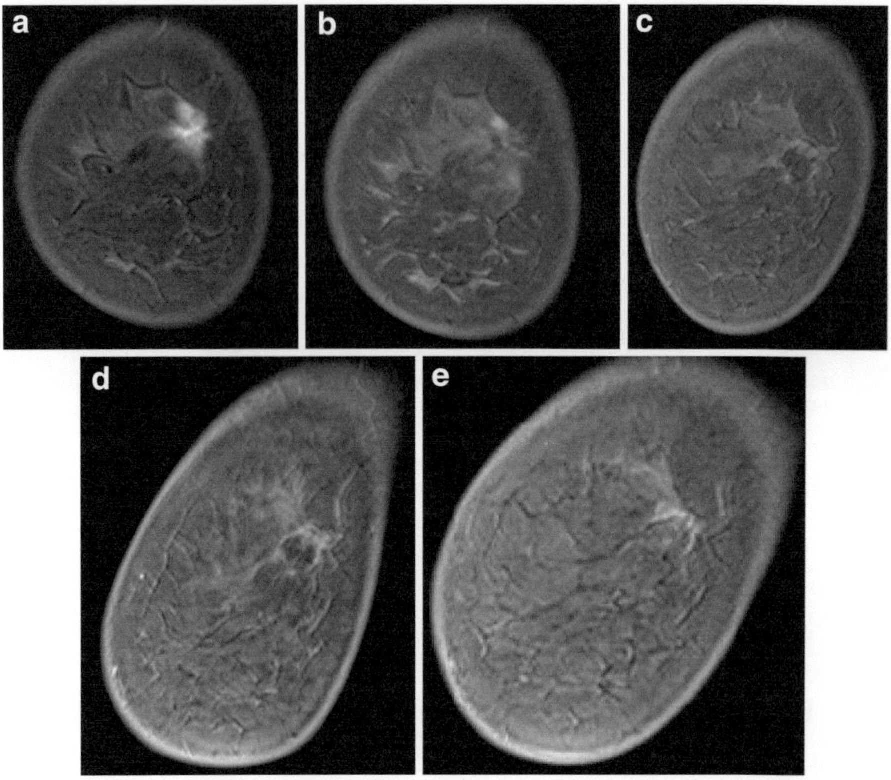

Fig. 9.1 (**a**) Representative preoperative coronal T1-weighted magnetic resonance imaging (MRI) demonstrating a 15 × 10 mm-sized enhanced mass without surrounding intraductal extensions. (**b**) MRI performed 1 month after radiofrequency ablation (RFA). A small de novo enhanced lesion at the caudal end of the tumor may be observed, as compared to the preoperative enhanced tumor. (**c**) MRI performed 6 months after RFA. The enhanced lesion noted 1 month after RFA is absent, and slightly hypo-reflective lesions can be observed in the ablation zone. (**d**) MRI performed 1 year after RFA. The hypointense region in the ablation zone is reduced. A ring-shaped hyperintense region appears in the surrounding tissue outside the ablation zone. (**e**) Two years after RFA, normal mammary gland structures have appeared in the interior of the ablation zone

The high sensitivity and specificity of MRI to identify intraductal spread of breast cancer have been well established [18, 19], and periodic MRI examinations have been demonstrated to improve the specificity further, compared to the previous MRI examination. In cases of inflammatory cell infiltration, enhanced MRI may be capable of detecting nodules in the margins of the ablation zone after RFA therapy, and the differential diagnosis of inflammatory cell infiltration and remaining tumor cells can be easily established by comparing the MRI findings before and after surgery (Figs. 9.1 and 9.2).

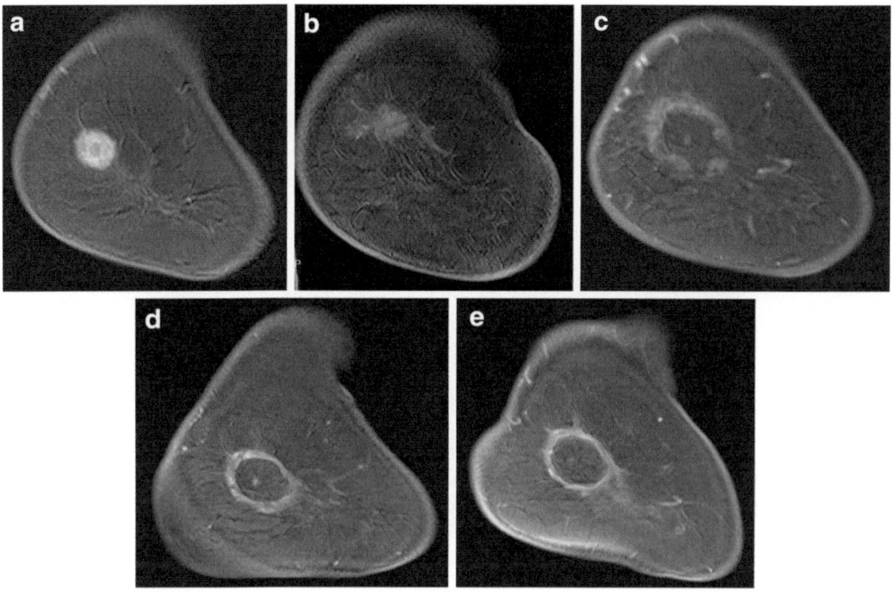

Fig. 9.2 (**a**) Representative preoperative magnetic resonance imaging (MRI) demonstrating an irregular 15 × 10 mm-sized enhanced mass (**b**) MRI performed 1 month after radiofrequency ablation (RFA). A slightly enhanced region can be observed in the ablation zone. (**c**) MRI performed 1 year after RFA showing a hypointense tumor in the ablation zone with peripheral enhancement. (**d**) Two years after RFA. The ring-shaped peripheral enhancement outside the ablation zone appears more conspicuous and clearer, and a hyperintense nodule can be detected within the ablation zone. (**e**) Three years after RFA. The hyperintense nodule within the ablation zone has diminished

9.4 Periodic Post-RFA Follow-Up Imaging

There is currently a lack of evidence of the usefulness of postoperative imaging studies for the ipsilateral breast after breast-conserving surgery. The most important aspect of postoperative follow-up imaging for early detection of tumor recurrences in the breast is to understand the recurrence pattern and the characteristic imaging findings after RFA.

The causes of breast cancer recurrence after RFA are considered to be the following: (1) an insufficiently ablated tumor, (2) unexpected extensive ductal spread of the carcinoma due to underdiagnosis based on preoperative imaging, (3) establishment of an entry wound and insertion route, and (4) the development of a de novo lesion.

Accordingly, we consider it necessary to take the four abovementioned causes of recurrence into consideration when performing postoperative imaging studies. Accordingly, the sites confirmed by the postoperative imaging study must include (1) the inside of the ablation zone, (2) the margins of the ablation zone, (3) the

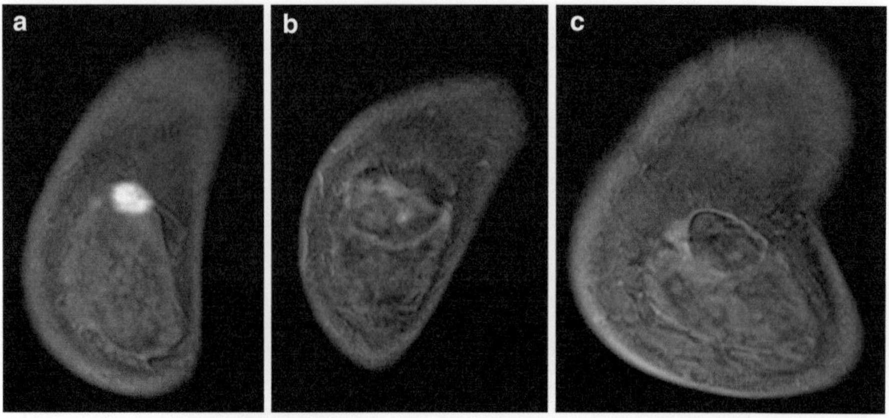

Fig. 9.3 (**a–f**) Coronal views on MRI scans before (*Pre*) and 1, 6, 12, 24, 36, and 60 months in a 44-year-old woman with a 15 mm invasive ductal cancer who underwent RFA followed by whole-breast irradiation. The mass is no longer enhanced after RFA. The peripheral enhancement was seen 6 months after RFA. And an ablation zone with peripheral ring enhancement has gradually decreased in size. The long-axis diameters measured on each view were 50, 45, 40, and 10 mm, respectively

insertion route into the mammary fat pad and the skin punctured by the RFA needle, and (4) the whole mammary gland.

Figures 9.3, 9.4, 9.5, 9.6, 9.7, 9.8, 9.9, and 9.10 show representative MMG, US, and MRI scans pre- and post-RFA. One month post-RFA, breast MRI clearly shows an ablated zone without surrounding rim enhancement, and the fat in the breast gland is hypodense due to fluid components such as necrotic tissue (Fig. 9.3). Moreover, no changes in the normal mammary gland are observed (Fig. 9.4). The destruction caused by the ablation shows findings similar to an intracystic tumor, both upon MRI and US (Figs. 9.4 and 9.5). Color Doppler US showing the absence of blood flow in the ablation zone (Figs. 9.6 and 9.7). Post-RFA, increased blood flow, fibrosis, and ring-shaped enhancement in the marginal zone of the ablation can be observed (Fig. 9.8). Subsequently, the liquid component is absorbed and reduced, but the necrotic tissue remains (Fig. 9.8). Moreover, in some cases, dystrophic calcification is observed in the ablation zone (Fig. 9.9). MMG shows an increase in coarse calcification, which is easily differentiated from the calcification findings of malignant disease (Fig. 9.9). MRI shows a slightly enhanced lesion, which is difficultly differentiated from the findings of malignant disease.

Furthermore, at our hospital, there were very few cases of implantation recurrence in the skin, largely owing to the fact that breast irradiation was performed after RFA. Conversely, we experienced a case of local recurrence in the skin at the punctured site 4 years after surgery; accordingly, the risk of recurrence in the insertion route of the RFA needle has to be carefully considered. In this case, the tumor was a palpable nodule, 15 mm in diameter, which was easily confirmed by MMG (Fig. 9.10).

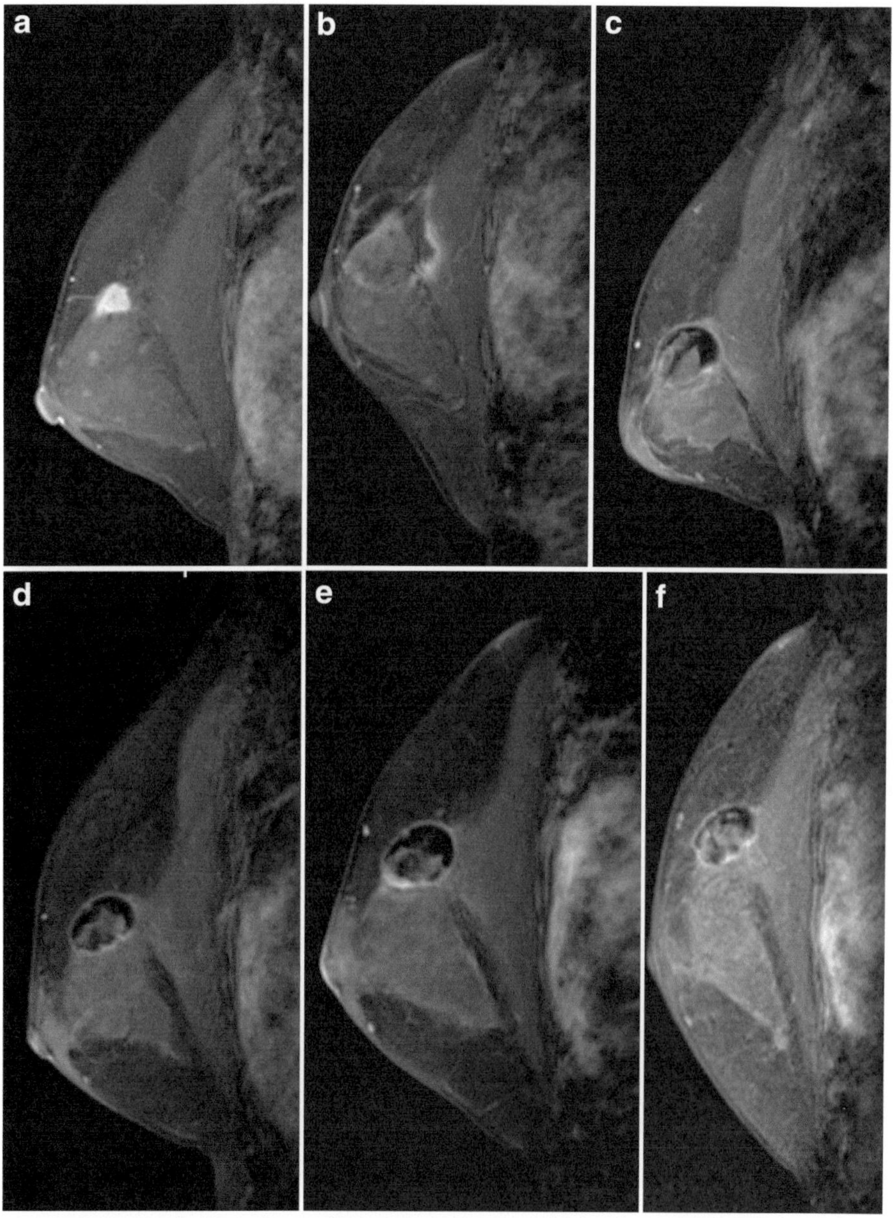

Fig. 9.4 (**a–f**) Sagittal views on MRI scans before (*Pre*) and 1, 6, 12, 24, and 36 months in a 65 -year-old woman with a 15 × 10 mm-sized invasive ductal cancer who underwent RFA followed by whole-breast irradiation and endocrine therapy

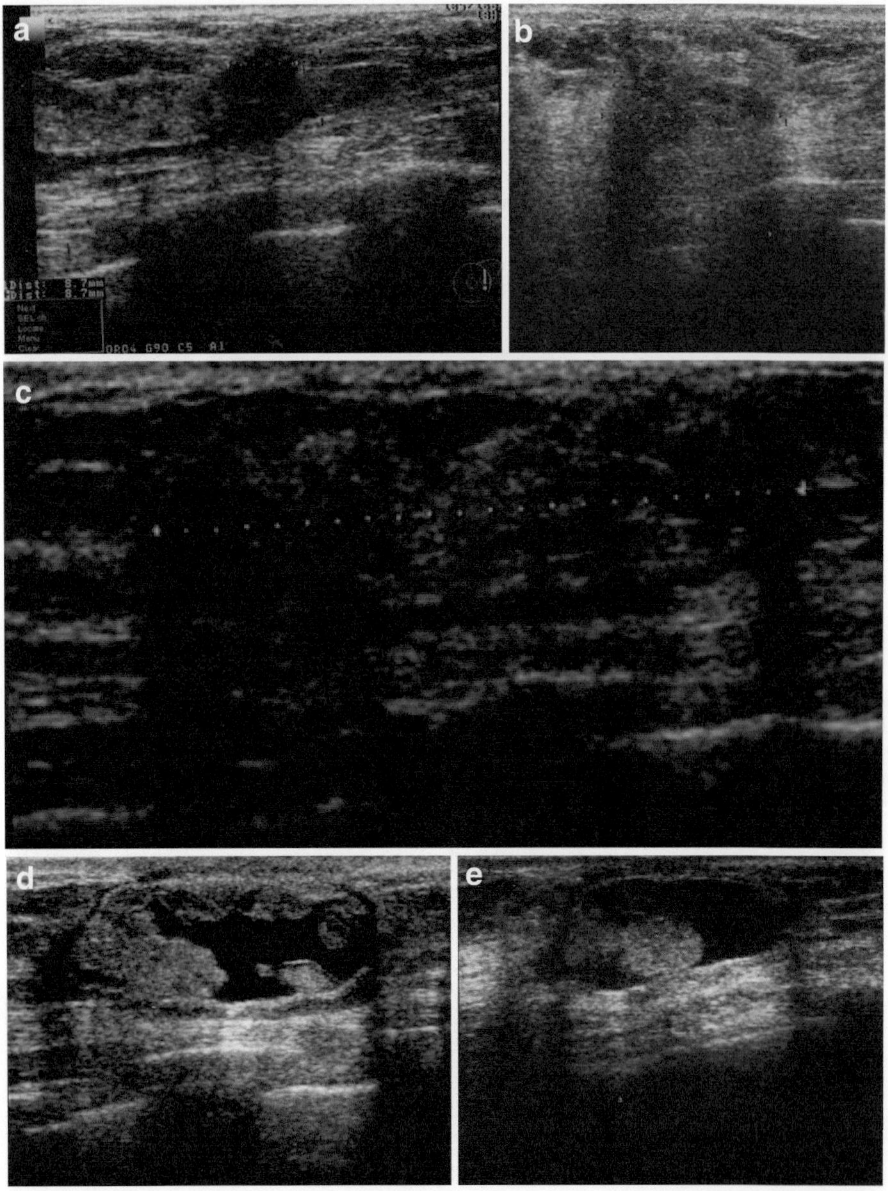

Fig. 9.5 (**a**) Representative preoperative ultrasonography (US) demonstrating an 8 × 8 mm-sized hypoechoic mass without intraductal extension. (**b**) US performed 1 month after radiofrequency ablation (RFA) demonstrating a 20 × 15 mm-sized hypoechoic lesion with an unclear boundary. (**c**) US obtained 1 year after RFA. The boundary of the ablation zone is recognized as a mass with a hypoechoic belt. (**d**) US performed 2 years after RFA. The ablation zone is showed as a 20 × 10 mm-sized cystic and solid tumor. (**e**) US performed 5 years after RFA. The ablation zone is reduced, and increases in the internal hypoechoic region and the circular solid mass with clear boundaries can be observed as lateral shadows

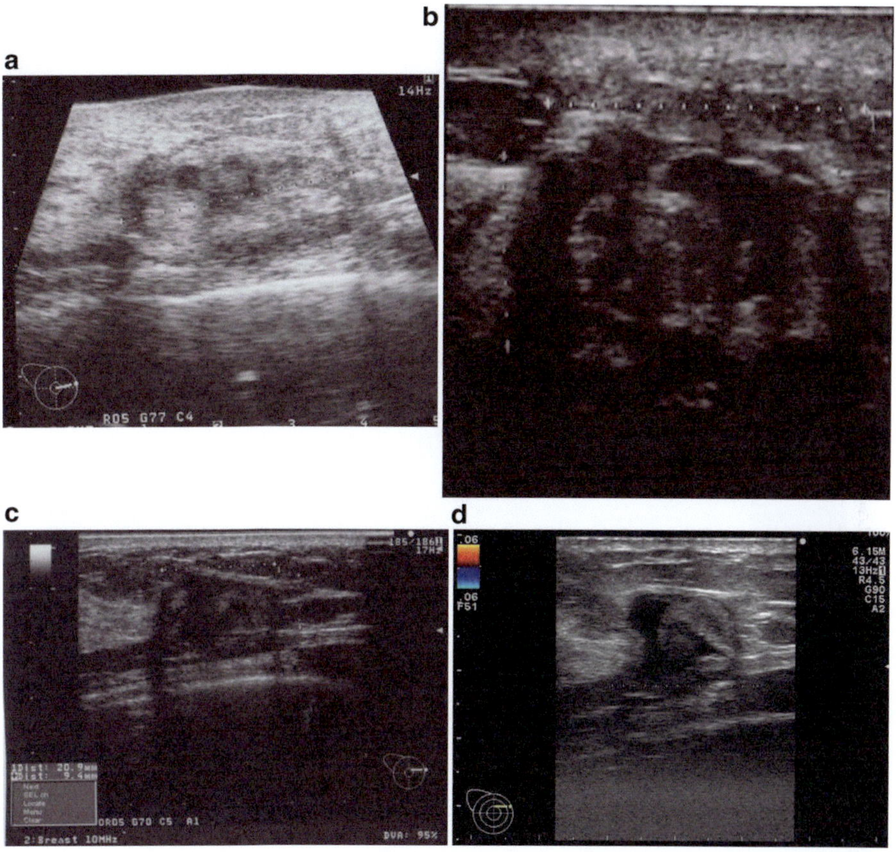

Fig. 9.6 (**a**) Representative ultrasonography (US) image obtained 1 month after radiofrequency ablation (RFA) showing a 20 mm-sized isoechoic ablation zone. The boundary of the ablation zone showed slightly low echogenicity, and the ablation zone is recognized as an oval shape. (**b**) US performed 3 months after RFA showing a hypoechoic area around the ablation zone. The boundary of the ablation zone is slightly hyperechoic compared to the surrounding fat tissue. (**c**) US performed 1 year after RFA revealing that the hypoechoic regions have spread widely and now appear as a lateral shadow. (**d**) US obtained 5 years after RFA revealing a cyst-like appearance of the ablation zone. Color Doppler US showing the absence of blood flow in the ablation zone. The hyperechoic components within the ablation zone appeared to be fluid, as determined by vibration of the US probe, and subsequent needle biopsy examination showed that the contents were necrotic tissue

There are two main challenges in the follow-up imaging of breast-conserving surgery: first, it is difficult to distinguish between primary and recurrent mammary gland tumors after RFA therapy as well as after standard breast-conserving surgery, and second, it is still necessary to verify the utility of MRI and MMG as follow-up examination methods.

The mammary gland after RFA is less deformed, and structural deformation of the mammary gland is unlikely. This is a great advantage when performing follow-

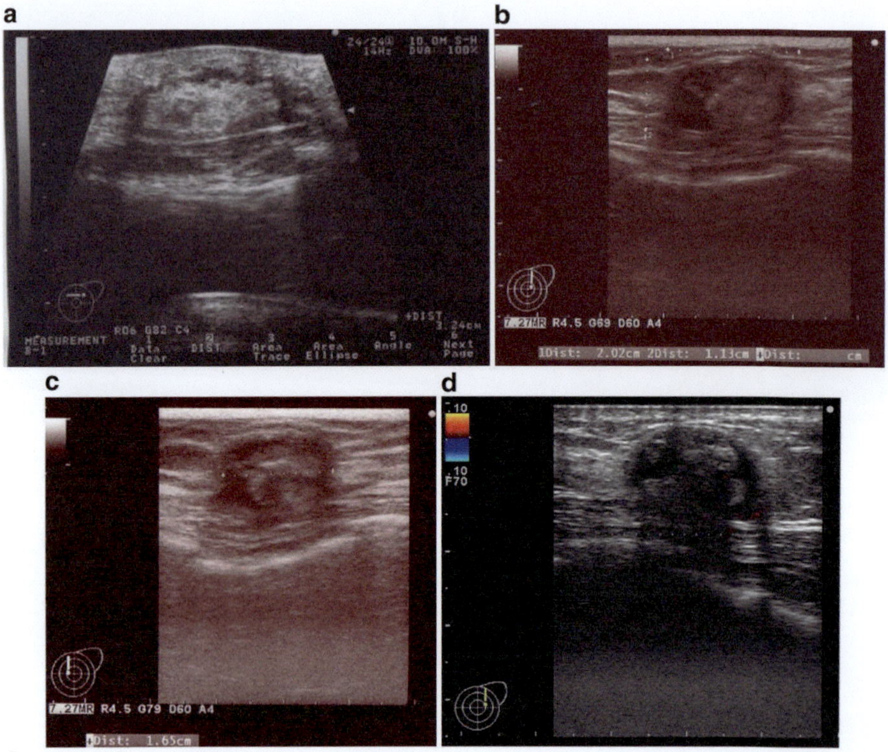

Fig. 9.7 (**a**) Representative ultrasonography (US) findings obtained 1 month after radiofrequency ablation (RFA) showing a 30 mm-sized hyperechoic oval mass. (**b**) US performed 3 years after RFA. The ablation zone appears as a 20 × 10 mm-sized cystic and solid tumor. (**c**) US performed 4 years after RFA. The ablation zone has reduced to 16 mm in size. (**d**) Color Doppler ultrasonography performed 5 years after RFA. The ablation zone has been further reduced to 12 × 10 mm in size, and blood flow is absent within the internal hyperechoic region

up MMG after RFA. Accordingly, postoperative MMG after RFA may be promising in the detection of early breast recurrences, as is the case for MMG examinations in healthy women.

9.5 Treatment Results in Our Hospital: A Pilot Study

Our study [20] was approved by the institutional review board for ethical issues at Chiba Cancer Center Hospital, Japan, and all patients provided written informed consent for study participation.

RFA was performed under ultrasound guidance using the 17-gauge Valleylab RF Ablation System with Cool-tip Technology. A US system (model SSD 5500; Aloka, Tokyo, Japan) with a 7.5- to 13.0-MHz broadband liner-array probe was

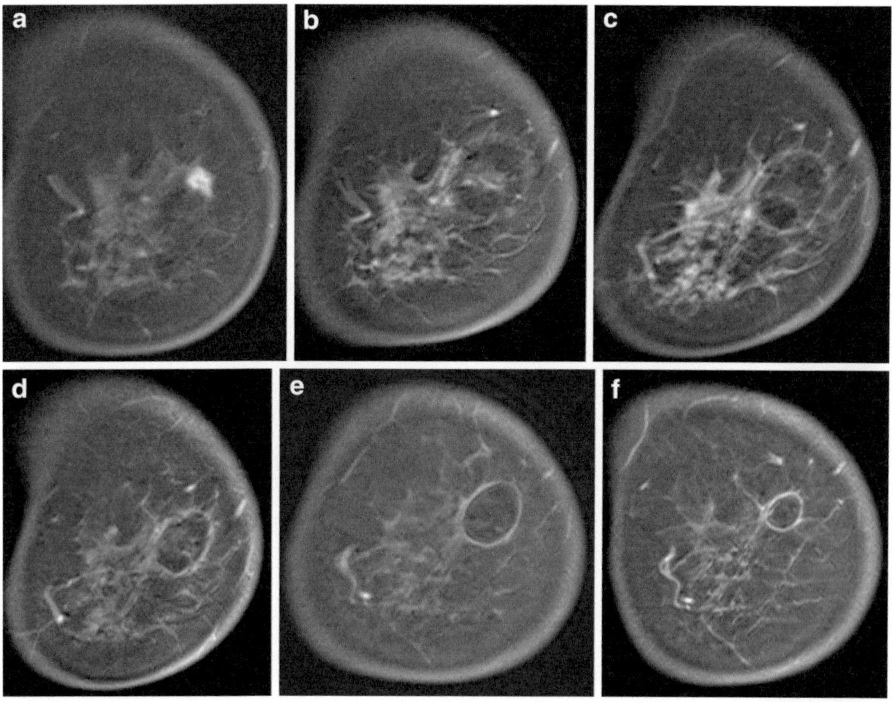

Fig. 9.8 (**a**) Representative preoperative magnetic resonance imaging (MRI) demonstrating an irregular 10 × 8 mm-sized enhanced mass without surrounding intraductal extension. (**b**) One month after radiofrequency ablation (RFA), a slightly enhanced region can be observed within the rounded ablation zone. The left region outside the ablation zone is a hyperintense area. This site is not present within the range of the tumor observed on preoperative MRI but rather represents marginal inflammatory cell infiltration outside the ablation zone. (**c**–**e**) MRI performed 6 months, 1 year, 3 years, and 5 years after RFA. The ablation zone has been further reduced to 6 × 5 mm in size, and a slightly enhanced region is absent within the ablation zone

used to identify the breast lesion for guiding the RFA probe into the lesion and monitoring thermocoagulation during RFA.

Postoperative MRI and US assessments and histological examinations were performed 4 weeks after RFA and before radiotherapy. Follow-up US was performed every 6 months after RFA, and MRI and MMG were performed every year after RFA.

Fifty patients undergoing RFA between February 2006 and December 2013 were enrolled in the study. Their mean age was 53.8 years (range, 38–78 years). Axillary lymph node dissection was performed in eight patients due to metastasis in the sentinel lymph node. RFA was performed for 50 breast tumors, including bilateral breast tumors in one patient, both of which met the eligibility criteria.

The mean tumor diameter was 1.2 cm (range, 0.5–2.0 cm) and the median observation period was 59.8 months (range, 6–100 months). The imaging and histopathological examinations were judged to be insufficient in three patients,

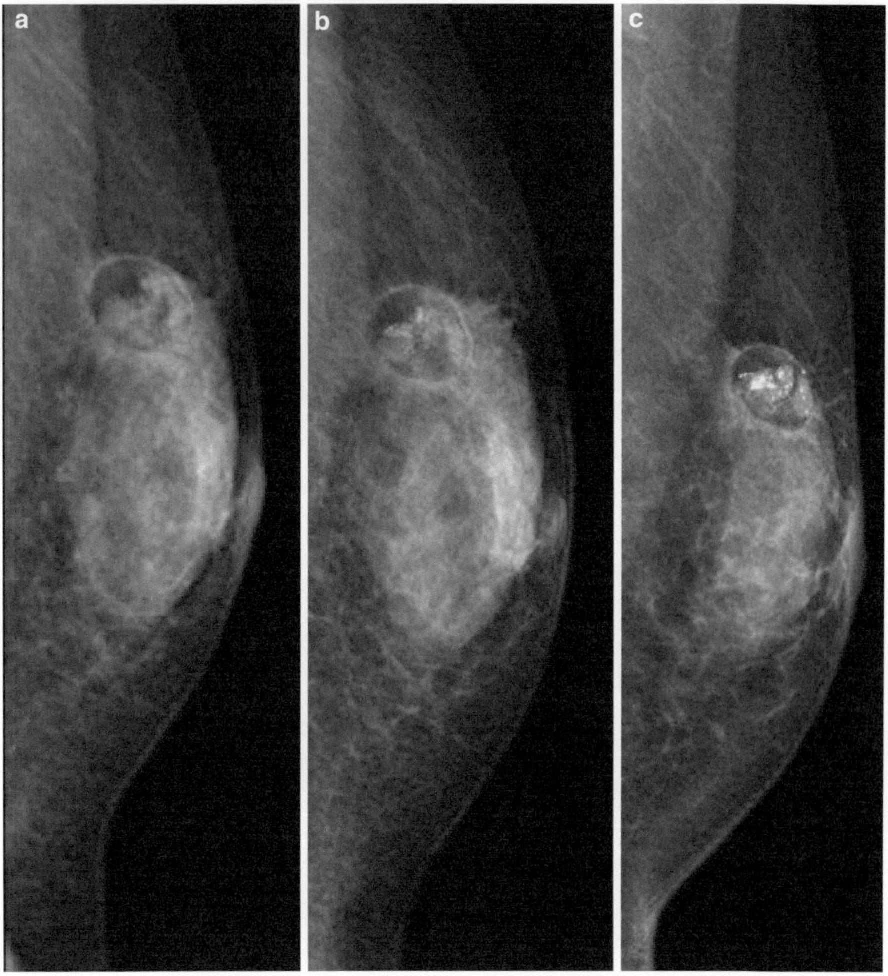

Fig. 9.9 (**a**: 2 years) (**b**: 3 years) (**c**: 5 years) Left mediolateral oblique mammographic views 2, 3, and 5 years after RFA in a 55-year-old woman with a 15 mm invasive ductal cancer. The roundish lucent area that was surrounded by the ring has gradually decreased in size. The coarse calcifications have gradually increase in the roundish lucent area

and their tumors were surgically resected. In two out of these three patients, viable tumor cells were observed at the ablated zone, and one patient was found to have residual cancer cells histopathologically.

One of the 50 patients (2 %) experienced breast tumor recurrence after RFA.

These results are similar to those of a previous multicenter retrospective study [21]. On 497 Japanese cases, the mean tumor diameter was reported to be 1.6 cm and the mean observation period was 50 months. In addition, when comparing patients with tumors >2 cm and those with tumors ≤ 2 cm, the incidence of local recurrence was found to be significantly lower for patients with tumors <2 cm in

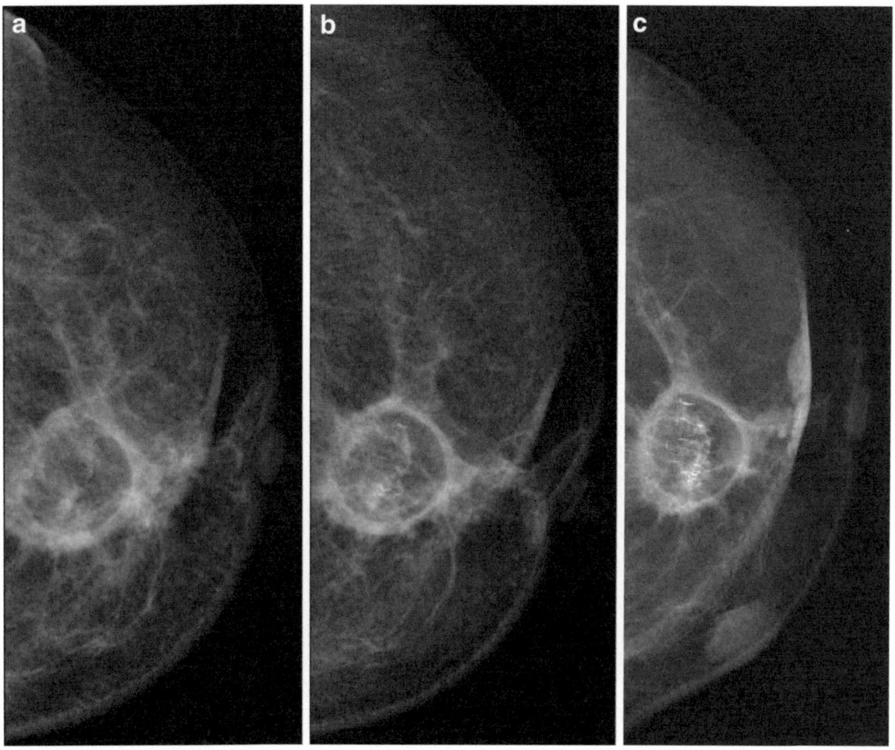

Fig. 9.10 (**a**) Representative mammography (MMG) image obtained 2 years after radiofrequency ablation (RFA) showing a ring-shaped low-density 20 × 20 mm-sized mass with high-density peripheral tissue. Calcification is absent within the ablation zone. (**b**) Three years after RFA. Coarse calcification has appeared within the ablation zone. The ring-shaped high-density region is narrower and clearer. (**c**) Local recurrence in the subcutaneous tissue at 4 years after RFA. The region of coarse calcification within the ablation zone has increased. A round high-density mass can be observed under the skin and outside the mammary gland

diameter (3 % vs. 18 %, $p < 0.01$). However, this report, as well as many others on the topic, did not mention the utility of postoperative imaging studies. Thus, understanding the imaging findings and the characteristics of RFA is important to ensure careful and effective follow-up of the patients.

9.6 Conclusions

Here, we explain the importance of postoperative imaging studies in the evaluation of RFA for breast cancer. Based on the findings of our pilot study, a multicenter clinical trial of RFA is ongoing in Japan since 2012 [22]. The purpose of this trial is to verify and compare the results of RFA to those of conventional breast-conserving therapy in terms of local control and survival. The secondary purpose of this study is to verify the utility of postoperative examinations, such as MMG, US, and MRI. We hope that this clinical trial will help establish the appropriate post-RFA follow-up diagnostic imaging methods.

References

1. Veronesi U, Cascinelli N, Mariani L, et al. Twenty-year follow-up of a randomized study comparing breast-conserving surgery with radical mastectomy for early breast cancer. N Engl J Med. 2002;347:1227–32.
2. Fisher B, Anderson S, Bryant J, et al. Twenty-year follow-up of a randomized trial comparing total mastectomy, lumpectomy, and lumpectomy plus irradiation for the treatment of invasive breast cancer. N Engl J Med. 2002;347:1233–41.
3. Smith RA, Duffy SW, Gabe R et al. The randomized trials of breast cancer screening: what have we learned?. Radiol Clin North Am. 2004;42:793–806.
4. Belli P, Costantini M, Romani M, et al. Magnetic resonance imaging in breast cancer recurrence. Breast Cancer Res Treat. 2002;73:223–35.
5. Coulthard A, Beveridge CJ, Potterton AJ. MRI in routine breast cancer follow-up: correlation with clinical outcome. Clin Radiol. 1999;54(7):459–61.
6. Veronesi U, Luini A, Galimberti V, et al. Conservation approaches for the management of stage I/II carcinoma of the breast: Milan Cancer Institute trials. World J Surg. 1994;18:70–5.
7. El-Tamer MB, Ward BM, Schifftner T, Neumayer L, Khuri S, Henderson W. Morbidity and mortality following breast cancer surgery in women: national benchmarks for standards of care. Ann Surg. 2007;245:665–71.
8. Arvold ND, Taghian AG, Niemierko A, et al. Age, breast cancer subtype approximation, and local recurrence after breast-conserving therapy. J Clin Oncol. 2011;29:3885–91.
9. Clarke M, Collins R, Darby S, et al. Effects of radiotherapy and of differences in the extent of surgery for early breast cancer on local recurrence and 15-year survival: an overview of the randomised trials. Lancet. 2005;366:2087–106. Review.
10. Schiller DE, Le LW, Cho BC, et al. Factors associated with negative margins of lumpectomy specimen: potential use in selecting patients for intraoperative radiotherapy. Ann Surg Oncol. 2008;15:833–42.
11. Waljee JF, Hu ES, Newman LA, et al. Predictors of re-excision among women undergoing breast-conserving surgery for cancer. Ann Surg Oncol. 2008;15:1297–303.
12. Kurniawan ED, Wong MH, Windle I, et al. Predictors of surgical margin status in breast-conserving surgery within a breast screening program. Ann Surg Oncol. 2008;15:2542–9.
13. Davis PL, Staiger MJ, Harris KB, et al. Breast cancer measurements with magnetic resonance imaging, ultrasonography, and mammography. Breast Cancer Res Treat. 1996;37:1–9.
14. Susini T, Nori J, Olivieri S, Livi L, Bianchi S, Mangialavori G, et al. Radiofrequency ablation for minimally invasive treatment of breast carcinoma: a pilot study in elderly inoperable patients. Gynecol Oncol. 2007;104:304–10.
15. Jeffrey SS, Birdwell RL, Ikeda DM, Daniel BL MD, Nowels KW, Dirbas FM, et al. Radiofrequency ablation of breast cancer: first report of an emerging technology. Arch Surg. 1999;134:1064–8.
16. Oura S, Tamaki T, Hirai I, Yoshimasu T, Ohta F, Nakamura R, et al. Radiofrequency ablation therapy in patients with breast cancers two centimeters or less in size. Breast Cancer. 2007;14:48–54.
17. Kinoshita T, Iwamoto E, Tsuda H, et al. Radiofrequency ablation as local therapy for early breast Carcinomas. Breast Cancer. 2011;18:10–7.

18. Nagashima T, Sakakibara M, Nakamura R, Arai M, Kadowaki M, Kazama T, et al. Dynamic enhanced MRI predicts chemosensitivity in breast cancer patients. Eur J Radiol. 2006;60:270–4.
19. Nagashima T, Suzuki M, Yagata H, Hashimoto H, Shishikura T, Imanaka N, et al. Dynamic-enhanced MRI predicts metastatic potential of invasive ductal breast cancer. Breast Cancer. 2002;9:226–30.
20. Yamamoto N, Fujimoto H, Nakamura R, et al. Pilot study of radiofrequency ablation therapy without surgical excision for T1 breast cancer: evaluation with MRI and vacuum-assisted core needle biopsy and safety management. Breast Cancer. 2011;18:3–9.
21. Ito T, Oura S, Yamamoto N, et al. Radiofrequency ablation of breast cancer. A multicenter retrospective analysis. J Clin Oncol 2012;30(15):suppl;abstr 1119.
22. Clinical Trial Registration URL:http://www.umin.ac.jp/ctr/index.htm. Unique identifier: UMIN000008675

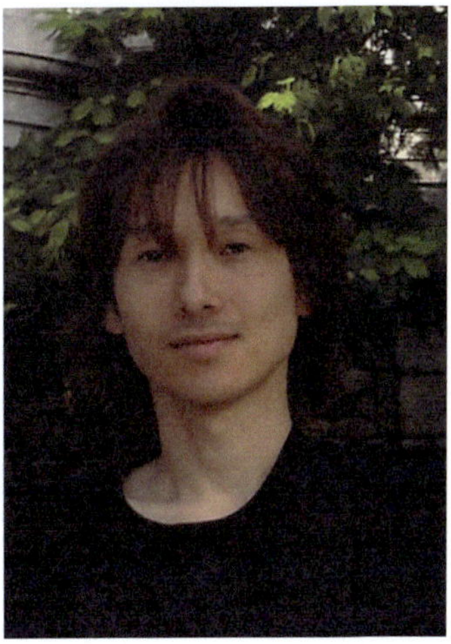

Rikiya Nakamura

Chapter 10
Cosmetic Evaluation of RFA

Tomomi Fujisawa

10.1 The Evaluation of Appearance After Radiofrequency Ablation

10.1.1 Cosmetics for the Breast Cancer Patient

Breast-conserving therapy (BCT) is now a well-established alternative methods to modified radical mastectomy (MRM) for the treatment of early-stage breast cancer [1, 2]. Several randomized clinical trials have confirmed that BCT and more radical procedures yield similar results for survival. An overview, which included almost 5000 patients, demonstrated that the 10-year survival was approximately equivalent for BCT and MRM. BCT is superior to MRM in the cosmetic, physical, psychological, social, occupational, and sexual point of view. And satisfaction of each views due to operation can continue for a long time after treatment. In many multicenter, randomized studies, BCT improved the evaluation of the patients' body image, resulted in higher treatment satisfaction, and yielded no significant difference from MRM with respect to fear of recurrence. The cosmetic outcome of such a treatment is very important for the psycho-socio-sexual functioning of most women.

T. Fujisawa (✉)
Department of Breast Oncology Gunma Prefectural Cancer Center, Takabayashi-nishi cho, 617-1, Ota-shi, Gunma 373-8550, Japan
e-mail: fujisawa@gunma-cc.jp

T. Kinoshita (ed.), *Non-surgical Ablation Therapy for Early-stage Breast Cancer*,
DOI 10.1007/978-4-431-54463-0_10

10.2 Previous Evaluation Methods for Cosmetics After Breast-Conserving Surgery

For this reason, cosmetic evaluation of treatments such as BCT is an important aspect of early-stage breast cancer treatments along with impact on overall survival. For this reason, many authors have established evaluation methods for BCT. Calle et al. distinguished the cosmetic result as excellent to good, good to fair, and poor, for treated lumpectomy, followed by irradiation or exclusive irradiation (radical radiotherapy without lumpectomy) [3]. Pezner et al. presented a method of objectively evaluating one aspect of cosmesis: breast retraction. Breast retraction assessment (BRA) is performed using a qualitative measurement grid. A clear acrylic sheet is supported vertically at chest height by a stand. The sheet is marked as a grid at 1-cm intervals. The Y-axis is at the midline and the X-axis is at the top of the grid. The observer locates the x- and y-coordinates for the nipple of each breast. BRA values are then calculated by simple vector geometry employing the Pythagorean theorem: $\mathrm{BRA} = \sqrt{(X_R - X_L)^2 + (Y_R - Y_L)^2}$ [4].

However, although this evaluation method reveals the difference in the position of nipples, it cannot assess the volume of residual breast.

Van Limbergen evaluated the placement of the nipple following BCT compared with the normal breast. Patients were scored as follows by global qualitative scoring by a three-member panel: El, good (slight sequelae); E2, moderate (marked sequelae detracting from cosmetic success, but still acceptable); E3, bad (severe fibrosis, telangiectasia, or breast contour deformation, unacceptable); and E4, complications (skin necrosis). Quantitative measurements consisted of the measurement of the relative upward (⊿A) and medio-lateral (⊿M) nipple displacement and the measurement of the retraction of the inferior (⊿I) and lateral (⊿L) breast contour. This was done on photographs taken under standard conditions. This study evaluated the correlation between scoring of the appearance and measurement [5].

Sacchini et al. evaluated tumorectomy and quadrantectomy by an analysis for symmetry using a computer. The following were noted: (1) difference in height between the two nipples, (2) difference in height between the mammary inferior profiles, (3) difference in the distance from the median line to the nipples, and (4) difference in the distance from the sternal notch to the nipples [6].

Rowland et al. used universal instruments to assess the physical and emotional outcomes as well as appearance after BCT. RAND 36-Item Health Survey, Medical Outcomes Study Social Support Survey, Center for Epidemiologic Studies Depression Scale, Revised Dyadic Adjustment Scale, the Watts Sexual Function Questionnaire, and a Cancer Rehabilitation Evaluation System were used to extract the evaluation of physical and emotional outcomes [7].

In 2000, the success of the operation was assessed not only for BCT but also for mastectomy with breast reconstruction. Nano et al. evaluated the cosmetic outcomes of mastectomy with breast reconstruction using FACT–B, Functional Assessment of Cancer Therapy–Breast and FACT–G, Functional Assessment of Cancer Therapy–General [8].

10.3 Evaluation Method of Cosmetics

The cosmetic outcomes for a surgical technique are an important factor to consider, as well as those of survival. The cosmetic and the functional outcome after postoperative breast radiotherapy depend on numerous patient- and therapy-related factors. The age, menopausal status, weight and general health status of the patient, the stage of the tumor, and the surgical intervention clearly influence the results.

In our study, we used the evaluation method for BCT about cosmetic outcomes produced by the TaskForce of the Japanese Breast Cancer Society (not published).

Each of the following categories was scored: size of the breast compared with the unaffected breast (0, severely different; 1, slightly different; 2, almost equal), deformity of the breast compared with the unaffected breast (0, severely different; 1, slightly different; 2, almost equal), scarring of the breast (0, severely conspicuous; 1, slightly conspicuous; 2, barely noticeable), hardness of the breast (0, severe; 1, slight; 2, normal, soft), shape of the nipple and areola (0, laterality; 1, no laterality), color of the nipple and areola (0, laterality; 1, no laterality), the distance of the sternum notch to the nipple (0, more than 2 cm; 1, less than 2 cm), and the laterality of the inferior margin of the breast (0, more than 2 cm; 1, less than 2 cm) (Fig. 10.1).

Total scores were graded as follows: 12–11 (excellent), 10–8 (good), 7–5 (fair), and 4–0 (poor). All scoring was done at 12 months after the operation, so this can be applied to the evaluation of the cosmetic outcomes of RFA, 12 months after the ablation procedure.

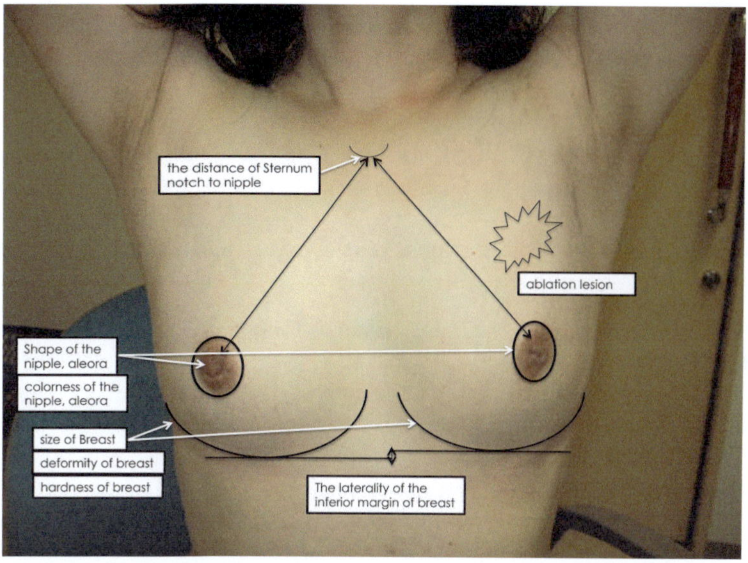

Fig. 10.1 The evaluation method for BCT

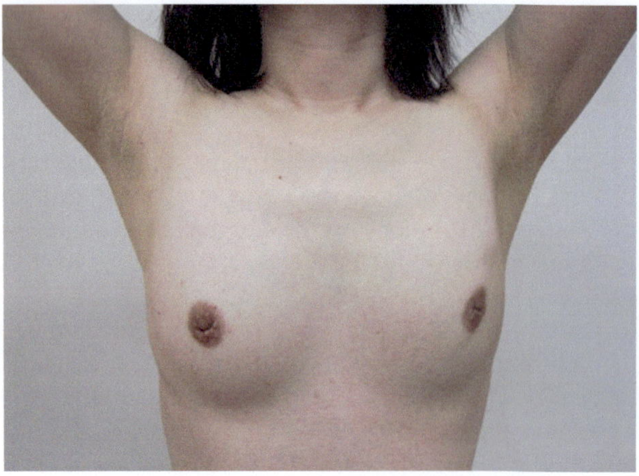

Fig. 10.2 Case 1; 45 years old, lt. C lesion, tumor size 1.1 cm T1N0M0 stage

10.3.1 Cosmetic Outcomes After RFA

The cosmetic outcomes of the following cases after RFA were evaluated at our institute:

Case 1; 45 Years Old, lt. C lesion, Tumor Size 1.1 cm, T1N0M0 Stage I (Fig. 10.2)

After 5 years, regarding the RFA lesion, the laterality of the inferior margin of the breast could be distinguished (i.e., it was slightly deformed compared to the contralateral side), but was almost comparable. Thus, it was scored 11 out of 12 and was considered excellent. In premenopausal women, breast tissues contain much protein, which is coagulated by the ablation heat. In this case, the coagulating tissue in the area of spreading heat due to RFA remained for 5 years, as a 3-cm diameter mass. It was difficult to distinguish the residual tumor or coagulated protein tissue by palpation; in order to do so, it was necessary to use magnetic resonance imaging.

In addition, vacuum-assisted biopsy can reveal if the residual tissue contains tumor and reduced coagulated protein tissue.

Case 2; 84 Years Old, lt. D lesion, Tumor Size 1 cm, T1N0M0 Stage I (Fig. 10.3-1)

Viewed from the front, there appears to be no problem. However, from the side, it is apparent that the skin over the area of the RFA was tight (Fig. 10.3-2). At the edge of the breast, the distance between the skin and deep muscle was too close, so adhesion of the skin and coagulated tissue has occurred. Such adhesion cannot be resolved by vacuum-assisted biopsy.

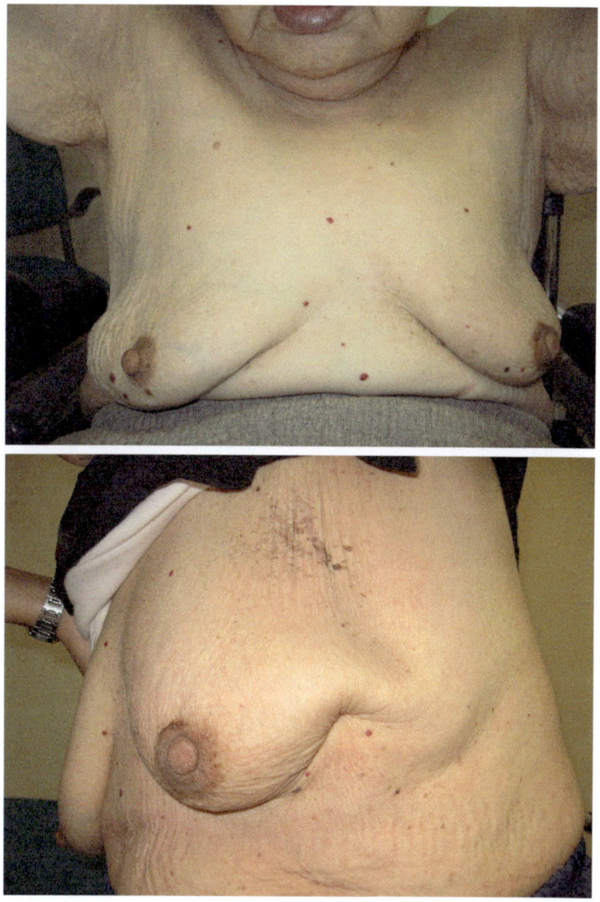

Fig. 10.3 Case 2; 84 years old, lt. D lesion, tumor size 1 cm T1N0M0 stage

Case 3; 77 Years Old, rt. C lesion, Tumor Size 1.5 cm, T1N0M0 Stage I (Fig. 10.4)

In this case, RFA heat had affected the skin, such that it was hard and wrinkled. As generally seen in older women, the breast was drooping and lay close to the tissue and skin below the breast.

Case 4; 75 Years Old, lt. DE lesion, Tumor Size 0.5 cm, T1N0M0 Stage I (Fig. 10.5)

In this case, the tumor size was very small, but it was located near to the nipple. During the operation, the distance between the nipple and the range of ablation heat was measured and found to be adequate. However, after ablation, the nipple collapsed. Although the ablation heat was not the direct cause of this problem,

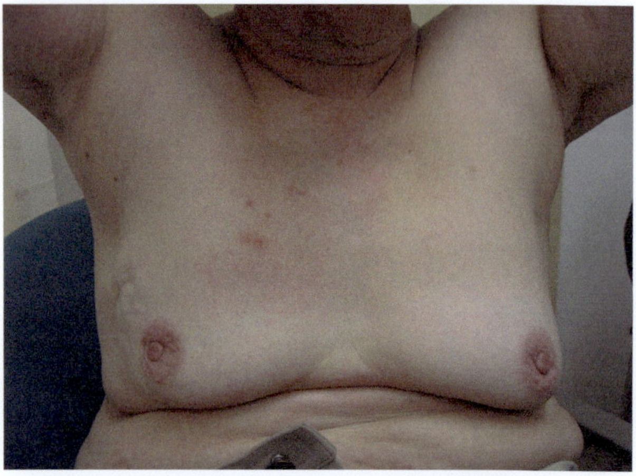

Fig. 10.4 Case 3; 77 years old, rt. C lesion tumor size 1.5 cm T1N0M0 stage

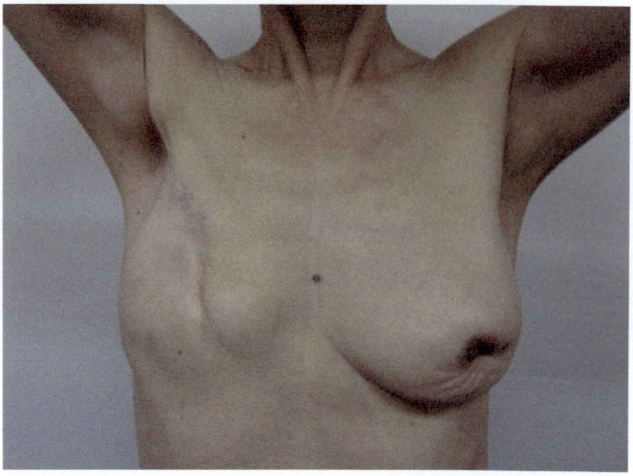

Fig. 10.5 Case 4; 75 years old, lt. DE lesion tumor size 0.5 cm T1N0M0 stage (Photo caption : Tomomi Fujisawa)

indirectly it had caused a coagulated mass to develop, which had pulled up the breast duct and led to the collapse of the nipple.

10.3.2 Contribution of Cosmetics to Successful Outcome After Ablation

To summarize the points that help to contribute to successful cosmetic outcomes after ablation of the breast:

1. Tumors less than 1.5 cm in diameter are suitable for ablation.

It is important to avoid adverse events. For example, adverse events resulting from ablation heat is severe. To avoid heat injury, a substantial distance between the

RFA needle and the skin and the needle and deep muscle is needed. Furthermore, the size of RFA needle will affect the range of heat reached. Because the breast of Japanese women have tendency to less small than that of other countries, so to undergo RFA for Japanese patients, 2-cm size of RFA needles are suitable.

2. Location of tumor.

For tumors located at the edge of the breast tissue or near the nipple, skin burn or deformity induced by the ablation heat can occur. To avoid this, it is important to measure the range spread *of* the ablation heat.

3. Menopausal status.

In premenopausal status, the breast tissue contains much protein and can cause a coagulated mass due to the ablation heat. Thus, in premenopausal cases, vacuum-assisted biopsy after RFA and radiotherapy is effective in reducing the coagulation tissue and improving the cosmetic outcome. In postmenopausal women, it is not a significant issue because the breast tissue contains more fat than protein. So after ablation, there is minimal coagulation mass due to necrosis of the fatty tissue.

References

1. Fisher B, Bauer M, Margolese R, Poisson R, Pilch Y, Redmond C, Fisher E, Wolmark N, Deutsch M, Montague E, Saffer E, Wickerham L, Lerner H, Glass A, Shibata H, Deckers P, Ketcham A, Oishi R, Russell I. Five-year results of a randomized clinical trial comparing total mastectomy and segmental mastectomy with or without radiation in the treatment of breast cancer. N Engl J Med. 1985;312(11):665–73.
2. Veronesi U, Banfi A, Del Vecchio M, Saccozzi R, Clemente C, Greco M, Luini A, Marubini E, Muscolino G, Rilke F, et al. Comparison of Halsted mastectomy with quadrantectomy, axillary dissection, and radiotherapy in early breast cancer: long-term results. Eur J Cancer Clin Oncol. 1986;22(9):1085–9.
3. Calle R, Pilleron J, Schlienger P, Vilcoq J. Conservative management of operable breast cancer. Ten years experience at the Foundation Curie. Cancer. 1978;42(4):2045–53.
4. Pezner RD, Patterson MP, Hill LR, Vora N, Desai KR, Archambeau JO, Lipsett JA. Breast retraction assessment: an objective evaluation of cosmetic results of patients treated conservatively for breast cancer. Int J Radiat Oncol Biol Phys. 1985;11(3):575–8.
5. Van Limbergen E, Rijnders A, Van der Schueren E, Lerut T, Christiaens R. Cosmetic evaluation of breast conserving treatment for mammary cancer. 2. A quantitative analysis of the influence of radiation dose, fractionation schedules and surgical treatment techniques on cosmetic results. Radiother Oncol. 1989;16(4):253–67.
6. Sacchini V, Luini A, Tana S, Lozza L, Galimberti V, Merson M, Agresti R, Veronesi P, Greco M. Quantitative and qualitative cosmetic evaluation after conservative treatment for breast cancer. Eur J Cancer Clin Oncol. 1991;27(11):1395–400.

7. Rowland JH, Desmond KA, Meyerowitz BE, Belin TR, Wyatt GE, Ganz PA. Role of breast reconstructive surgery in physical and emotional outcomes among breast cancer survivors. J Natl Cancer Inst. 2000;92(17):1422–9.
8. Nano MT, Gill PG, Kollias J, Bochner MA, Malycha P, Winefield HR. Psychological impact and cosmetic outcome of surgical breast cancer strategies. ANZ J Surg. 2005;75(11):940–7.

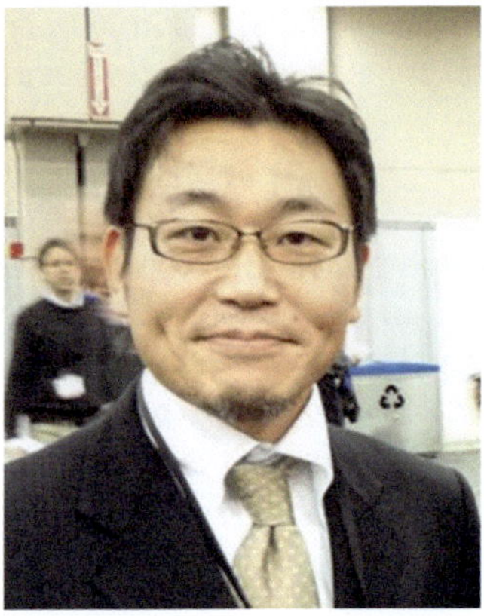

Tomomi Fujisawa

Chapter 11
RFA of Breast Cancer: A Multicenter Retrospective Analysis

Toshikazu Ito

11.1 Introduction

Clinical research on various minimally invasive therapies for breast cancer has been conducted in the past 10 years. There are reports of mastectomy or lumpectomy after radiofrequency ablation (RFA) for early-stage breast cancer [1–11], as well as those without mastectomy or lumpectomy after RFA [12–14], with the success rate of RFA being high in both scenarios. The purpose of the present study is to retrospectively investigate the safety and appropriateness of RFA without lumpectomy or mastectomy at ten institutions in Japan that belong to the Breast Cancer Society for Minimally Invasive Therapy.

11.2 Patients and Methods

11.2.1 Patients

A total of 520 patients with breast cancer who were treated with RFA were retrospectively recruited from ten Japanese institutes participating in the retrospective multicenter study conducted by the Breast Cancer Society for Minimally Invasive Therapy. Because of the retrospective nature of the study, various factors such as the criteria for RFA treatment and the pre- and postoperative pathological and imaging modalities used differed among the ten institutions. Core needle biopsy and/or vacuum-assisted biopsy was performed preoperatively in some

T. Ito (✉)
Department of Surgery, Rinku General Medical Center, 2-23 Rinku, Izumisano, Osaka 598-8577, Japan
e-mail: t-ito@rgmc.izumisano.osaka.jp

T. Kinoshita (ed.), *Non-surgical Ablation Therapy for Early-stage Breast Cancer*,
DOI 10.1007/978-4-431-54463-0_11

patients who had undergone primary systemic therapy, to evaluate the viability of regressed or disappeared tumors and to detect the presence of tumor tissues around the regressed or disappeared tumors. To evaluate the viability of tumor tissues after RFA, hematoxylin and eosin (H&E) staining and/or nicotinamide adenine dinucleotide-diaphorase (NADH-diaphorase) staining was used for examination of ultrasound-guided core needle biopsy and/or vacuum-assisted biopsy or fine needle aspiration cytology. Written informed consent was obtained from all patients according to institutional review board guidelines.

11.2.2 RFA Procedure

With respect to the RFA methods and criteria for assessing response used at the ten study sites, there are some minor differences such as the electrodes used and the methods for collecting tumor tissue samples before and after RFA, but they are generally the same.

11.2.3 Factors Assessed for Local Recurrence

The intraoperative factors evaluated were the type of RFA needle used, the total ablation time, and the temperature of the tumor just after ablation. The postoperative factors evaluated were imaging and pathological modalities, the timing of tissue sampling for the assessment of tumor viability, lymph node status, adjuvant systemic therapy, and adjuvant radiotherapy.

11.2.4 Statistical Analysis

The chi-square test or Fisher's exact test was used to evaluate the association between each factor and local recurrence. Local recurrence-free survival (IBRFS) was estimated using the Kaplan-Meier method and was compared among subgroups using the log-rank test. The level of significance was set at $p < 0.05$ (two tailed). All statistical analyses were performed using SPSS software version 17.0.

11.3 Results

The Cool-tip radiofrequency system, LeVeen needle electrode system, and RITA system were used for RFA treatment of breast cancer. Of the 520 patients, 487 received RFA using the Cool-tip system.

Table 11.1 Patient characteristics

Age (years)	53.6 ± 12.0
Follow-up (months)	45.4 ± 19.7
Tumor size (cm)	1.59 ± 1.09
Multicentricity solitary/multicentric	516/5
Histology	0.41 ± 0.60
Invasive ductal carcinoma	457
Invasive lobular carcinoma	13
Others	51
Lymph node −/+	418/103
ER +/−/unknown	473/79/5
PgR +/−/unknown	368/144/9
HER2 +/−/IHC2+&FISH not performed/unknown	412/75/5/29
Radiotherapy +/−/unknown	463/56/2
Primary systemic therapy −/+	386/135
Type of electrode Cool-tip/LeVeen/RITA	488/16/17

ER estrogen receptor, *PgR* progesterone receptor, *HER2* human epidermal growth factor receptor type-2, *IHC* immunohistochemistry, *FISH* fluorescent in situ hybridization, *RFA* radiofrequency ablation, *VAB* vacuum-assisted biopsy

Mean patient age was 54 years (range, 22–92 years). Mean tumor size was 1.6 cm in diameter. Four hundred and twenty-five tumors (86 %) were ≤2 cm in diameter. The median follow-up period was 50 months (range, 3–92 months). The mean time required for ablation was 19 min (range, 4–72 min), and the average temperature of the tumor after ablation was 91 °C.

A total of 134 patients (25.8 %) had received primary systemic therapy before RFA. Four patients had multicentric tumors and 63 patients had ductal spreading tumors with an average length of 0.4 cm. Twelve patients had lobular carcinoma and 55 patients underwent RFA treatment without adjuvant radiotherapy (Tables 11.1 and 11.2).

The local recurrence rate after RFA was higher in tumors negative for estrogen receptors (8 of 78, 10 %) than in tumors positive for estrogen receptors (17 of 437, 4 %; $p < 0.05$) and was higher in tumors positive for HER2/neu than in tumors negative for HER2/neu (14.9 % vs. 3.2 %; $p < 0.01$). The local recurrence rate after RFA was higher in tumors with positive nodes than in tumors with negative nodes (9.8 % vs. 3.6 %) and was higher in tumors without irradiation than in tumors with irradiation (18.2 % vs. 3.2 %; $p < 0.001$). The local recurrence rate after RFA was higher in tumors >2 cm (13 of 72, 18 %) than in tumors ≤2 cm (11 of 425, 3 %; $p < 0.001$) (Fig. 11.1) in diameter. RFA-related adverse events observed were local pain (17 patients), skin burn (14 patients), and nipple retraction (four patients).

Table 11.2 Factors related to local recurrence and distant metastasis

Factor	Local recurrence	p-value X^2 test (Fisher's exact test)	Distant metastasis	No recurrence
Tumor size				
≦2.0 cm	11 (2.5 %)	<0.0001	9 (2.1 %)	410 (94.5 %)
>2.0 cm	14 (16.3 %)		0 (0 %)	96 (97.0 %)
Nodal status (−)	15 (3.6 %)	<0.001	7 (1.7 %)	(94.7 %) 84
(+)	10 (9.8 %)		8 (7.8 %)	(82.4 %) 67
ER (−)	8 (10.3 %)	0.042	3 (3.8 %)	(85.9 %) 408
(+)	17 (3.9 %)		12 (2.7 %)	(93.4 %) 126
PgR (−)	12 (8.4 %)	0.063	5 (3.5 %)	(88.1 %) 345
(+)	13 (3.5 %)		10 (2.7 %)	(93.8 %) 387
HER2 (−)	13 (3.2 %)	0.008	12 (2.9 %)	(93.9 %) 60
(+)	11 (14.9 %)		3 (4.1 %)	(81.1 %) 5
Unknown	1 (7.7 %)		0 (0 %)	(92.3 %) 43
Radiotherapy (−)	10 (18.2 %)		2 (3.6 %)	(78.2 %) 435
(+)	15 (3.2 %)	<0.0001	13 (2.8 %)	(94.0 %)

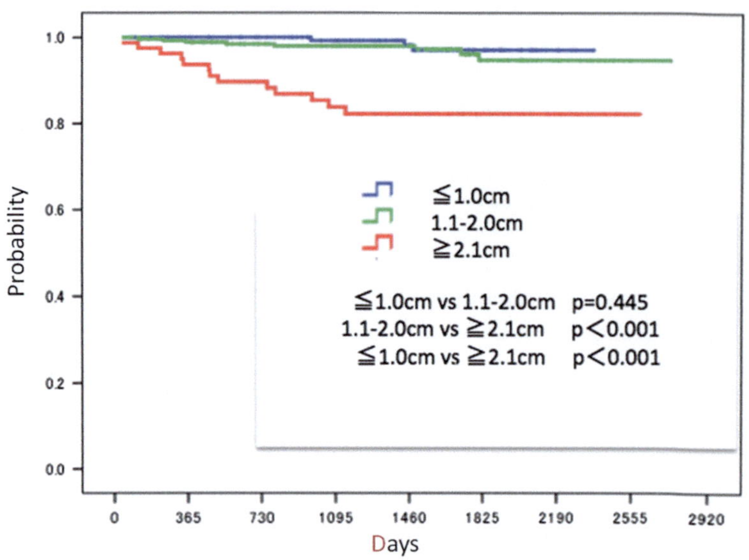

Fig. 11.1 Local recurrence-free survival after RFA treatment

11.4 Conclusions

RFA is considered to be a safe and promising minimally invasive treatment of small breast cancer ≤2 cm in diameter. Further studies are necessary to optimize the technique and evaluate its future role as local therapy for breast cancer.

References

1. Jeffrey SS, Birdwell RL, Ikeda DM, et al. Radiofrequency ablation of breast cancer. Arch Surg. 1999;134:1064–8.
2. Singletary SE. Radiofrequency ablation of breast cancer. Am Surg. 2003;69:37–40.
3. Burak WE, Agnese DM, Povoski SP, et al. Radiofrequency ablation of invasive breast carcinoma followed by delayed surgical excision. Cancer. 2003;98:1369–76.
4. Noguchi M, Earashi M, Fujii H, et al. Radiofrequency ablation of small breast cancer followed by surgical resection. J Surg Oncol. 2006;93:120–8.
5. Khatri VP, McGahan JP, Ramsamooj R, et al. A phase II trial of image-guided radiofrequency ablation of small invasive breast carcinomas: use of saline-cooled tip electrode. Ann Surg Oncol. 2007;14:1644–52.
6. Medina-Franco H, Soto-Germes S, Ulloa-Gómez JL, et al. Radiofrequency ablation of invasive breast carcinomas: a phase II trial. Ann Surg Oncol. 2008;15:1689–95.
7. Imoto S, Wada N, Sakemura N, et al. Feasibility study on radiofrequency ablation followed by partial mastectomy for stage I breast cancer patients. Breast. 2009;18:130–4.
8. Manenti G, Bolacchi F, Perretta T, et al. Small breast cancers: in vivo percutaneous US-guided radiofrequency ablation with dedicated cool-tip radiofrequency system. Radiology. 2009;251:339–46.
9. Motoyoshi A, Noguchi M, Earashi M, et al. Histopathological and immunohistochemical evaluations of breast cancer treated with radiofrequency ablation. J Surg Oncol. 2010;102:385–91.
10. Kinoshita T, Iwamoto E, Tsuda H, et al. Radiofrequency ablation as local therapy for early breast carcinomas. Breast Cancer. 2011;18:10–7.
11. Ohtani S, Kochi M, Ito M, et al. Radiofrequency ablation of early breast cancer followed by delayed surgical resection—a promising alternative to breast-conserving surgery. Breast. 2011;20:431–6.
12. Oura S, Tamaki T, Hirai I, et al. Radiofrequency ablation therapy in patients with breast cancers two centimeters or less in size. Breast Cancer. 2007;14:48–54.
13. Earashi M, Noguchi M, Motoyoshi A, Fujii H. Radiofrequency ablation therapy for small breast cancer followed by immediate surgical resection or delayed mammotome excision. Breast Cancer. 2007;14:39–47.
14. Yamamoto N, Fujimoto H, Nakamura R, et al. Pilot study of radiofrequency ablation therapy without surgical excision for T1 breast cancer: evaluation with MRI and vacuum-assisted core needle biopsy and safety management. Breast Cancer. 2011;18:3–9.

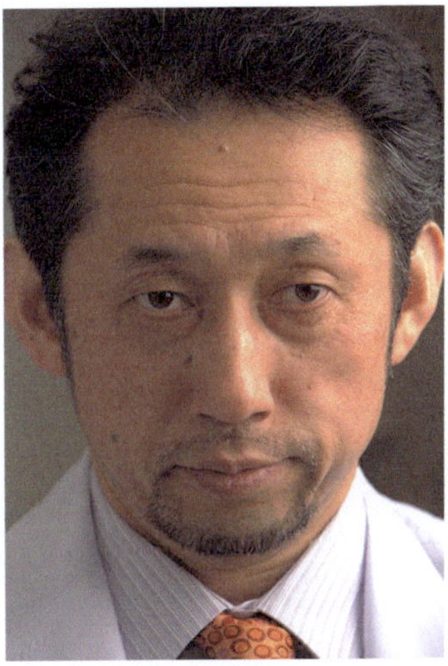

Toshikazu Ito

Chapter 12
RFA with a Cool-Tip Electrode in Early Breast Cancer

Takayuki Kinoshita

12.1 Background of Our Study

There has been a change in the management of cancer patients with localized disease, from total mastectomy to lumpectomy complemented by adjuvant radiotherapy and chemo-endocrine therapy, without significant outcome [1, 2]. Early detection of small breast lesions may further change the attitude toward less invasive and even noninvasive management [3].

A major goal of breast-conserving treatment is the preservation of a cosmetically acceptable breast. Although a variety of patient and treatment factors have been reported to influence the cosmetic result, the amount of breast tissue resected appears to be a major factor [4]. Several investigators are studying the feasibility of percutaneous minimally invasive techniques to ablate breast tumors. Several modalities such as cryosurgery, laser ablation, thermoablation, and high-intensity-focused ultrasound have been investigated [5]. By minimizing damage and disruption to normal surrounding tissue, the morbidity of local treatment, such as scarring and deformity, can be reduced, and cosmetic result can potentially be improved. With the widespread application of screening mammography, the mean size of the breast tumors detected has continued to decrease which further emphasize the need for less invasive means for achieving local tumor destruction such as RF ablation [6].

This phase I/II study was to determine the safety and efficacy of radiofrequency ablation of early breast carcinomas using saline-cooled electrode. Our secondary goal was to determine the size, configuration, and pathological features of acute RF ablative treatment of breast carcinomas.

T. Kinoshita (✉)
Division of Breast Surgery, National Cancer Center Hospital, 5-1-1, Tsukiji Chuo-ku, Tokyo 104-0045, Japan
e-mail: takinosh@ncc.go.jp

T. Kinoshita (ed.), *Non-surgical Ablation Therapy for Early-stage Breast Cancer*,
DOI 10.1007/978-4-431-54463-0_12

12.2 RFA Study with a Cool-Tip Electrode in Early Breast Cancer

12.2.1 Patients

All patients had prior histological diagnosis of breast cancer established by stereotactic or ultrasound-guided core biopsy. Core biopsy had to be adequate for routine pathological evaluations (grade, estrogen receptor, progesterone receptor, Her 2-neu) because after RF ablation has been performed, viable tumor may not be available for these analyses.

Eligibility criteria included age between 20 and 90 years, tumor size less than or equal to 3.0 cm in diameter on ultrasound examination. Patients were excluded if there was evidence of diffuse calcification suggestive of extensive of multifocal ductal carcinoma in situ more than 3.0 cm in size.

MRI was performed to all the patients to evaluate the lesions more precisely and compared with the results of RF ablation. Patients treated with preoperative chemotherapy were excluded. This study was approved by the National Cancer Center, Japan Institutional Review Board, and all patients provided written informed consent.

12.2.2 Treatment

All patients underwent breast ultrasound and MRI preoperatively to determine if the tumor was visible, as it would facilitate ultrasound-guided RF ablation. The patient could elect to undergo either a lumpectomy or a mastectomy as in both situations the RF-ablated tissue would be available for pathological review. Sentinel lymph node biopsy (SLNB) was performed for axillary staging. Tracers for SLNB were injected into subareolar parenchyma to prevent the air/fluid interfering with intraoperative ultrasound imaging.

After general anesthesia was induced and SLNB was completed, the breast tumor was identified with intraoperative ultrasound using the Toshiba Aplio XG SSA-790A (Toshiba Medical Systems Corporation, Otawara, Japan) with a PLT-1204AT (2D, 12 MHz) and a PLT-1204MV (4D, 14 MHz) probe. Under ultrasound guidance, the 17-gauge, Valleylab™ RF Ablation System with Cool-tip™ Technology (Covidien, Energy-Based Devices, Interventional Oncology, Boulder, CO, USA) was inserted in the center of the tumor (Fig. 12.1). With ultrasound imaging in the two planes, we ensured that the electrode was located in the center of the lesions using linear 2D probe for the vertical image and 4D probe for the coronary image (Fig. 12.2). In all cases, a 2-cm active tip electrode was used. Before ablation, we injected 20–40 ml of 5 % glucose to avoid skin or

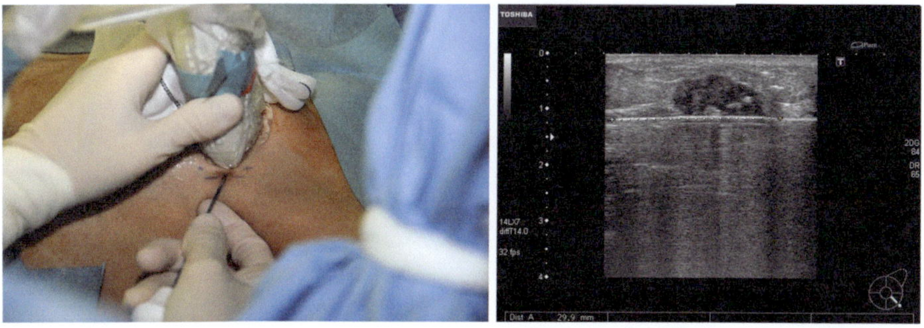

Fig. 12.1 Technique of performing breast radiofrequency ablation (RFA). Under ultrasound guidance, the RF electrode is percutaneously inserted into the breast tumor. The needle is seen transversing the target tumor

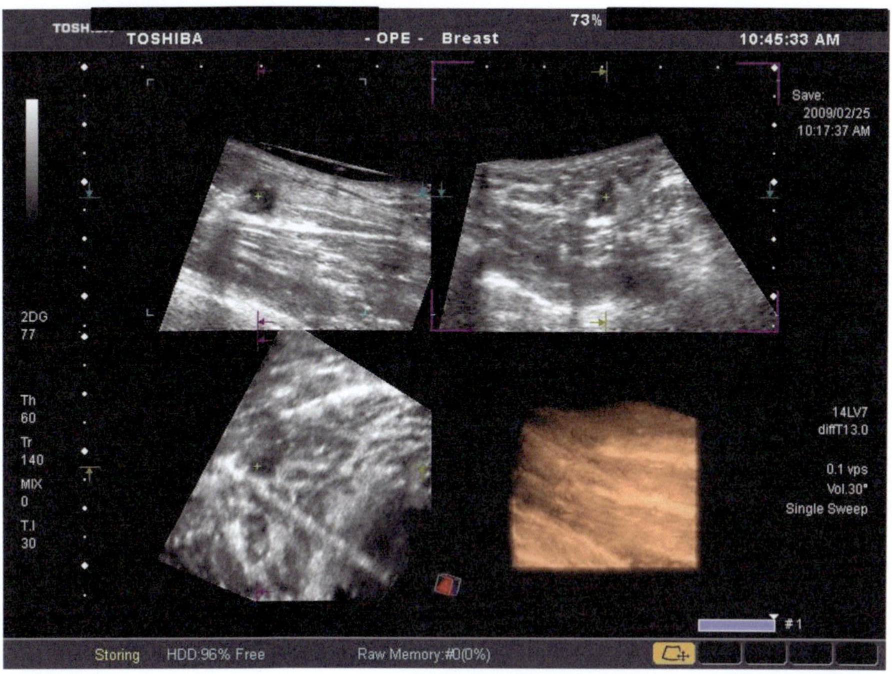

Fig. 12.2 Confirmation of the location of the needle using 4D probe. With ultrasound imaging in the two planes, we ensured that the electrode was located in the center of the lesions using linear 2D probe for the vertical image and 4D probe for the coronary image

muscle burn. The needle electrode was attached to a 500-kHz, monopolar RF generator capable of producing 200 W power. Grounding was achieved by attaching two grounding pads to the patient's thighs before the producer. Tissue impedance was monitored continuously using circuitry incorporated into the

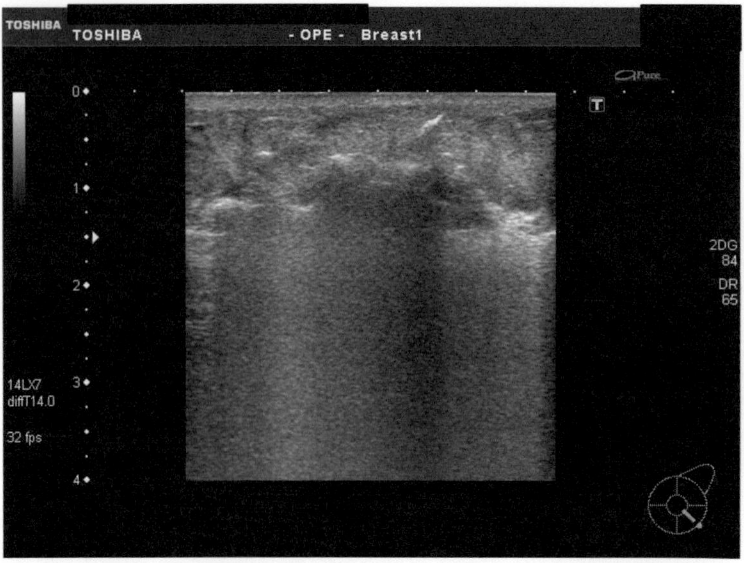

Fig. 12.3 Intraoperative breast ultrasound. Radiofrequency was applied until the tumor was completely hyperechoic

generator. A peristaltic pump (Watson-Marlow, Medford, MA) was used to infuse 0 °C normal saline solution into the lumen of the electrode at a rate of sufficient to maintain a tip temperature of 15–25 °C.

RF energy was applied to tissue with an initial power setting of 10 W and subsequently increased with increments of 5 W each minute to a maximum power of 55 W. Saline circulating internally within the electrode cools the adjacent tissue, maximizing energy deposition and reducing tissue charring. The power setting was left at this point until power "roll-off" occurred. Power roll-off implies that there is an increase in the tissue impedance caused by loss of sodium chloride, which occurs with tissue coagulation around the monopolar electrode. When this occurs, the power generator will shut off, stopping the flow of current and further tissue coagulation. After waiting 30–60 s, second phase was started at 75 % of the last maximum power until a second roll-off occurs. The appearance and progression of hyperechogenicity on ultrasound was used to guide the therapy. Radiofrequency was applied until the tumor was completely hyperechoic (Fig. 12.3). To minimize thermal injury to the skin, sterile ice packs were placed on the breast during the ablation procedure (Fig. 12.4). Following RF ablation, standard tumor resection achieved with either a wide local excision or mastectomy according to the preference of the patient. The surgical specimen was obtained and immediately sent fresh to pathology department.

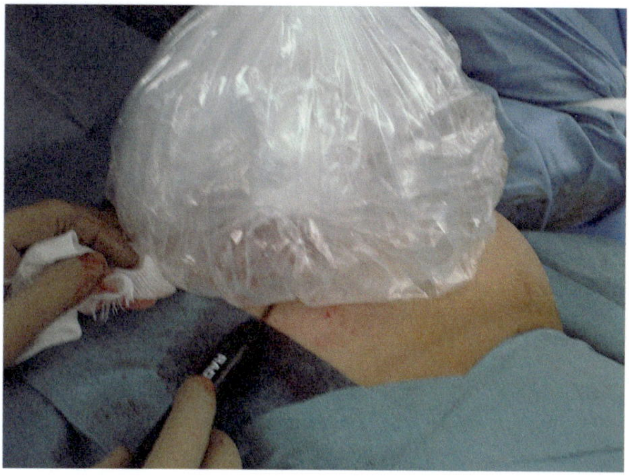

Fig. 12.4 Skin protection. The skin is protected by placing an ice pack during the RFA procedure

12.2.3 Pathological Evaluation for RFA

12.2.3.1 Frozen Section

The surgical specimen were submitted to the pathologists for NADH-diaphorase cell viability analysis and routine histopathological examination. A tissue slice including the representative cut surface of the tumor and non-ablated mammary glands was removed and subjected to frozen section preparation.

One to two pieces of representative tumor tissue and another piece of non-ablated mammary glands were snap frozen in liquid nitrogen and cut into 5-μm-thick sections using a cryostat (Shiraimatsu, Tokyo, Japan). One of the sections was stained with hematoxylin and eosin (H&E) and was microscopically confirmed to contain the representative tumor tissue and non-ablated mammary gland tissue. Other sections were stored at −20 °C until NADH-diaphorase assay.

12.2.3.2 Histological Analysis

From residual tissue specimens, an entire representative cut surface of the ablated tumor and surrounding tissue were taken as tissue blocks for histopathological examination. The blocks were formalin-fixed, paraffin-embedded, and cut into 3- to 4-μm-thick sections. These sections were stained with H&E. Histopathologically, viability of tumors was evaluated in consideration of thermocautery artifact. When the degeneration was marked in cancer cells, the effect of thermocautery was effective. The tumor area with marked degeneration was calculated for each case.

Immunohistochemically, expression of estrogen receptor (ER, clone ID5 clone, Dako, Grostrup, Denmark), progesterone receptor (PR, clone IA6 Dako), and HER2 (Herceptest, Dako) was examined. For ER and PgR, a tumor was judged as positive if 10 % or more of tumor cells with positive nuclear immunoreactions irrespectively of intensity of the immunoreactions. For HER2, judgment of immunoreactions was performed according to the recommendation of ASCO/CAP guideline.

12.2.3.3 NADH-Diphorase Cell Viability Analysis

The enzyme histochemical analysis of cell viability was performed based on the reduction of nitroblue tetrazolium chloride, a redox indicator, by NADH-diphorase, resulting in an intense blue cytoplasmic pigmentation. The activity of this enzyme has been shown to subside immediately upon cell death. For this analysis, 5-μm cryostat-cut unfixed sections were placed on a coplin staining jar, incubated in 0.05 M Tris-buffered saline (TBS, pH 7.4) containing 500 mg/L tetranitro blue tetrazolium and 800 mg/L β-NADH (Sigma-Aldrich Corp., St. Louis, MO) for 30 min at 37 °C. Thereafter, the sections were fixed in 10 % formalin for 30 min, washed with distilled water for 2 min, and mounted with cover glass. Based on the area of cells with blue cytoplasmic staining, the viability of tumor cells and non-ablated mammary gland cells as control was evaluated.

12.2.4 Results of the Study

Fifty patients were enrolled in the study and 49 completed RF ablation therapy. For one patient, the ablation system had some trouble, and we decided not to proceed with the therapy. The demographics of 50 patients who were enrolled in the RF ablation study were shown in Table 12.1. Their median age was 61 years (range, 36–82). The median breast tumor size based on the ultrasonographic maximum dimension was 1.70 cm (range 0.5–3.0). The histology was invasive ductal carcinoma for 43 patients (86 %).

RF ablation time ranged from 3 to 18 min (mean, 8.7 min). Mean tumor impedance was 195.1 Ω, and in 4 of 49 patients, there was reduction in the impedance during treatment by a mean of 53.4 Ω.

A median of 1 cycle and a mean power of 48.5 W (range, 5–118 W) were used to achieve tumor ablation.

RFA of the breast tumor was monitored with ultrasonography every 3 min.

In 49 patients, as tumor heating around the multiple array electrodes developed, an ill-defined, hyperechoic zone developed. The size of the ablation measured by ultrasonography ranged 15–50 mm (mean, 27.3 mm).

RFA-related adverse events were observed in five cases (10 %): two with skin burn and three with muscle burn. The entire skin burn area was excised during the breast tumor resection, and the patient had no further sequelae. These events occurred in initial cases. So, in order to avoid these burns, 10 ml of 5 % glucose was injected between skin and tumor and also between muscle and tumor. Since then, no skin burns were observed.

Table 12.1 Patient demographics of 50 patients

	Number of patients
Age (years)	
Median	61
Range	36–82
Method of diagnosis	
Mammogram screening	33 (66 %)
Palpable mass ± mammogram	17 (34 %)
Tumor classification	
Tis	2 (4 %)
T1	34 (68 %)
T2	14 (28 %)
Tumor location	
Upper outer	18 (36 %)
Lower outer	6 (12 %)
Upper inner	18 (36 %)
Lower inner	7 (14 %)
Central	1 (2 %)
Tumor size on US (cm)	
Median	1.70
Range	0.5–3.0
Tumor size on MRI (cm)	
Median	1.70
Range	0.7–4.5
Lymph node status	
N0	45 (90 %)
N1	5 (10 %)

There was no bleeding from the needle track upon removal of the RFA needle electrode in any of the 49 patients.

Surgical resection consisted of total mastectomy in 27 patients, while 23 patients underwent wide local excision. In the early stages of this study, we select the patients with a small breast cancer who prefer to be treated by mastectomy.

On H&E examination, the tumor architecture was maintained despite ablation, which allowed pathologic size to be accurately assessed. The RFA-treated carcinomas showed a range of pathologic findings. All of the treated tumors showed elongated nuclei with smudged chromatin (Fig. 12.5c). All cases showed extensive electrocautery changes with densely eosinophilic stromas.

In resected samples ablated with a 2.0 cm active tip of electrode, the results of H&E and NADH examination showed that mean diameter of major axis was 3.0 cm (range 0–6.6 cm) and one of minor axis was 2.2 cm (range, 0–6.6 cm) (Table 12.2).

The NADH viability staining was available for 38 patients, and in 29 (76.3 %), there were no evidence of viable malignant cells (Fig. 12.5d).

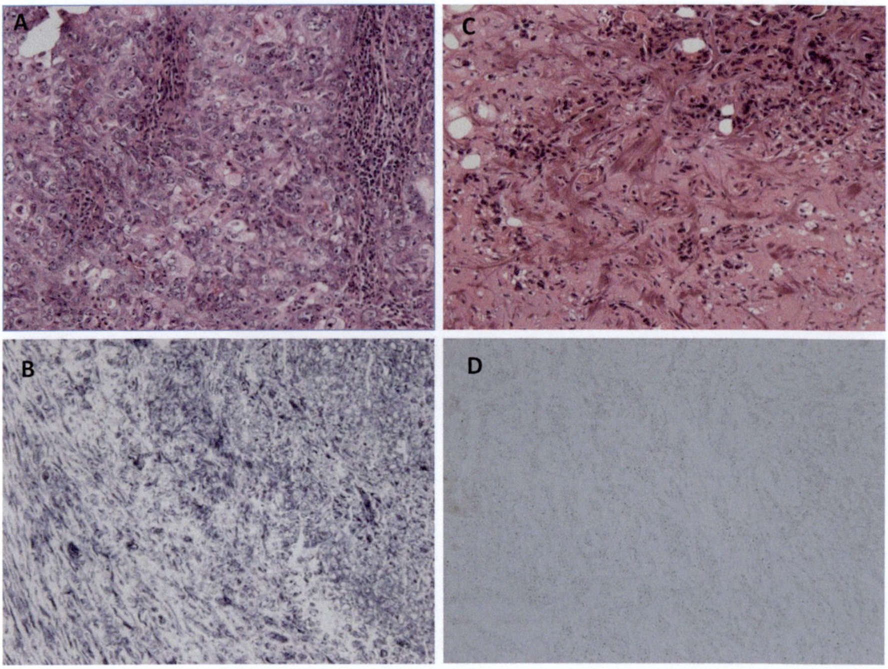

Fig. 12.5 NADH viability study. (**a**) H&E section of non-ablated breast tumor. (**b**) NADH viability study of non-ablated breast tumor T. (**c**) H&E section of ablated breast tumor. (**d**) NADH viability study demonstrating nonviable ablated tumor (magnification 200×)

Among cases of tumor diameter less than 2 cm in pathological examination, the NADH viability staining was available for 22 patients, and in 20 (90.9 %), there were no evidence of viable malignant cells. The two viable cases were due to insufficient ablation; the reason of one case was defective device, and another case was that impedance was too high for tumor to be ablated completely.

In H&E examination, all tumors diagnosed as non-viability with NADH staining were confirmed changes with some characteristics, i.e., amorphism in interstitial cells, linear form, rarefaction and inspissation in nucleus of epithelial cell, and so on.

Among most of cases diagnosed viable malignant cell with NADH staining, each tumor diameter was nearly 3 cm. Only one case had incomplete ablation of the index tumor, as a result of the tumor being eccentric within the RFA zone.

In total, on H&E and/or NADH staining, 17 patients (34 %) in 50 RFA cases had some viable invasive or in situ disease seen in surgical excision specimen.

Table 12.3 shows treatment result is depending on the pathological tumor size including both invasive and intraductal lesions measured in surgical excision specimen. In 28 cases of tumor diameter equal or less than 2 cm in pathological examination, 25 cases (89 %) were confirmed complete ablation. In 22 cases of tumor diameter more than 2 cm, only 8 cases (36 %) were confirmed complete

Table 12.2 Pathological findings of 49 patients

	Number of patients
Tumor type	
Invasive ductal	43 (86 %)
Invasive lobular	1 (2 %)
Mucinous	2 (4 %)
Medullary	2 (4 %)
DCIS	2 (4 %)
Tumor grade	
1	24 (48 %)
2	15 (30 %)
3	11 (22 %)
Pathological nodal status	
Negative	41 (82 %)
Positive	9 (18 %)
Pathologic tumor size (cm)	
Median	1.7
Range	0.1~8
Extended intraductal component (EIC)	
Present	15 (30 %)
Absent	35 (70 %)
Pathologic response to RFA	
Longest diameter of ablation zone (cm)	
Median	3.0
Range	0~6.6
Shortest diameter of ablation zone (cm)	
Median	2.0
Range	0~5.5
Incomplete tumor ablation	17 (34 %)
Residual INV	8 (16 %)
Residual DCIS	9 (18 %)

RFA radio frequency ablation

Table 12.3 Correlation between pathological tumor size and tumor ablation

Pathological tumor size (cm)[a]	No. of pts.	Complete tumor ablation (%)	Incomplete tumor ablation (%)
≦2 cm	28	25 (89 %)	3 (11 %)
>2 cm	22	8 (36 %)	14 (64 %)

[a]Size of invasive and DCIS

ablation. And Table 12.4 indicates treatment result is also depending on the existence of extended intraductal component (EIC) of the tumor in surgical excision specimen. In 35 cases of tumor without EIC in pathological examination, 31 cases (89 %) were confirmed complete ablation. In 15 cases of tumor with EIC, only 2 cases (13 %) were confirmed complete ablation.

Table 12.4 Correlation between existence of EIC and tumor ablation

	No. of pts.	Complete tumor ablation (%)	Incomplete tumor ablation (%)
EIC present	15	2 (13 %)	13 (87 %)
EIC absent	35	31 (89 %)	4 (11 %)

EIC extended intraductal component

As these results, pre-RFA MRI detection with ultrasonography should be examined to detect the EIC of the tumor, and appropriate cases for RFA must be focused.

12.3 Discussion

Radiofrequency ablation (RFA) is mainly used in clinical practice to treat unresectable hepatic tumors, and, so far, experience with breast carcinomas is limited [7–19].

RFA causes local tumor cell destruction by thermal coagulation and protein denaturation [5, 9, 20]. The higher the target temperature, the less exposure time is needed for cellular destruction [21, 22]. Cell death approximately occurs above 45–50 °C. The target temperature mostly used at the tip of the prongs 95 °C and was maintained around 15 min [23]. It is conceivable this setting could result in melting the fatty tissue, with bad cosmetic results. However, the lesions might be destroyed equally well with a lower target temperature and shorter ablation time [12].

Clearly, more research on the radiofrequency dose and effect is necessary to optimize RFA in breast carcinomas.

The shape, size, and design of the RF electrode determine the shape of the ablation zone and, in the end, the success of the procedure. Because the size of thermal lesion is limited using a single-needle electrode, multiarray electrode has been developed that can produce thermal lesion of 3–5 cm in diameter.

In our trials, the area of ablation zone with a 2-cm active tip of electrode was following: mean diameter of major axis was 3.0 cm (range 0–6.6 cm) and one of minor axis was 2.0 cm (range 0–5.5 cm).

Some study reported that the distance between the tumor and the skin and the chest wall should be at least 1 cm, because of possible burn to normal tissue. Lateral compression of the breast during the entire ablation procedure or ice cooling in cases of borderline distance to the skin is also essential to prevent possible skin burns [9, 12].

Although according to 5 % glucose injection between the skin and tumor, and between the chest wall and tumor, and the skin cooled with ice in order to avoid these burns, tumor diameter less than 1 cm could be performed with RFA.

The difficulty in assessing the margin of the ablated lesions is a limitation in all percutaneous ablation techniques. To minimize the risk of local recurrence and to make sure the whole tumor and safe margin is ablated, the lesions need to be excised with a rim of at least 1 cm.

After excision, tumor viability is tested by NADH-diaphorase. Almost every study immediately excised the ablated lesion [7, 8, 12, 13]. Burak et al. and Hayashi et al. had an interval of 1–3 weeks before excising the ablated zone [9, 11]. It was hypothesized that due to the effect of local vessel thrombosis and necrosis of surrounding tissue, the ablated zone expands in the period of time and provides a more accurate excision. In the end, the two trials did not have higher percentages of complete tumor ablation compared to the other studies, concluding that an interval time between ablation and excising the tumor might not be necessary [9, 11].

In cases of tumor diameter less than 2 cm, the NADH viability staining was available for 22 patients, and in 20 (90.9 %), there were no evidence of viable malignant cells. The other two viable cases were due to insufficient ablation; the reason of one case was defective device, and another case was that impedance was too high for tumor to be ablated completely. The breast cancer tissue is usually composed of tumor, normal tissue, fat, vessel, and so on and heterogeneous. The fat tissue is one of the highest electrical resistance. And high resistance means less effect from electrical power such as radiofrequency. So, we suspect that the component in our cases with high impedance against RFA might be fatty.

Up until now, only one pilot study has been performed that tested RFA in three elderly patients with breast cancer without excision of the ablated zone [24]. All three patients completed the treatment without complications, and after 18 months of follow-up, no recurrence occurred. In the future, if RFA is to be used as a replacement for surgery, CNB might also be an option to confirm successful ablation. Fornage et al. suggested that multiple core-needle biopsies through and periphery of the ablated lesion should be obtained 3–4 weeks after the RFA procedure.

Indication for RFA can be early breast cancer (T≦2 cm). In 28 cases of tumor diameter equal or less than 2 cm, 25 cases (89 %) were confirmed complete ablation (Table 12.3). In 35 cases of tumor without EIC in pathological examination, 31 cases (89 %) were confirmed complete ablation. In 15 cases of tumor with EIC, only 2 cases (13 %) were confirmed complete ablation. According to MRI detection, tumor diameter and the EIC could be evaluated more accurately. Appropriate cases for RFA should be selected deliberately after enough diagnosis with ultrasound and MRI detection on diameter, type, EIC, multiple lesions, and so on.

The optimal conditions for RFA collates result with the following conditions: (1) tumor diameter less than 2 cm diagnosed with ultrasound and (2) less than 2 cm except for multiple lesions and extended intraductal spread lesion more than 2 cm diagnosed with MRI detection.

Also, in two cases, tumor body couldn't be ablated sufficiently. Effects of RFA depend on tissue resistivity, so fatty tissue and tumor components can affect these effects. Components of breast carcinoma are different in each patient, and further studies are needed. And in cases of that, initial resistance is too high and roll-off occurs immediately as our study showed, and target temperature can't be reached, procedures should be changed from RFA to lumpectomy for patients' safety, and the reasons of these incidents need to be examined with resected samples.

In Japan, radiofrequency ablation is a popular treatment method in liver cancer.

Half of liver cancer patients is treated by radiofrequency ablation. This system is familiar to many physicians even in local hospitals and clinics.

Although the cryo-ablation and the HIFU haven't been approved by the Japanese government, only radiofrequency ablation has been approved and has the possibility to be admitted as option for local treatment.

RFA seems to be a promising new tool for minimally invasive procedure of small breast carcinoma. However, follow-up data regarding local effects on the surrounding breast tissue or recurrence rates are hardly available. Further research will be necessary to establish the optimal technique and to demonstrate the long-term oncologic and cosmetic effects of radiofrequency ablation.

Acknowledgment of Research Support of this Study These studies were supported in part by a Grant for Project Promoting Clinical Trials for Developing of New Drugs and Medical Devices from the Japan Agency for Medical Research and Development (AMED).

References

1. Fisher B, Remand C, Poisson R, et al. Eight year results of a randomized clinical trail comparing total mastectomy and lumpectomy with or without radiation in treatment of breast cancer. N Engl J Med. 1989;320:822–8.
2. Veronessi U, Salvatori B, Luini A, et al. Conserving treatment of early breast cancer: long term results of 1232 cases treated with quadrantectomy, axillary dissection and radiotherapy. Ann Surg. 1990;211:250–9.
3. Olsen O, Gotzche PC. Cochrane review on screening for breast cancer with mammography. Lancet. 2001;358:1340–2.
4. Vreling C, Collette L, Fourquet A, et al. The influence of patient tumor and treatment factors on the cosmetic results after breast-conserving therapy in the EORTC7 'boost vs. no boost' trial. EORTC Radiotherapy and Breast Cancer Cooperative Groups. Radiother Oncol. 2000;55:219–32.
5. Singletary SE. Minimally invasive techniques in breast cancer treatment. Semin Surg Oncol. 2001;20:246–50.
6. Cady B, Stone MD, Schuler JG, et al. The new era in breast cancer. Invasion, size, and nodal involvement dramatically decreasing as a mammographic screening. Arch Surg. 1996;131:301–8.
7. Jeffrey SS, Birdwell RL, Ikeda DM. Radiofrequency ablation of breast cancer: first report of an emerging technology. Arch Surg. 1999;134:1064–8.
8. Izzo F, Thomas R, Delrio P. Radiofrequency ablation in patients with primary breast carcinoma: a pilot study in 26 patients. Cancer. 2001;92:2036–44.
9. Burak WE, Agnese DM, Pozoski SP. Radiofrequency ablation of invasive breast carcinoma followed by delayed surgical excision. Cancer. 2003;98:1369–76.
10. Singletary SE. Feasibility of radiofrequency ablation for primary breast cancer. Breast Cancer. 2003;10:4–9.
11. Hayashi AH, Silver SF, van der Westhuizen NG. Treatment of invasive breast carcinoma with ultrasound-guided radiofrequency ablation. Am J Surg. 2003;185:429–35.
12. Fornage BD, Sneige N, Ross MI. Small (< or = 2-cm) breast cancer treated with ultrasound-guided radiofrequency ablation. Am J Surg. 2004;231:215–24.
13. Noguchi M, Earashi M, Fujii H. Radiofrequency ablation of small breast cancer followed by surgical resection. J Surg Oncol. 2006;93:120–8.

14. Khatri VP, McGahan JP, Ramsamooj R, Griffey S, Brook J, Cronan M, et al. A phase II trial of image-guided radiofrequency ablation of small invasive breast carcinoma: use of saline-cooled tip electrode. Ann Surg Oncol. 2007;14:1644–52.
15. Medina-Franco H, Soto-Germes S, Ulloa-Gomez JL, Romero-Trejo C, Uribe N, Ramirez-Alvarado CA, et al. Radiofrequency ablation of invasive breast carcinoma: phase II trial. Ann Surg Oncol. 2008;15:1689–95.
16. Imoto S, Wada N, Sakemura N, Hasebe T, Murata Y. Feasibility study on radiofrequency ablation followed by partial mastectomy for stage I breast cancer patients. Breast. 2009;18:130–4.
17. Wiksell H, Lofgren L, Schassburger KU, Grundstorm H, Janicijevic M, Largerestedt U, et al. Feasibility study on treatment of small breast carcinoma using percutaneous US-guided preferential radiofrequency ablation (PRFA). The Breast. 2010;19:216–25.
18. Kinoshita T, Iwamoto E, Tsuda H, Seki K. Radiofrequency ablation as local therapy for early breast carcinomas. Breast Cancer. 2011;18:10–7.
19. Ohtani S, Kochi M, Ito M, Higaki K, Takada S, et al. Radiofrequency ablation of early breast cancer followed by delayed surgical resection- a promising alternative to breast-conserving surgery. The Breast. 2011;20:431–6.
20. Van den Bosch MAAJ, Daniel BL. MR-guided interventions of the breast. Magn Reson Imaging Clin N Am. 2005;13:505–17.
21. Curley SA. Radiofrequency ablation of malignant liver tumors. Oncologist. 2001;6:14–23.
22. Dickson JA, Calderwood SK. Temperature range and selective sensitivity of tumors to hyperthermia: a critical review. Ann Ny Acad Sci. 1980;335:180–205.
23. Dickson JA, Calderwood SK. Thermosensitivity of neoplastic tissues in vivo. In: Storm F, editor. Hyperthermia in cancer therapy. Boston: GK Hall Medical; 1983. p. 63–140.
24. Susini T, Nori J, Olivieri S. Radiofrequency ablation for minimally invasive treatment of breast carcinoma. A pilot study in elderly inoperable patients. Genecol Oncol. 2006;26:304–10.

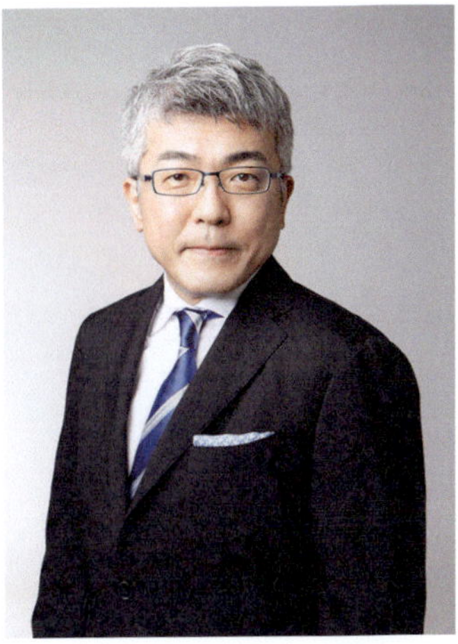

Takayuki Kinoshita

Chapter 13
RFA with a LeVeen Needle Electrode in Early Breast Cancer

Shigeru Imoto

13.1 Current Status of RFA in the Era of Breast-Conserving Treatment of Breast Cancer

Since breast cancer arises from terminal duct lobular units, it often shows extensive intraductal components (EIC). EIC is defined as intraductal carcinoma that is present prominently in invasive carcinoma or clearly extends from the tumor margin [1]. Holland et al. examined the relationship between EIC and intraductal carcinoma at 1 cm intervals from the tumor margin in 217 cases of breast cancer treated with total mastectomy. Among them, 151 cases had EIC-positive tumor and 66 were EIC-negative. About one-third of the EIC-positive tumors had intraductal carcinoma 2 cm from the tumor margin, which was a much higher percentage than that in EIC-negative tumors (2 %). To make the surgical margin negative in EIC-positive tumor, breast tissues have to be adequately resected.

Modern breast-conserving treatment consists of breast-conserving surgery (BCS), breast irradiation, and adjuvant therapy based on the intrinsic subtype of breast cancer. In a meta-analysis by the Early Breast Cancer Trialists' Collaborative Group, breast irradiation reduced isolated local recurrence and breast-specific mortality in node-negative breast cancer as well as node-positive breast cancer [2]. Absolute risk reductions due to BCS followed by breast irradiation compared with BCS alone were 19 % and 3 % in 10 years in 6097 node-negative cases and 33 % and 9 % in 1024 node-positive cases, respectively. Breast irradiation is effective for locoregional management after BCS.

To determine the prognostic impact of ipsilateral breast tumor recurrence (IBTR) after BCS, Japanese investigators retrospectively analyzed 1901 cases with tumors

S. Imoto (✉)
Department of Breast Surgery, School of Medicine Kyorin University, 6-20-2 Shinkawa, Mitaka, Tokyo 181-8611, Japan
e-mail: imoto@ks.kyorin-u.ac.jp

T. Kinoshita (ed.), *Non-surgical Ablation Therapy for Early-stage Breast Cancer*,
DOI 10.1007/978-4-431-54463-0_13

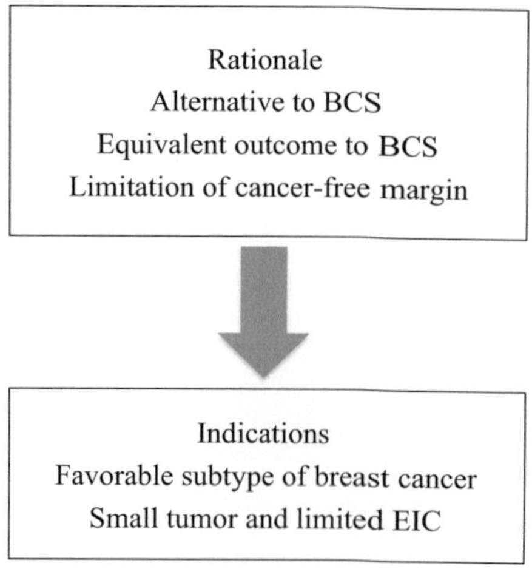

Fig. 13.1 Background of RFA in breast cancer (*BCS* breast-conserving surgery, *EIC* extensive intraductal components)

3 cm or less in diameter [3]. At a median follow-up of 107 months, the 10-year disease-free survival, overall survival, and IBTR were estimated to be 84 %, 78 %, and 8.5 %, respectively. IBTR was significantly associated with younger age, positive surgical margin, and no breast irradiation. IBTR was an independent prognostic factor of distant metastasis. Appropriate surgical resection is essential for reducing IBTR after BCS. In addition, breast irradiation and adjuvant therapy based on the intrinsic subtype are also necessary for controlling locoregional and distant recurrence after BCS.

RFA is a standard treatment for liver cancer in Japan and Western countries. Hepatitis B or C viral infection can lead to the development of multiple cancer lesions in the liver. More than half of the cases show recurrence even with adequate primary therapy of liver cancer. Since liver surgery tends to be invasive, RFA is an appropriate therapy in liver cancer to minimize surgical stress. On the other hand, RFA has a completely different background in breast cancer (Fig. 13.1). First, RFA should be preferable to BCS. Second, RFA should control IBTR as well as BCS. Third, ablated lesions are limited in the breast, since breast cancer often has some degree of EIC. Extensive ablation may burn the skin or pectoral muscle. Fourth, primary chemotherapy is recommended for early breast cancer with an aggressive phenotype. Overall, RFA is a promising alternative to BCS in favorable breast cancer. Its feasibility and curative potential in breast cancer should be confirmed as a possible breast-conserving treatment.

13.2 RFA with a LeVeen Needle Electrode in Early Breast Cancer

With regard to RFA in breast cancer, Jeffrey et al. first reported the feasibility of RFA in five cases with a LeVeen needle electrode (Boston Scientific Corporation, USA) in 1999 [4]. Izzo et al. demonstrated RFA in 26 cases with the same device in

2001 [5]. In this report, all patients with invasive breast carcinoma underwent RFA followed by immediate resection. Tumor viability was examined by hematoxylin and eosin (HE) and nicotinamide adenine dinucleotide (NADH) diaphorase staining. There were 20 cases with T1 tumor and 6 with T2 tumor, which ranged in size from 0.7 to 3.0 cm. The mean treatment time with RFA was about 15 min. Coagulation necrosis was found in 25 of the 26 cases (96 %). The skin of one patient (4 %) was burned due to RFA. This pilot study was sufficiently promising to support a trial of RFA alone in breast cancer.

13.3 Feasibility Study on RFA Followed by BCS at the NCCHE

To develop an RFA technique and to examine cell viability in ablated tissues, a feasibility study was conducted at the National Cancer Hospital East (NCCHE), where the author had worked previously [6]. This study was approved by the ethics committee at the NCCHE. The eligibility criteria were as follows: tumor of 2 cm or less in diameter measured by caliper, clinically negative axillary lymph nodes, no diffuse calcification according to mammography, and no evidence of EIC on magnetic resonance (MR) mammography.

Our procedure for RFA was based on Izzo's protocol (Fig. 13.2). Briefly, under general anesthesia, a LeVeen needle electrode or a co-access-type sheath was inserted under ultrasound guidance. A needle electrode of this type has a 10-tine multiple array. An array diameter of 2 cm or 3 cm is suitable for RFA in breast cancer. The tip of the needle electrode must be located in the center of the tumor, and the array is deployed. To avoid burning the skin or pectoral muscle, 5 % glucose was injected into the subdermal tissues and retromammary space. RFA was performed using an RF-2000 generator (Boston Scientific Corporation, USA). At the first ablation, the initial electrical power was 10 W (Fig. 13.3). After 2 min, the power was increased in steps of 5 W each minute until roll-off, which was defined as the maximum impedance of tissue coagulation. When roll-off was not observed

Fig. 13.2 RFA procedure with a LeVeen needle electrode

T1N0 BC without EIC
Under general anesthesia
Sentinel node biopsy (± axillary lymph node dissection)
Insertion of LeVeen™ electrode (Array diameter 2cm or 3cm)
Injection of 5%-gulcose into the subdermal and retromammary tissues
RFA using Generator RF2000
1st RFA: 10 W for 2 minutes, increased in step of 5 W/minute until roll-off
(80 W was maintained until roll-off)
2nd RFA: 10 W for 1 minute and in the same manner
Cooling of ablated breast during and after RFA for 6 hours

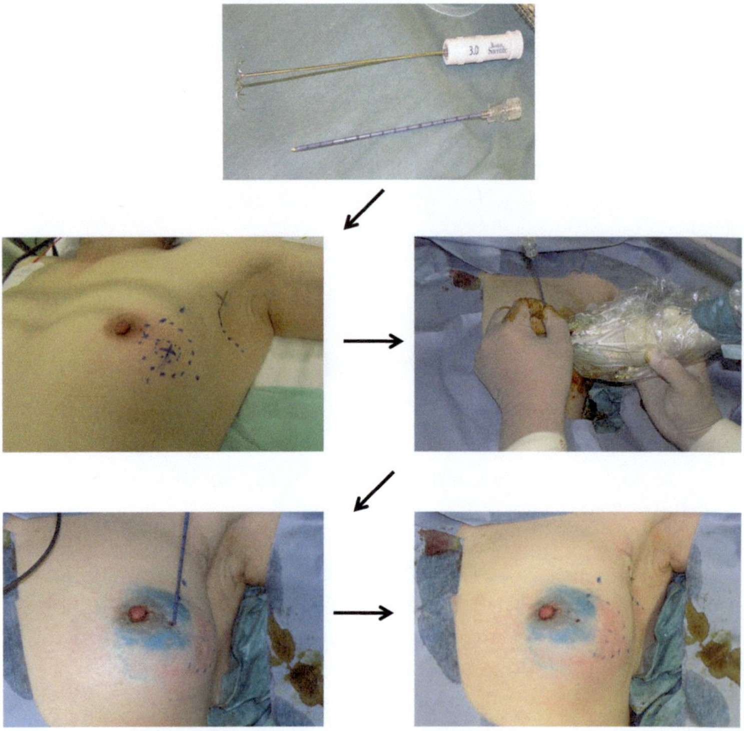

Fig. 13.3 Initial experience of RFA with a LeVeen needle electrode

even at 80 W, the same electric power was applied until roll-off. Ablated breast was cooled with an ice pack during RFA.

The primary endpoint was adverse events due to the RFA procedure. Table 13.1 shows the main results of our initial experience. Ultimately, 30 patients were enrolled. The ablation time ranged from 8 to 41 min. The initial impedance at the first ablation ranged from 85 to 237 Ω. The highest impedance was recorded in a case of RFA failure, since the tip of the needle electrode was located outside of the objective tumor. RFA-related adverse events were observed in nine cases: two skin burn and seven muscle burn. Twenty-six cases (87 %) had pathological degenerative changes in tumor specimens by HE staining. Two of the remaining four cases had unexpected EIC beyond the ablated breast tissues. The other two cases had viable cancer tissues: in one case the needle electrode was not inserted appropriately, as mentioned above, and in the other the increase in electrical power was modified. In 24 of the 26 cases (92 %) examined by NADH diaphorase staining, cancer tissues were completely ablated. Our experience demonstrated that RFA was reliable and feasible in clinical stage I breast cancer with no EIC.

Table 13.1 Initial experience with a LeVeen needle electrode system

No. of cases	30
Tumor size (cm)	0.9–2.4
Ablation time (minutes)	8–41
Initial impedance (Ω) (range, median)	
First ablation	85–237, 136
Second ablation	83–220, 114
Maximum electric power (W) (range, median)	
First ablation	15–89, 45
Second ablation	7–50, 20
Adverse events	
Skin burn	2
Pectoral muscle burn	7
Degenerative changes with HE staining	28
No ductal components beyond ablated breast tissues	26
Ductal components beyond ablated breast tissues	2
Viable tumor cells with HE staining	2
Tumor cell viability with NADH diaphorase staining	
Negative (not viable)	24
Positive (viable)	2
Not examined	4

Table 13.2 shows the results of RFA followed by breast surgery reported previously [4–15]. In all cases, the sample size was quite small and complete ablation rates ranged between 60 % and 100 %. Burn was a common adverse event (4 %). Two hundred thirty-four of the 282 cases examined (83 %) had complete ablation. If we only consider cases with T1BC, the complete ablation rate is 86 % (152/177). When RFA followed by breast irradiation and adjuvant therapy is considered, nonsurgical treatment may be a promising strategy for breast cancer.

13.4 Phase II Study on RFA Alone at Kyorin University Hospital

A phase II study on RFA alone in T1N0BC was started in 2009. The eligibility criteria were similar to those in the above feasibility study. Figure 13.4 shows the scheme of this study. The primary endpoint was breast deformity after RFA, and the secondary endpoints were IBTR and quality of life. This study was planned to register 30 cases over 3 years. Unfortunately, only 20 cases were registered because of the strict eligibility criteria, and enrollment was closed in March 2013. In all

Table 13.2 RFA followed by breast surgery

Author (year)	No.	T	Electrode	Ablation rate	Complications (No.)
Jeffrey (1999) [4]	5	T2-3	LeVeen	80 %	None
Izzo (2001) [5]	26	T1-2	LeVeen	96 %	Skin burn (1)
Burak (2003) [7]	10	T1	LeVeen	90 %	None
Singletary (2003) [8]	29	T1-2	RITA	86 %	Skin burn (1)
Hayashi (2003) [9]	22	T1	RITA	64 %	Skin burn (1)
Noguchi (2006) [10]	10	T1	RITA	100 %	None
Khatri (2007) [11]	15	T1	Cool-tip	93 %	Skin puckering (2) Wound infection (1)
Medina-Franco (2008) [12]	25	T1-2	Elektrotom	76 %	Skin burn (3) Wound infection (1)
Imoto (2009) [6]	30	T1	LeVeen	87 %	Skin burn (2) Muscle burn (7)
Hung (2011) [13]	20	T1	LeVeen or Cool-tip	90 %	None
Kinoshita (2011) [14]	49	T1-2	Cool-tip	61 %	Skin burn (2) Muscle burn (3)
Ohtani (2011) [15]	41	T1	Cool-tip	88 %	Skin burn (1)
Total	282	T1-3	Various	83 %	Skin burn (11) Miscellaneous (18)

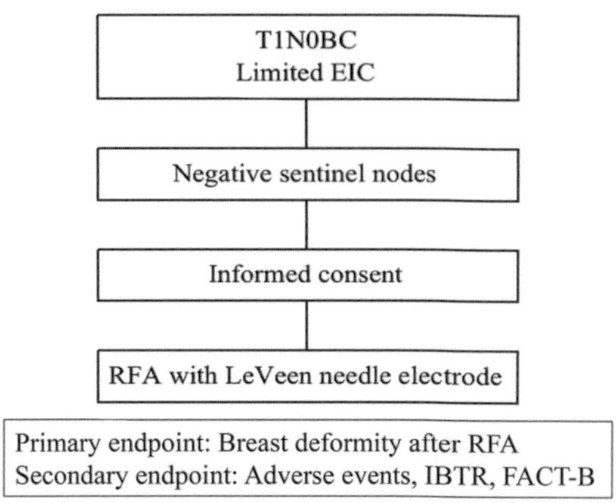

Fig. 13.4 Phase II study at Kyorin University Hospital (2009–2013)

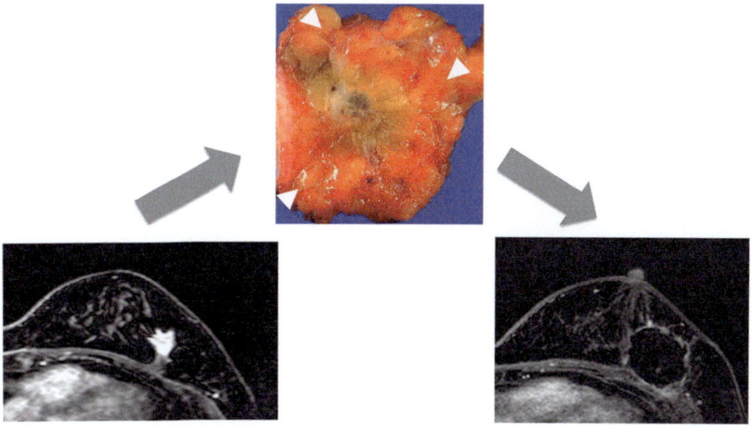

Fig. 13.5 Correlation between red ring formation and MR mammogram in ablated breast tissues. A congestive margin (*arrowhead*) was seen in ablated specimens. An enhanced primary tumor on MR mammogram changed to no enhancement after RFA

cases, the ablated lesions were followed-up periodically by mammography, breast ultrasound, and MI mammography. As a preliminary result, all of these cases were disease-free at a median follow-up of 35 months.

MI mammography has been reported to be useful after RFA in breast cancer [16]. We found that completely ablated tissues had no enhanced lesions by MR mammography. Interestingly, the margin of the ablated lesions in the previous feasibility study suggested congestive breast tissues in resected specimens, which were referred to as "a red ring formation" (Fig. 13.5).

13.5 Future Prospects

RFA with a LeVeen needle electrode is feasible and reliable for the ablation of early breast cancer without EIC. Ideally, a randomized phase III trial will be needed to compare RFA with BCS in patients with breast cancer. However, a phase III study is very unlikely. First, eligible cases are very limited in early breast cancer. Second, the sample size would have to be very large because the rate of IBTR is very low. From our initial experience at the NCCHE, eligible cases were estimated to comprise only 4–5 % of patients with operable breast cancer. Nevertheless, this method may be useful for patients with EIC-negative breast cancer. We are currently conducting a multicenter phase II study on RFA with a Cool-tip electrode in early breast cancer. Recently, ACOSOG performed a multicenter phase II study on cryoablation followed by delayed surgical resection in breast cancer (ACOSOG Z1072). The complete cryoablation rate in this study will be reported elsewhere. In conclusion, thermal ablation therapy is a promising strategy in early breast cancer. In addition to further trials, programs to teach the skills required for RFA in breast cancer are needed to help spread this technique worldwide.

Acknowledgments The author thanks Dr. Noriaki Wada and Dr. Takahiro Hasebe, with whom he collaborated at the NCCHE, and Dr. Hirotsugu Isaka, Dr. Hiroki Ito, Dr. Kentaro Imi, and Dr. Kaisuke Miyamoto of Kyorin University Hospital for performing our studies.

These studies were supported in part by a Grant for Project Promoting Clinical Trials for Developing of New Drugs and Medical Devices from the Japan Agency for Medical Research and Development (AMED).

References

1. Holland R, Connolly JL, Gelman R, et al. The presence of an extensive intraductal component following a limited excision correlates with prominent residual disease in the remainder of the breast. J Clin Oncol. 1990;8:113–8.
2. Early Breast Cancer Trialists' Collaborative Group. Effects of radiotherapy and of differences in the extent of surgery for early breast cancer on local recurrence and 15-year survival: an overview of the randomised trials. Lancet. 2005;366:2087–106.
3. Komoike Y, Akiyama F, Iino Y, et al. Ipsilateral breast tumor recurrence (IBTR) after breast-conserving treatment for early breast cancer. Cancer. 2006;106:35–41.
4. Jeffrey SS, Birdwell RL, Ikeda DM, et al. Radiofrequency ablation of breast cancer. Arch Surg. 1999;134:1064–8.
5. Izzo F, Thomas R, Delrio P, et al. Radiofrequency ablation in patients with primary breast carcinoma. Cancer. 2001;92:2036–44.
6. Imoto S, Wada N, Sakemura N, et al. Feasibility study on radiofrequency ablation followed by partial mastectomy for stage I breast cancer patients. Breast. 2009;18:130–4.
7. Burak WE, Angese DM, Povoslo SP, et al. Radiofrequency ablation of invasive breast carcinoma followed by delayed surgical excision. Cancer. 2003;98:1369–76.
8. Singletary SE. Feasibility of radiofrequency ablation for primary breast cancer. Breast Cancer. 2003;10:4–9.
9. Hayashi AH, Silver SF, van der Westhuizen NG, et al. Treatment of invasive breast carcinoma with ultrasound-guided radiofrequency ablation. Am J Surg. 2003;185:429–35.
10. Noguchi M, Earashi M, Fujii H, et al. Radiofrequency ablation of small breast cancer followed by surgical resection. J Surg Oncol. 2006;93:120–8.
11. Khatri VP, McGahan JP, Ramsamooj R, et al. A phase II trial of image-guided radiofrequency ablation of small invasive breast carcinoma: use of saline-cooled tip electrode. Ann Surg Oncol. 2007;14:1644–52.
12. Medina-Franco H, Soto-Germes S, Ulloa-Gomez JL, et al. Radiofrequency ablation of invasive breast carcinoma: a phase II trial. Ann Surg Oncol. 2008;15:1689–95.
13. Hung WK, Mak KL, Ying M, et al. Radiofrequency ablation of breast cancer: a comparative study of two needle designs. Breast Cancer. 2011;18:124–8.
14. Kinoshita T, Iwamoto E, Tsuda H, et al. Radiofrequency ablation as local therapy for early breast carcinomas. Breast Cancer. 2011;18:10–7.

15. Ohtani S, Kochi M, Ito M, et al. Radiofrequency ablation of early breast cancer followed by delayed surgical resection – a promising alternative to breast-conserving surgery. Breast. 2011;20:431–6.
16. Nagashima T, Sakakibara M, Sangai T, et al. Surrounding rim formation and reduction in size after radiofrequency ablation for primary breast cancer. Jpn J Radiol. 2009;27:197–204.

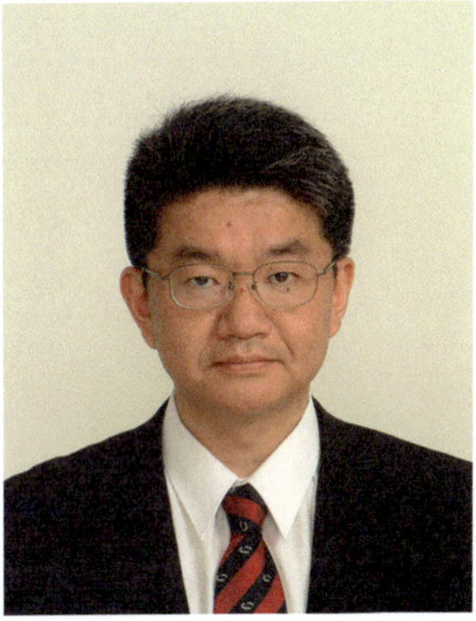

Shigeru Imoto

Chapter 14
RFA of Early Breast Cancer Followed by Delayed Surgical Resection

Shoichiro Ohtani

14.1 Why Did We Perform RFA Followed by Delayed Surgical Resection?

This study [1] investigated delayed surgical resection performed 1–2 months after RFA to better assess tumour cell death over the entire ablated area; most RFA feasibility studies have investigated resection performed immediately after RFA, although one study reported on delayed surgical resection undertaken 1–3 weeks after RFA [2]. At the beginning of our study, we also performed immediate resection after RFA; however, pathological HE evaluation failed to demonstrate tumour cell death within the ablated zone. A delay in resection facilitates more physiological assessment. Therefore, we decided to excise the ablated area 1–-2 months after RFA. To our best knowledge, no report has estimated tumour cell death in specimens resected 1–2 months after RFA. In specimens examined 1–-2 months after RFA, complete tumour cell death could not be demonstrated by HE staining alone, whereas this was demonstrated by NADH staining in the same specimens. NADH staining is easy and reliable in this study field. Interestingly, the cell nuclei disappearance was observed both from the centre and the ablated zone periphery by HE staining, and a cell death area was clearly demarcated from the surrounding viable tissue by a band of foam cells, which we termed the protein degenerative ring. Following resection of the ablated area 6 months after RFA, all cell nuclei in that area will disappear; complete tumour cell death may be demonstrated by HE staining alone if resection is performed over 6 months after RFA.

S. Ohtani (✉)
Department of Breast Surgery, Hiroshima City Hiroshima Citizens Hospital, 7-33, Motomachi, Naka-ku, Hiroshima 730-8518, Japan
e-mail: sho_ohtani@hotmail.com

T. Kinoshita (ed.), *Non-surgical Ablation Therapy for Early-stage Breast Cancer*,
DOI 10.1007/978-4-431-54463-0_14

14.2 Materials and Method

14.2.1 Enrollment

Forty-one patients, with pathologically proven invasive or non-invasive breast carcinoma less than 2 cm and clinically lymph node negative, were enrolled in this pilot study, conducted between March 2007 and February 2009. Core needle biopsy or vacuum-assisted biopsy was performed to determine tumour grade, lymphovascular invasion, hormone receptor status and HER2/neu status. The other inclusion criteria were as follows: tumour easily imaged by ultrasound and lumpectomy planed as the initial treatment. Exclusion criteria included more than one tumour in the same breast and the presence of extensive suspicious microcalcifications surrounding the tumour mass. Patients with pacemakers, sensitivity to lidocaine or coagulopathy, or who were pregnant or lactating were also excluded. Pretreatment evaluation consisted of a complete history and physical examination, pathological review of the carcinoma and laboratory evaluation including a complete blood count and coagulation profile. Furthermore, bilateral mammography, enhanced breast MRI and positron emission tomography-CT were performed within 2 months of RFA. This study was approved by the institutional review board at Hiroshima City Hospital. All enrolled patients were informed about this study and signed a written consent for participation.

14.2.2 Breast MRI Scans

Breast MRI scans were performed before ablation and within 48 h before surgical resection. The 3-T system (Signa; G.E. Medical Systems, Japan) was utilized. Patients were imaged in the prone position with a dedicated double breast coil. Axial and sagittal T1- and T2-weighted images were obtained by the following protocol: (1) axial, T1-weighted spin-echo (500–700/16–17 [repetition time in milliseconds/echo time in milliseconds]) sequence with a 32–36 cm field of view, 3 mm section, 1 mm gap and 512×256 matrix for both breasts; (2) axial, T2-weighted fast spin-echo with fat saturation sequence of the affected breast, 12–18 cm field of view, 3 mm section, 1 mm gap and 128 or 192 matrix; and (3) sagittal T1-weighted spin-echo with fat saturation sequence after the intravenous gadodiamide administration (0.5 M, Omniscan; Nycomed, Japan). A 20 ml gadodiamide bolus was administered, regardless of body weight, followed by a 20 ml physiological saline bolus. Imaging was initiated during saline injection.

14.2.3 Radiofrequency Ablation

RFA was performed under either general anaesthesia or local anaesthesia and sedation. In the local anaesthesia group, intravenous sedation with midazolam-titrated doses was administered in preparation for RFA. Under local anaesthesia and sedation, sentinel lymph node biopsy was first performed, and then, under ultrasound guidance, 0.5 % lidocaine was injected around the tumour. For analgesia, a sufficient volume of lidocaine injected over the pectoralis major is important. A small skin incision was made with a number 11 surgical blade. A 3 cm Cool-tip RF needle electrode (Valleylab, Boulder, CO, USA) was inserted at the centre of the tumour under ultrasound guidance. For prevention of skin burn, 5 % glucose liquid with a higher electrical resistance than saline was injected between the skin and tumour to increase the space between. The needle electrode was attached to a 500 kHz monopolar RF generator capable of producing 200 W. Grounding was achieved by attaching two grounding pads to the patient's thighs before the procedure. Tissue impedance was monitored continuously using circuitry incorporated in the generator. Radiofrequency energy was applied only once not exceeding 15 min. Power was set at 5 W and increased by 10 W intervals every 1 min until a rapid increase in impedance occurred (so-called roll-off). For prevention from skin burn, a sterile ice bag was placed on the skin over the ablated area. The core temperature of the ablated area was measured immediately after roll-off. Under general anaesthesia, the abovementioned procedure was performed but without using lidocaine and midazolam.

14.2.4 Surgery

Breast-conserving surgery (Bp 1.5 cm) was performed immediately after RFA (immediate surgical resection) under general anaesthesia or 1–2 months after RFA (delayed surgical resection) under local anaesthesia.

14.2.5 Pathological Evaluation

After the specimen removal, pathological evaluation with hematoxylin-eosin (HE) staining was performed to evaluate the therapeutic effect according to the response criteria of the Japanese Breast Cancer Society [3] and to estimate the tumour size and marginal status. Moreover, to accurately evaluate tumour cell death, histochemical analysis of tumour viability with nicotinamide adenine dinucleotide diaphorase (NADH) staining was performed [7].

14.2.6 Follow-Up

Decisions regarding adjuvant chemotherapy or hormonal therapy were made based on the pretreatment tumour size measured by breast MRI. Axillary lymph node metastasis was determined by sentinel lymph node biopsy results. Furthermore, prognostic indications such as estrogen receptor status, progesterone receptor status, HER2/neu status, lymphovascular invasion and grade were determined by pretreatment core biopsy. According to each patient's risk category, adjuvant therapy was administered in all patients. Whole breast irradiation was also performed in every case.

14.3 Results

14.3.1 Patient Characteristics

Of the 41 patients in this pilot study, nine initially underwent breast-conserving surgery immediately after RFA under general anaesthesia (immediate surgical resection). RFA was subsequently performed under local anaesthesia and sedation in the remaining 32, following which breast-conserving surgery was performed under local anaesthesia 1–2 months after RFA (delayed surgical resection). All but one patient completed one RFA session. Patient characteristics are summarized in Table 14.1 (median tumour size as assessed by enhanced MRI scan, 13 mm [range, 5–18 mm]; median volume of 0.5 % lidocaine administered, 42 ml [range, 32–55 ml]; median RFA application time, 9 min [range, 6–15 min]; median tumour core temperature immediately after RFA, 85 °C [range, 64–100 °C]). There were no treatment-related complications other than that of a superficial burn in one case right above the ablated area.

14.3.2 Breast MRI Imaging

On post-RFA MRI scans, 29/30 studies (96 %) in which the patient had pre-RFA enhancement displayed no residual enhancement of the breast lesion. In one case (4.1 %), in which intolerable pain prevented completion of one RFA session, post-MRI scans demonstrated residual enhancement consistent with residual invasive and intraductal tumour, which was confirmed histologically. Therefore, a post-ablation MRI scan appears to predict therapeutic effect by RFA for breast cancer. An ablation zone, characterized by altered signal intensity and architectural distortion, with a minor degree of peripheral enhancement was easily visible in all cases.

Table 14.1 Characteristic of patients and primary tumour characteristics ($n = 41$)

		No. of cases
Age (years)		
Range		38–92
Median		59
Tumour size on MRI		
Median (mm)		13
<10 mm		6
10 mm >=		35
Histology		
IDC		36
DCIS		5
Tumour grade	1	26
	2	3
	3	2
ER	+	38
	–	3
PgR	+	35
	–	6
HER2	+	1
	–	40
Anaesthesia		
General		9
Local		32
Ablation time (minutes)		
Range		6–15
Median		9
Core temperature (°C)		
Range		65–100
Median		85
Complication		
Superficial skin burn		1
None		40

IDC invasive ductal carcinoma, *DCIS* non-invasive ductal carcinoma

This ablation zone measured 3.0–6.1 cm at its greater diameter (median, 3.7 cm) and 1.8–5.5 cm at its lesser diameter (median, 2.5 cm). We termed this peripheral enhancement the protein degenerative ring, within which NADH staining demonstrated complete cell death. Representative pre- and post-RFA MRI scans demonstrating successful ablation and the protein degenerative ring are shown in Fig. 14.1. Residual cancer, which was suspected on MRI in one case, was confirmed pathologically (Fig. 14.2).

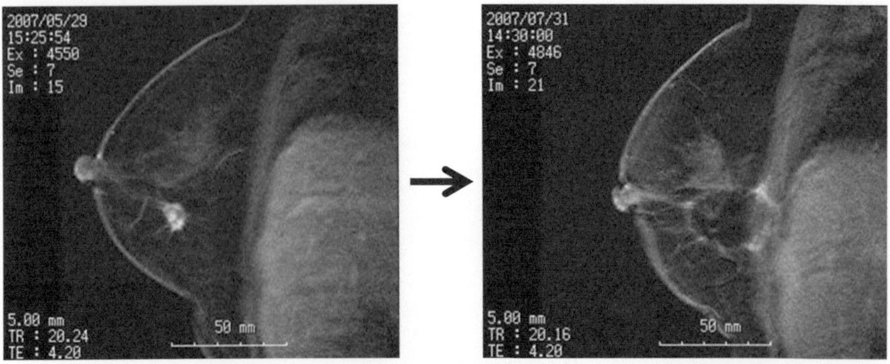

Fig. 14.1 Enhanced MRI scans demonstrate successful RFA ablation. (**a**) An irregular, enhancing lesion is observed in the pre-RFA image. (**b**) After RFA, the tumour is no longer enhanced. A zone of ablation within the protein degenerative ring is demonstrated

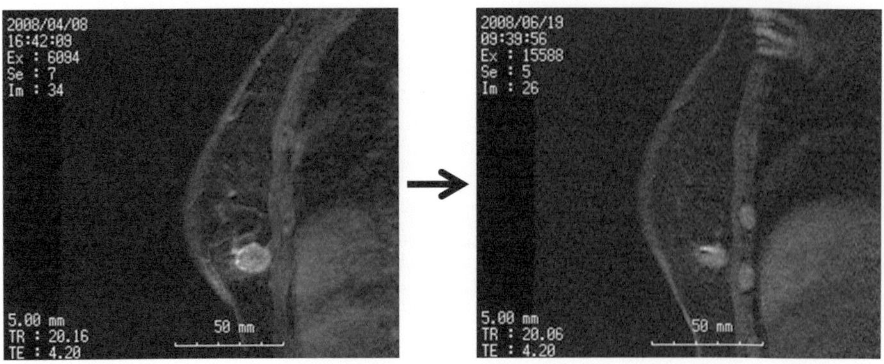

Fig. 14.2 The post-RFA MRI demonstrates residual enhancement consistent with a residual invasive and intraductal tumour, which was confirmed histologically. (**a**) Before RFA, (**b**) 1.5 months after RFA

14.3.3 Pathological Evaluation

HE staining of the ablated lesion removed immediately after RFA could not demonstrate complete tumour cell death, because cancer cell was diagnosed as viable cell only by HE staining. According to the response criteria of the Japanese Breast Cancer Society [3], no pathological complete response (Grade 3) was observed in specimens removed immediately after RFA; however, it was observed in 4 (12.5 %) specimens removed by delayed surgical resection. As times elapse after ablation, tumour cell death in a tissue sample by delayed surgical resection could be more easily diagnosed than in resection immediately after RFA. However, even in delayed surgical resection specimens, HE staining alone could not reveal all pathological complete cell death (Table 14.2). Therefore, to evaluate more accurate tumour cell death, NADH staining was performed in specimens from 12 patients, in

Table 14.2 Histological analysis of ablated area by RFA

Resection immediately after RFA (9 cases)	Delayed surgical resection (32 cases)
Grade 1a: 4 cases (44.4 %)	Grade 1a: 1 case (3.3 %)
Grade 1b: 1 case (11.1 %)	Grade 1b: 6 cases (18.7 %)
Grade 2: 2 cases (22.2 %)	Grade 2: 22 cases (68.7 %)
Grade 3: 0 case (0 %)	Grade 3: 4 cases (12.5 %)
Evaluation by response criteria of Japanese Breast Cancer Society	

Response criteria of Japanese Breast Cancer Society	
Grade 0	No response
	Almost no change in cancer cells after treatment
Grade 1	Slight response
Grade 1a	Mild response
	Mild change in cancer cell regardless of the area or marked changes in cancer call seen in less than one third of cancer cells
Grade 1b	Moderate response
	Marked changes in one third or more but less two thirds of tumour cells
Grade 2	Marked response
	Marked changes in two thirds or more of tumour cells
Grade 3	Complete response
	Necrosis or disappearance of all tumour cells. Replacement of all cancer cells by granuloma-like and/or fibrous tissue. In the case of complete disappearance of cancer cells, pretreatment pathological evidence of the presence of cancer is necessary

Table 14.3 Comparison of pathological evaluation by NADH and HE staining

NADH staining	HE staining
No viable cell: 12 cases (100 %)	Grade 1a: 0 case (0 %)
Viable cell: 0 case (0 %)	Grade 1b: 1 case (8.3 %)
	Grade 2: 9 cases (75 %)
	Grade 3: 2 cases (16.6 %)

all (100 %) of whom no viable cancer cells (i.e., complete cell death) within the whole ablated area and surgical margins were demonstrated. Of these 12 cases, only two showed complete pathological response by HE staining (Table 14.3). Therefore, NADH staining is indispensable for evaluating tumour cell death, even in delayed surgical resection specimens. The macroscopic and histological findings are shown in Fig. 14.3. In five cases, complete histological ablation could not be achieved, with only non-invasive components remaining in four cases. Complete ablation was indicated on imaging examination in these four cases, yet pathological evaluation revealed residual non-invasive ductal cancer outside the degenerative protein ring. This may indicate the limitations of imaging-based diagnosis (in particular with regard to the extent of ductal spread, accurate diagnosis of which is not easy). Invasive and non-invasive components were found in one case (Fig. 14.2), where uncontrolled pain resulted in treatment failure. Adequate analgesia is also essential for successful ablation. Overall, a complete ablation rate of 87.8 % (36/41) was observed, based on the findings of HE and NADH staining.

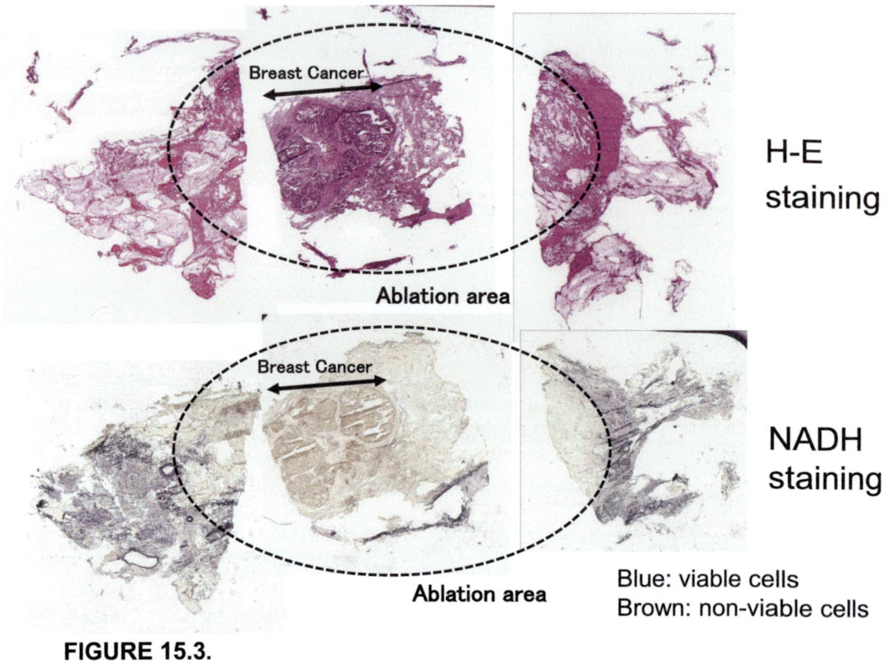

Fig. 14.3 NADH staining showed pathological complete cell death in a whole ablated area including surgical margin. HE staining of ablated lesion removed immediately after RFA could not demonstrate complete cancer cell death

14.4 Discussion

Many investigators have attempted feasibility studies on RFA followed by resection, as shown on Table 14.4, whose results support the use of RFA in the treatment of localized breast cancer [1, 2, 5–14]. The experience of RFA of early breast cancer followed by delayed surgical resection is much more limited. In these studies, only two studies including our study [1] and Burak's study [2] have performed delayed surgical resection and have evaluated the complete tumour cell death after RFA. Burak's delayed surgical resection was undertaken 1–3 weeks after RFA. We excised the ablated area 1–2 months after RFA. A longer waiting period after ablation could provide important information regarding the true ablated zone. A delay in resection facilitates more physiological assessment. Therefore, a delay in the assessment of the ablated zone might allow the zone to expand, due to the effects of local vessel thrombosis and subsequent necrosis of the surrounding tissue. This clearly could not be assessed on an evaluation immediately after completing ablation. To our best knowledge, no report has estimated tumour cell death in specimens resected 1–2 months after RFA. Complete tumour cell death could not be shown only by HE staining. On the other hand, NADH staining

Table 14.4 Feasibility studies on radiofrequency ablation followed by surgical resection

First author (year) Ref.	No. of cases	T	Electrode	Application time	Power (W)	Time (min)	Complete ablation	Complications
Jeffrey (1999) [5]	5	T2–T3	LeVeen	2 times	20–60	12–28	80 %	None
Izzo (2001) [6]	26	T1–T2	LeVeen	2 times	25–80	7–25	96 %	Skin burn (1 case)
Burak (2003) [2]	10	T1	LeVeen	Over 2 times	–	7–21	90 %	None
Singletary (2003) [7]	29	T1–T2	RITA	1 time	–	30–45	86 %	skin burn (1 case), wound infection (4 cases)
Hayashi (2003) [8]	22	T1	RITA	1 time	–	–	64 %	Skin burn (1 case)
Noguchi (2006) [9]	10	T1	RITA	Over 2 times	–	–	100 %	None
Khatri (2007) [10]	15	T1	Cool-tip	Over 2 times	14–53	7–36	93 %	Skin puckering (2 cases), wound infection (1 case)
Medina-Franco (2008) [11]	25	T1–T2	Elektrotom	1 time	30–55	–	76 %	Skin burn (3 cases), wound infection (1 case)
Imoto (2009) [12]	30	T1	LeVeen	2 times	7–89	5–42	87 %	Skin burn (2 cases), muscle burn (7 cases)
Wiksell (2010) [13]	31	T1	NeoDynamics AB	1 time	–	6.5–11	84 %	Skin burn (1 case), muscle burn (1 case), pneumothorax (1 case)
Kinoshita (2011) [14]	49	T1–T2	Cool-tip	2 time	5–118	–	85 %	Skin burn (2 cases), muscle burn (3 cases)
Present study [1]	41	T1	Cool-tip	1 time	50–110	6–15	88 %	Skin burn (1 case)
Total	293	T1–T3	Various	1-over 2 times	–	–	84 %	Skin burn (12 cases), muscle burn (11 cases)
								Pneumothorax (1 case), miscellaneous (8 cases)

demonstrated complete cancer cell death in same specimens. NADH staining is easy and reliable to estimate cancer cell death. NADH staining is indispensable for estimating breast cancer cell death in even specimens that was resected 1–2 months after RFA.

Our findings demonstrated that a single RFA session can eradicate breast cancer less than 1.5 cm by greater diameter with no extra-intraductal component (EIC); two or more sessions may be effective in tumours over 1.5 cm. Paradoxically, patient selection remains a very important factor in determining the suitability of RFA for breast cancer. NADH staining demonstrated complete cell death within the ablated area (the degenerative protein ring) by MRI scanning. Thus, when performing RFA without resection, if the tumour is located within this area, core needle biopsy is unnecessary to confirm cell viability. A post-ablation MRI scan can predict the therapeutic effect by RFA for breast cancer.

RFA represents a minimally invasive treatment option for the local therapy of early breast cancer instead of breast-conserving surgery. Despite the use of various RFA procedures, the overall total ablation rate in the literature is 84 % (Table 14.4) [1, 2, 5–14]. RFA followed by whole breast irradiation may be a promising protocol for the local control of breast cancer. To confirm that RFA is an alternative to breast-conserving surgery, a randomized control clinical trial is indispensable for comparing the two treatments.

14.5 Conclusion

We found that RFA for breast cancer could be safely applied in an outpatient setting with good patient tolerance and that only one RFA session could achieve total tumour cell death within the whole ablated area. RFA is a promising, minimally invasive alternative to breast-conserving surgery for local treatment in women with small ($\leq$1.5 cm) breast cancer.

References

1. Ohtani S, Kochi M, Ito M, et al. Radiofrequency ablation of early breast cancer followed by delayed surgical resection – a promising alternative to breast-conserving surgery. Breast. 2011;20:431–6.
2. Burak WE, Angese DM, Povoslo SP, et al. Radiofrequency ablation of invasive breast carcinoma followed by delayed surgical excision. Cancer. 2003;98:1369–76.
3. Kurosumi M, Akashi-Tanaka S, Akiyama F, et al. Histopathological criteria for assessment of therapeutic response in breast cancer (2007 version). Breast Cancer. 2008;15:5–7.
4. Neumann RA, Knobler RM, Pieczkowski F, Gebhart W. Enzyme histochemical analysis of cell viability after argon laser-induced coagulation necrosis of the skin. J Am Acad Dermatol. 1991;25:991–8.
5. Jeffrey SS, Birdwell RL, Ikeda DM, et al. Radiofrequency ablation of breast cancer. Arch Surg. 1999;134:1064–8.

6. Izzo F, Thomas R, Delrio P, et al. Radiofrequency ablation in patients with primary breast carcinoma. Cancer. 2001;92:2036–44.
7. Singletary SE. Feasibility of radiofrequency ablation for primary breast cancer. Breast Cancer. 2003;10:4–9.
8. Hayashi AH, Silver SF, van der Westhuizen NG, et al. Treatment of invasive breast carcinoma with ultrasound-guided radiofrequency ablation. Am J Surg. 2003;185:429–35.
9. Noguchi M, Earashi M, Fujii H, et al. Radiofrequency ablation of small breast cancer followed by surgical resection. J Surg Oncol. 2006;93:120–8.
10. Khatri VP, McGahan JP, Ramsamooj R, et al. A phase II trial of image-guided radiofrequency ablation of small invasive breast carcinoma: use of saline-cooled tip electrode. Ann Surg Oncol. 2007;14:1644–52.
11. Medina Franco H, Soto Germes S, Ulloa Gomez JL, et al. Radiofrequency ablation of invasive breast carcinoma: phase II trial. Ann Surg Oncol. 2008;15:1689–95.
12. Imoto S, Wada N, Sakemura N, et al. Feasibility study on radiofrequency ablation followed by partial mastectomy for stage I breast cancer patients. Breast. 2009;18:130–4.
13. Wiksell H, Lofgren L, Schassburger K, et al. Feasibility study on the treatment of small breast carcinoma using percutaneous US-guided preferential radiofrequency ablation (PRFA). Breast. 2010;19:219–25.
14. Kinoshita T, Iwamoto E, Tsuda H, et al. Radiofrequency ablation as local therapy for early breast carcinomas. Breast Cancer. 2011;18:10–7.

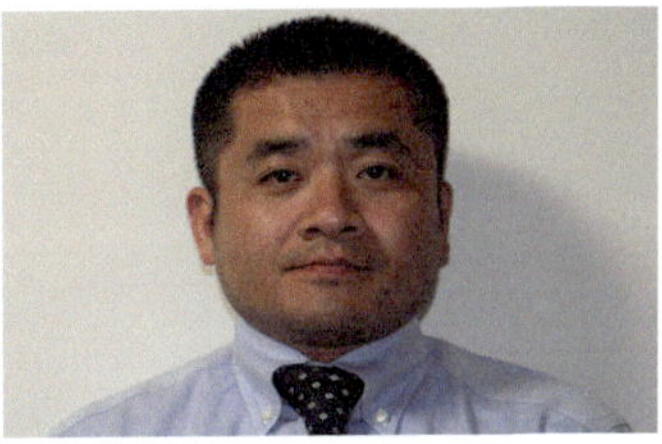

Shoichiro Ohtani

Chapter 15
RFA of Early Breast Cancer Without Resection

Masato Takahashi

15.1 Background

Breast-conserving surgery for small breast cancer has been accepted as one of the standard treatments. A major goal of breast-conserving surgery is to acquire both perfect local control and perfect preservation of a cosmetic acceptance [1]. However, there are some patients who are not satisfied with the cosmesis. Several investigators are studying minimally invasive techniques such as cryosurgery, laser ablation, high-intensity-focused ultrasound, and radiofrequency ablation (RFA) [2, 3].

RFA is a high-frequent current produced by frictional heating electrode tips placed in the lesion that flows into the surrounding tissue initiating ionic agitation, producing heat, and causing cell destruction. The radiofrequency probe is typically placed under ultrasound guidance. RFA has been demonstrated to be effective in the treatment of unresectable hepatic tumors [4].

Recently, minimally invasive surgery such as RFA is a novel application for small breast cancer and expected to bring an excellent cosmetic effect. So far, published data on RFA in breast cancer are limited.

15.2 Objective

The aim of this study is to verify the clinical safety and usefulness of the radiofrequency ablation (RFA) for small breast cancer without resection.

M. Takahashi (✉)
NHO Hokkaido Cancer Center, 2-3-54 Kikusui 4 Jo, Shiroishi-ku, Sapporo, Hokkaido 003-0804, Japan
e-mail: masatotk@sap-cc.go.jp

T. Kinoshita (ed.), *Non-surgical Ablation Therapy for Early-stage Breast Cancer*,
DOI 10.1007/978-4-431-54463-0_15

- To confirm the pathologic efficacy of RFA for small size (<1.5 cm) breast cancer
- To investigate the safety of RFA technique and the influence of patients' QOL
- To analyze factors which influenced the size of necrosis

15.3 Materials and Methods

Between January 2006 and October 2007, 20 breast cancer patients were performed RFA with cool-tip RF system after sentinel LN biopsy under general anesthesia. No tumor resection after RFA treatment was performed. All patients have consented as a clinical research, beforehand.

15.4 Eligibility Criteria

- Age between 20 and 80 years
- Tumor size less than or equal to 1.5 cm in diameter
- Histologically proven invasive ductal carcinoma or DCIS by mammotome biopsy
- Excluded if there was evidence of multifocal lesions or diffuse calcification by MMG or MRI
- Informed consent

RF generator is capable of producing 200 W power. These are two grounding pads. Tissue impedance was monitored continuously. A pump was used to infuse 0 °C normal saline solution into the lumen of the electrodes and maintain a tip temperature of 15–25 °C. We started RFA at 5 W and raised the output to 10 W 1 min later, until the generator stopped delivering radiofrequency energy by auto-stop mechanism.

At first, mammography, ultrasonography, and physical examination are performed. If the tumor is diagnosed as breast cancer, it is necessary to perform ultrasonographic-guided vacuum-assisted breast biopsy (VAB). The histopathological diagnosis of ductal carcinoma must be established in a tumor specimen obtained by VAB. Informed consent is absolutely needed because it is still an experimental procedure and not a standard treatment. MRI is very important to determine the precise size of the tumor. If the tumor size including ductal involvement is over 1.5 cm diameter, the case is excluded. Sentinel lymph node biopsy was performed before the RF ablation procedure. We perform MRI 3 and 6 months after RFA. We perform VAB to confirm complete necrosis 6 months after RFA.

Tumor viability after RFA was assessed by hematoxylin-eosin and ssDNA staining. QOL after RFA was assessed both subjectively (QOL-ACD score) and objectively (JBCS cosmesis criterion) (Fig. 15.1).

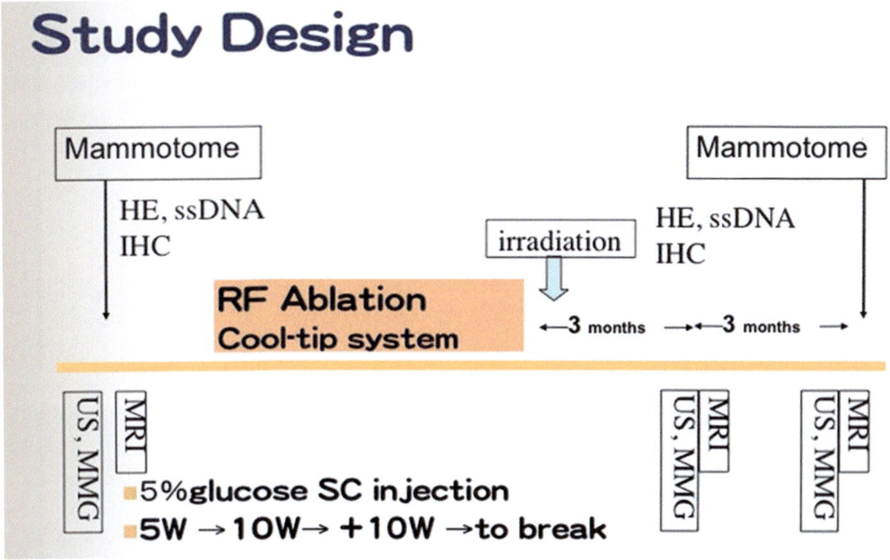

Fig. 15.1 Study design

15.5 Results

Preoperative mammotome revealed 4 patients had DCIS and 16 patients had IDC. The patient median age was 53 years old. The mean greatest dimension of tumors was 1.0 cm (range, 0.5–1.5 cm) (Fig. 15.2).

MRI showed the dimension of coagulation necrotic area by RFA treatment was 3.5 cm (range, 2.5–5.4 cm), suggesting that at least 10 mm margin was achieved around the 1.5 cm-sized primary tumor. Post-ablation MR imaging demonstrates well-defined zones of ablation and correlates well with pathological findings (Figs. 15.3 and 15.4).

Histological examination with H&E staining showed various changes, from coagulation necrosis and disappearance of tumor ductal structures to cytoplasmic vacuolation and swelling of nuclei with retention of the cancer duct structure (Fig. 15.5).

The degenerative changes after RF ablation increased gradually, and it took 6 months until the disappearance of all tumor cells. No patient was troubled with skin burn. Neither local nor distant recurrence has occurred in all patients (median follow-up was 34 months).

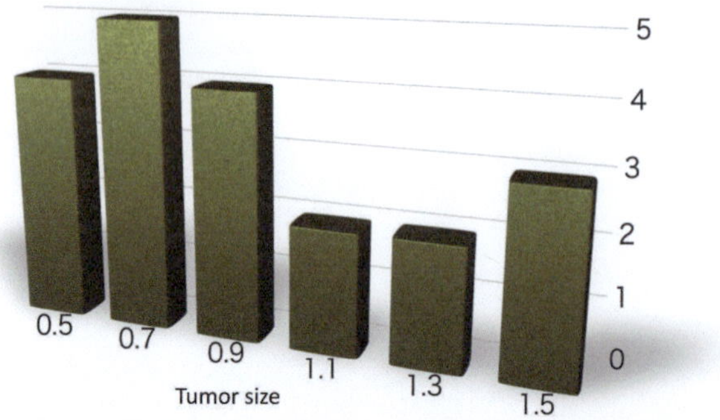

Fig. 15.2 Tumor size

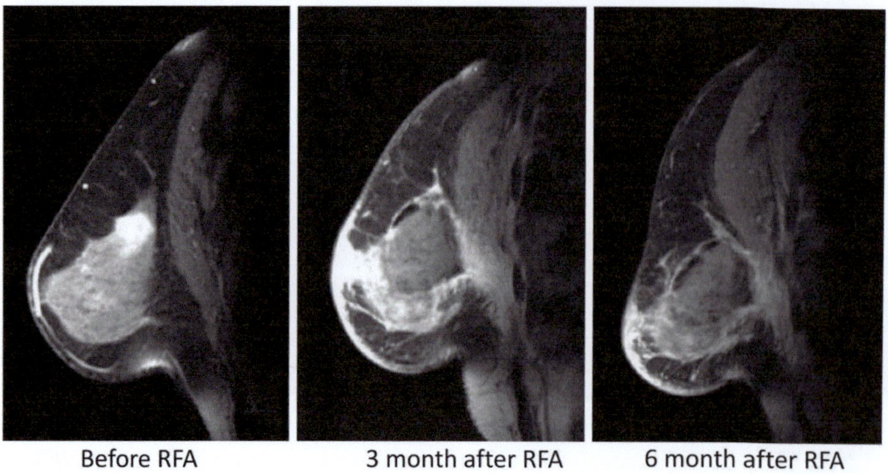

Fig. 15.3 MRI findings

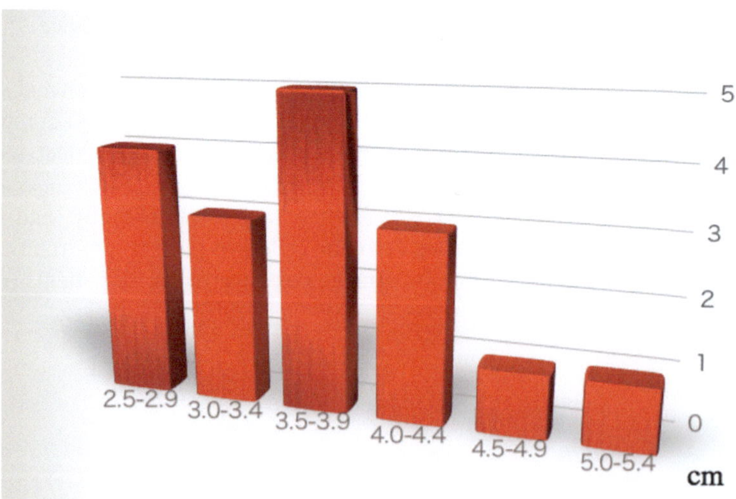

Fig. 15.4 Necrotic size measured by MRI

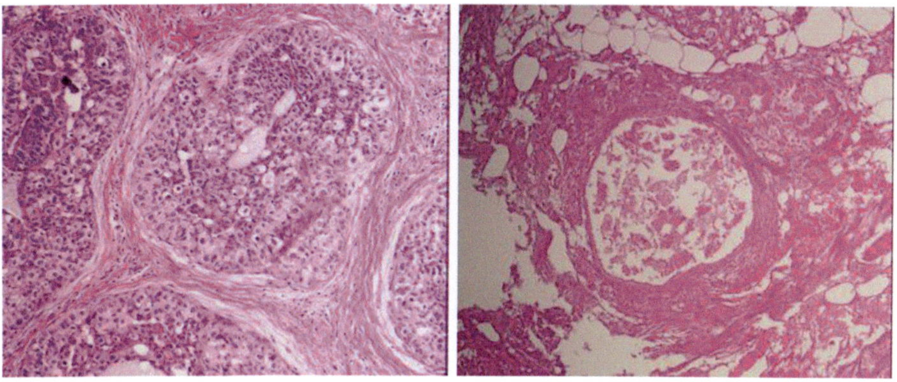

Fig. 15.5 Histological examination

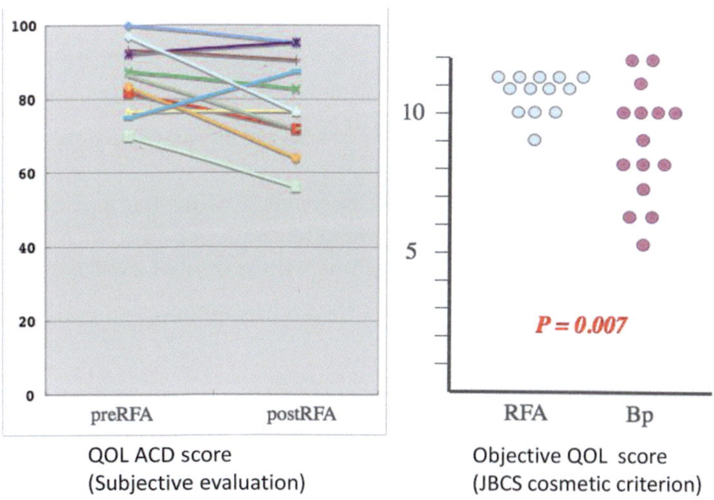

Fig. 15.6 QOL analysis

QOL after RFA was assessed both subjectively (QOL-ACD score) and objectively (JBCS cosmesis criterion). Most of patients were satisfied with the cosmesis of the RFA treated breast. Objective QOL score (JBCS cosmesis criterion) showed splendid cosmetic outcome (Fig. 15.6).

To treat RFA for breast cancer more safely, we analyzed factors which influenced the size of necrosis. Patient age, body mass index (BMI), background concentration measured by MMG, and fat involvement measured by CT did not influence the size of necrosis ($P = 0.21$, 0.17, 0.64, 0.40). The state of posterior

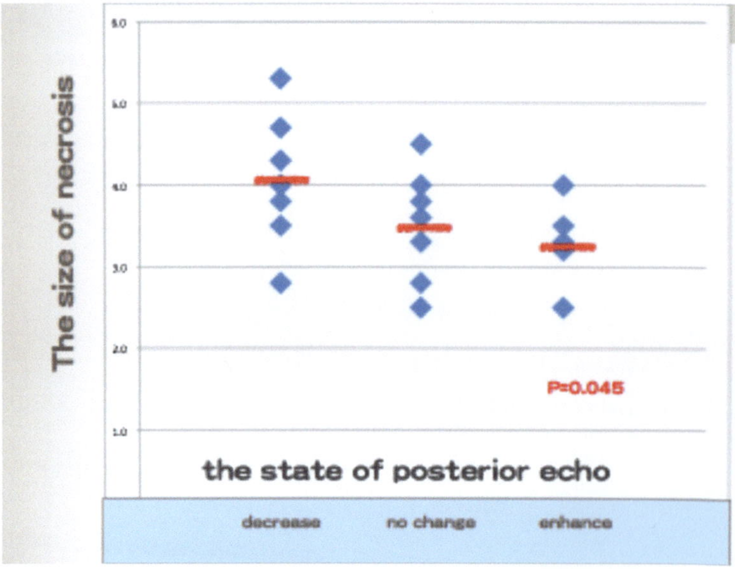

Fig. 15.7 Association between the state of posterior echo and the size of necrosis

echo detected by ultrasonography was associated with the size of necrosis ($p = 0.045$) (Fig. 15.7). Hence, RFA for the tumor with rich fiber such as scirrhous type tends to make necrosis wider than the one with poor fiber such as solid tubular type.

15.6 Conclusion

Radiofrequency ablation (RFA) is indicated only in patients with small, well-localized breast cancer. MR imaging has greater accuracy for determining the extent of disease, and post-ablation MRI demonstrates well-defined zones of ablation and correlates well with pathological findings.

Our pilot studies are encouraging with regard to cosmesis and local control. However, further studies are needed to determine whether the use of RF ablation for small breast cancer can provide local control and survival rates equivalent to those of conventional breast-conserving surgery.

References

1. Haloua MH, Krekel NM, Winters HA, et al. A systematic review of oncoplastic breast-conserving surgery: current weaknesses and future prospects. Ann Surg. 2013;257:609–20.
2. Singletary SE. Minimally invasive techniques in breast cancer treatment. Semin Surg Oncol. 2001;20:246–50.

3. Zhao Z, Wu F. Minimally-invasive thermal ablation of early-stage breast cancer: a systemic review. Eur J Surg Oncol. 2010;36:1149–55.
4. Sutherland LM, Williams JA, Padbury RT, et al. Radiofrequency ablation of liver tumors: a systematic review. Arch Surg. 2006;141:181–90.

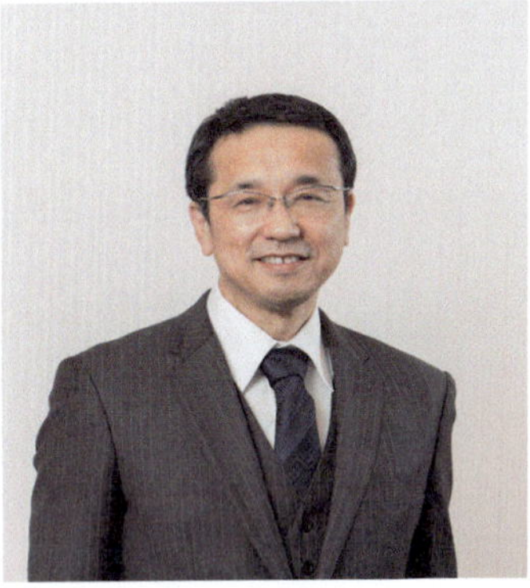

Masato Takahashi

Chapter 16
Prospective Study of RFA of Early Breast Cancer Without Resection

Sota Asaga and Takayuki Kinoshita

16.1 Introduction

Detection of early-stage breast cancer has recently increased by the wide spread of screening mammography, and the demand of minimally invasive breast surgery is also elevated. The current mainstream of breast surgery is modified radical mastectomy (Auchincloss) or partial mastectomy (breast-conserving surgery), which has changed from radical mastectomy. The alteration of surgical treatment was based on several large-scale, randomized clinical trials [1–4]. Radiofrequency ablation (RFA) is one of minimally invasive breast surgery which was recently launched. Several feasibility studies [5–10] demonstrated that complete coagulation and necrosis by RFA were observed in most patients of small breast tumors. These studies have a small number of patients and tumor resection was done immediately or 1 month after RFA to validate the tumor necrosis by thermocoagulation.

There are only two reports about RFA without tumor resection for early-stage breast cancer [11, 12]. One of these demonstrates that RFA can be a substitute for breast-conserving surgery in elderly patients with a single breast mass of less than 3 cm in diameter [11]. The study has 21 candidates, and the treatment efficacy is evaluated 1 year after RFA. However, as locoregional recurrence within 1 year after breast-conserving surgery is rare [3, 4], it is necessary to observe for the long term to conclude that RFA is effective as standard surgery. Although the other one was observed for a long time, as mean follow-up of 60 months, and reported favorable prognosis, the study protocol was including mandatory vacuum-assisted biopsy resection, and there was no description about the volume of excised specimen by

S. Asaga (✉) • T. Kinoshita
Breast Surgery Division, National Cancer Center Hospital, 5-1-1 Tsukiji, Chuo-ku, Tokyo 104-0045, Japan
e-mail: soasaga@ncc.go.jp

T. Kinoshita (ed.), *Non-surgical Ablation Therapy for Early-stage Breast Cancer*,
DOI 10.1007/978-4-431-54463-0_16

delayed vacuum-assisted biopsy [12]. In addition, both studies had small number of participants, and these studies are determined as phase I study. Therefore, novel large-scale multicenter prospective phase II study needs to be launched to demonstrate the effectiveness of RFA for early-stage breast cancer. We introduce the details of the study protocol.

16.2 Aim of Prospective Study

The aim of prospective study is to demonstrate that RFA can be an alternative treatment strategy for early-stage breast cancer to partial mastectomy. In order to show that the effectiveness and safety are equivalent between RFA and partial mastectomy, end points of prospective study should be disease-free survival in ipsilateral breast and adverse events.

We introduce our prospective trial of RFA without tumor resection as a substitute for breast-conserving surgery in patients with a small single breast mass.

16.3 Study Design

16.3.1 Study Overview

The study flow is described in Fig. 16.1. This prospective phase II study is planned as a single-arm study to compare with the results of previous randomized control study of lumpectomy or partial mastectomy. Informed written consent was obtained from each participant who is appropriate in the inclusion criteria and exception to the exclusion criteria. RFA is performed with sentinel lymph node biopsy followed by whole breast irradiation. The appropriate adjuvant therapy needs to be offered for all patients every according to the guidelines. The vacuum-assisted breast biopsy is done at 3 months after whole breast irradiation. Partial mastectomy or total mastectomy is mandatory for the patients with residual tumor diagnosed the vacuum-assisted biopsy. Thereafter, the programed examinations including breast ultrasonography, mammography, and contrast breast MRI will be performed for every patient to diagnose the ipsilateral breast tumor recurrence, which is described particularly in Sect. 17.3.7.7 and Table 16.1.

16.3.2 Primary End Point

The primary end point of this study is 5-year disease-free survival in ipsilateral breast.

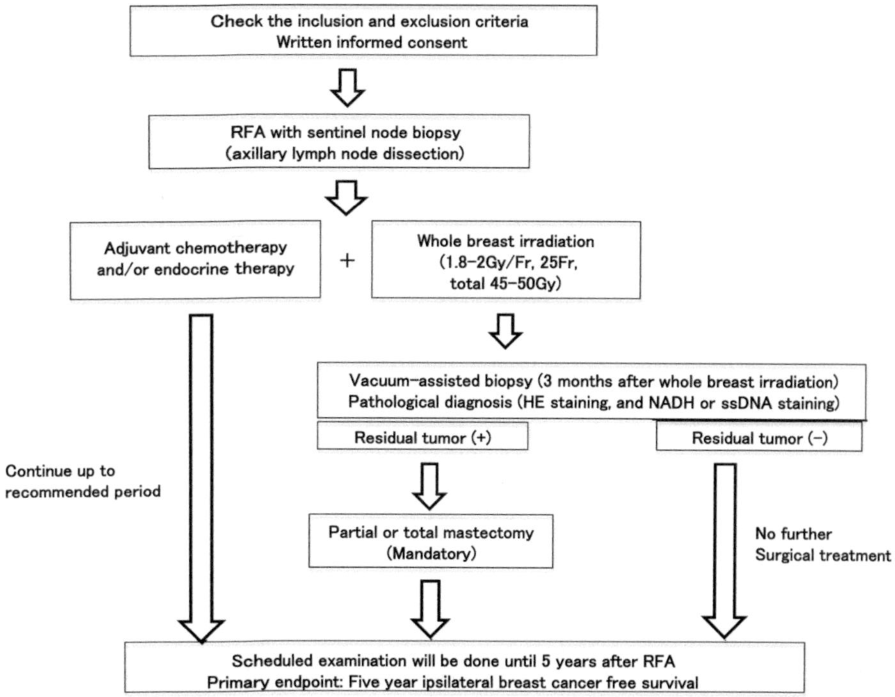

Fig. 16.1 This figure shows the flow of the study. The protocol treatment includes RFA itself as well as whole breast irradiation and vacuum-assisted biopsy at 3 months after the radiotherapy. If the residual tumor existed, the lesion must be treated by partial or total mastectomy. These is "one package" of breast RFA

16.3.3 Secondary End Point

The secondary end points of this study are overall survival, distant disease-free survival, adverse events of RFA, and tumor viability after RFA.

16.3.4 Inclusion Criteria

Small breast mass is suitable for RFA. Our data indicate that histologically complete tumor necrosis was significantly less frequent in tumors of more than 1.5 cm in diameter than those of under 1.5 cm in diameter [13]. Therefore, eligibility criteria were defined as a single breast mass of under 1.5 cm in diameter by radiological findings. In addition, the clinically node negative was also defined as eligibility criteria.

Table 16.1 The schedule of examinations before and after RFA

	Pre-RFA	Within 1 week after RFA	*	1 Y	1 Y 6 M	2 Y	2 Y 6 M	3 Y	3 Y 6 M	4 Y	4 Y 6 M	5 Y
Medical interview	○	○	○	○	○	○	○	○	○	○	○	○
Physical examination	○		○	○	○	○	○	○	○	○	○	○
Mammography	○			○		○		○		○		○
Needle biopsy (vacuum assisted)	○		○									
Breast ultrasonography	○		○	○	○	○	○	○	○	○	○	○
Contract MRI or CT	○		○	○		○		○		○		○
Chest X-ray	○			○		○		○		○		○
Blood test	○		○	○	○	○	○	○	○	○	○	○
Cosmetic evaluation	○		○	○		○		○		○		○
Questionnaire	○		○	○		○		○		○		○

Y year, *M* month, *MRI* magnetic resonance imaging, *CT* computed tomography

16.3.5 Exclusion Criteria

The patients who have contraindications of RFA should be excluded, for example, patients who have a cardiac pacemaker or implantable cardiac defibrillator. Patients who are pregnant are also excluded. Other factors which may affect end points should be excluded, for example, patients who suffer from other malignant diseases, severe cardiovascular disease, severe neural disease, or have bilateral breast cancers.

There are several types of breast carcinomas to avoid RFA. The existence of extensive intraductal component concomitant to invasive carcinoma and pure mucinous carcinoma should not be treated by RFA. In addition, ductal carcinoma in situ without mass lesion on ultrasonography, and multicentric or multifocal breast cancers should be excluded. Patients with metastatic breast cancers are also excluded. Skin burn may result in case tumors are located near the skin, but we do not consider the tumor location in the breast.

16.3.6 Informed Consent

In this study, protocol was approved by the institutional review boards of all participating institutions, and all participants provided written informed consent.

16.3.7 Treatment Procedure

16.3.7.1 Diagnosis of Breast Cancer

Diagnosis of breast cancer is done by both image diagnosis and pathology. All participants undergo bilateral breast mammography and breast ultrasonography. All patients unless they are allergic to contrast medium undergo thin-sliced chest-computed tomography or breast magnetic resonance imaging. These images are required to decide whether the lesion is suitable for RFA.

Tumor pathology is also mandatory. Tumor specimen is obtained by needle biopsy before RFA, and pathological diagnosis by hematoxylin and eosin staining and immunohistochemistry tests including estrogen receptor, progesterone receptor, HER2, and Ki67 index is performed to decide the adjuvant systemic therapy as tumor specimen cannot be obtained by RFA.

16.3.7.2 RFA

For the purpose of quality control in the multi-institutional trial, the same RFA needle, Cool-tip RF needle (COVIDIEN, Mansfield, MA, USA), is used in all institutions. RFA was performed under general anesthesia, and the ablation protocol is the same as previously described [14]. Five percent glucose solution was injected between the skin and tumor and the skin and pectoral muscle to prevent skin and muscle burn. We also cool the area just above the tumor with ice from beginning of ablation to pulling out the needle. In addition, overnight moderate cooling (be careful for frostbite) is recommended.

16.3.7.3 Sentinel Lymph Node Biopsy

Sentinel lymph node biopsy was done for all patients in this trial, unless incomplete local control may affect secondary end points. Patients with positive sentinel nodes undergo axillary lymph node dissection. Recently, the American College of Surgeons Oncology Group Z0011 trial demonstrated that among patients with limited SLN metastatic breast cancer treated with breast conservation and systemic therapy, treatment with sentinel lymph node dissection alone compared with axillary lymph node dissection did not result in inferior survival [15]. In this study, axillary lymph node dissection is mandatory for positive sentinel nodes (macrometastasis) because prediction of primary and secondary end points was based on historical control data of NSABP B-06.

16.3.7.4 Whole Breast Irradiation

In this study, whole breast irradiation is done for all patients regardless of sentinel lymph node involvement. Whole breast irradiation must start within 8 weeks after RFA (participants without adjuvant chemotherapy) or within 8 weeks after finishing adjuvant chemotherapy. The total exposure dose is 45–50 Gy, which consisted of 25 fractions of 1.8–2 Gy X-ray irradiation. The maximum 10 Gy electron beam irradiation focus to ablation site is allowed in this study. Both accelerated partial breast irradiation (APBI) and intraoperative radiotherapy (IORT) are not allowed in this study.

16.3.7.5 Adjuvant Therapy

Most patients undergo adjuvant treatment. The adjuvant chemotherapy is decided by each physician according to NCCN guideline and recommendation of St. Gallen Breast Cancer Conference. All patients who have estrogen or progesterone receptor-positive disease undergo adjuvant endocrine therapy with recommended dose and term.

16.3.7.6 Assessment of Complete Ablation and Additional Treatment

The assessment of complete ablation is performed at 3 months after finishing whole breast irradiation by ultrasonography-guided vacuum-assisted needle biopsy. The specimen obtained at least two which consisted of one from the center and one from peripheral area of the ablated lesion. Pathological diagnosis is done by both hematoxylin and eosin staining and nicotinamide adenine dinucleotide (NADH)-diaphorase staining. The conditions of NADH-diaphorase staining was the same as previously described [16]. In case tumor viability is confirmed, the participant undergo partial mastectomy as soon as possible. The rate of conversion to partial mastectomy is also recorded, and the participants who received partial mastectomy are included in the analysis of end points.

16.3.7.7 Assessment and Report of Events

After the needle biopsy performed after whole breast irradiation, the first physical and radiological examinations are performed at 1 year after RFA. The examinations contain mammography, breast ultrasonography, chest X-ray, blood test, and chest CT or breast MRI. Chest CT or breast MRI is done for all participants except contraindication of contrast medium.

After the 1-year full checkup, physical examination, breast ultrasonography, and blood test are done at every 6 months of follow-up visit, and chest or contrast breast MRI is done every 12 months until 5 years after RFA (Table 16.1). Physicians report the breast cancer-specific events or delayed adverse event related to RFA.

16.3.8 Statistical Analysis

The primary end point is ipsilateral breast tumor-free survival during 5 years from RFA, determined as proportion of participants who have any malignant disease in ipsilateral breast during the first 5 years after RFA treatment. The secondary end points are overall survival, distant disease-free survival, adverse events of RFA, and tumor viability rate after RFA. We calculated disease-free survival as the number of years from RFA until the first evidence of breast cancer relapse at any site and overall survival as the number of years from RFA to death from any cause. Tumor viability rate is defined as the proportion of incomplete ablation proved by pathological examination of both hematoxylin and eosin staining and NADH-diaphorase staining of specimen of the needle biopsy performed at 3 months after whole breast irradiation.

The target accrual of this study is 372 patients which are based on having 80 % power to detect non-inferiority of RFA with a one-sided statistical significance level of 10 % under the assumption that 5-year disease-free survival on ipsilateral breast with standard partial mastectomy was 94.3 %[17] and defining non-inferiority as a hazard ratio of less than 1.1. It is expected that lost follow-up will be 10 % of participants.

16.3.9 Assessment of Cosmetic Appearances After RFA

RFA provides excellent cosmetic appearances for patients as it is local treatment procedure for breast cancer without resection. Cosmetic appearances after RFA are evaluated as well as tumor control in this study by both questionnaires to patients and surgeon's analysis which is in comparison between treated breast and contralateral breast. The latter one consisted of eight items, which are size of breast, shape of breast, needle scar, induration of treated site, shape of nipple, color of nipple, location of nipple, and shape of inframammary fold. Patient's photograph is required to keep objectivity of the surgeon's analysis. (Of course, patient's face must be out of the photo.) Two photographs are taken from each patient: one is hands on the waist, and the other is hands on the back of the head.

The patient's questionnaire is important to justify the cosmetic evaluation. This study uses the body image scale which was previously reported [18]. Patients themselves access the exclusive website to answer the questionnaire. The schedule of taking photos to assess the cosmetic appearances and obtaining questionnaire are described in Table 16.1.

16.4 Current Status and Future

This study was done in accord with an assurance filed with and approved by the Ministry of Health, Labour and Welfare in Japan, as well as taking approval from local institutional review boards. Study has started at nine leading institutions for breast cancer in Japan. As, to date, there was no phase II prospective study to demonstrate the effectiveness of RFA for early-stage breast cancer, our multicenter phase II trial will make RFA to become alternative local treatment strategy for early-stage breast cancer as well as partial mastectomy . Our study will make new era of surgical procedure for early-stage breast cancer. After finishing our phase II study, a new phase III study to demonstrate the non-inferiority to the latest partial mastectomy needs to be started.

Acknowledgment These studies were supported in part by a Grant for Project Promoting Clinical Trials for Developing of New Drugs and Medical Devices from the Japan Agency for Medical Research and Development (AMED).

References

1. Turner L, Swindell R, Bell WG, et al. Radical versus modified radical mastectomy for breast cancer. Ann R Coll Surg Engl. 1981;63(4):239–43.
2. Maddox WA, Carpenter Jr JT, Laws HL, et al. A randomized prospective trial of radical (Halsted) mastectomy versus modified radical mastectomy in 311 breast cancer patients. Ann Surg. 1983;198(2):207–12.
3. Veronesi U, Cascinelli N, Mariani L, et al. Twenty-year follow-up of a randomized study comparing breast-conserving surgery with radical mastectomy for early breast cancer. N Engl J Med. 2002;347(16):1227–32.
4. Fisher B, Anderson S, Bryant J, et al. Twenty-year follow-up of a randomized trial comparing total mastectomy, lumpectomy, and lumpectomy plus irradiation for the treatment of invasive breast cancer. N Engl J Med. 2002;347(16):1233–41.
5. Izzo F, Thomas R, Delrio P, et al. Radiofrequency ablation in patients with primary breast carcinoma: a pilot study in 26 patients. Cancer. 2001;92(8):2036–44.
6. Jeffrey SS, Birdwell RL, Ikeda DM, et al. Radiofrequency ablation of breast cancer: first report of an emerging technology. Arch Surg. 1999;134(10):1064–8.
7. Burak Jr WE, Agnese DM, Povoski SP, et al. Radiofrequency ablation of invasive breast carcinoma followed by delayed surgical excision. Cancer. 2003;98(7):1369–76.
8. Kinoshita T, Iwamoto E, Tsuda H, et al. Radiofrequency ablation as local therapy for early breast carcinomas. Breast Cancer. 2011;18(1):10–7.
9. Hayashi AH, Silver SF, van der Westhuizen NG, et al. Treatment of invasive breast carcinoma with ultrasound-guided radiofrequency ablation. Am J Surg. 2003;185(5):429–35.
10. Fornage BD, Sneige N, Ross MI, et al. Small (< or = 2-cm) breast cancer treated with US-guided radiofrequency ablation: feasibility study. Radiology. 2004;231(1):215–24.
11. Palussiere J, Henriques C, Mauriac L, et al. Radiofrequency ablation as a substitute for surgery in elderly patients with nonresected breast cancer: pilot study with long-term outcomes. Radiology. 2012;264(2):597–605.
12. Noguchi M, Motoyoshi A, Earashi M, et al. Long-term outcome of breast cancer patients treated with radiofrequency ablation. Eur J Surg Oncol. 2012;38(11):1036–42.
13. Tsuda H, Seki K, Hasebe T, et al. A histopathological study for evaluation of therapeutic effects of radiofrequency ablation in patients with breast cancer. Breast Cancer. 2011;18 (1):24–32.
14. Oura S, Tamaki T, Hirai I, et al. Radiofrequency ablation therapy in patients with breast cancers two centimeters or less in size. Breast Cancer. 2007;14(1):48–54.
15. Giuliano AE, Hunt KK, Ballman KV, et al. Axillary dissection vs no axillary dissection in women with invasive breast cancer and sentinel node metastasis: a randomized clinical trial. JAMA. 2011;305(6):569–75.
16. Seki K, Tsuda H, Iwamoto E, et al. Histopathological effect of radiofrequency ablation therapy for primary breast cancer, with special reference to changes in cancer cells and stromal structure and a comparison with enzyme histochemistry. Breast Cancer. 2011;18(1):18–23.
17. Fisher B, Jeong JH, Anderson S, et al. Twenty-five-year follow-up of a randomized trial comparing radical mastectomy, total mastectomy, and total mastectomy followed by irradiation. N Engl J Med. 2002;347(8):567–75.
18. Hopwood P, Fletcher I, Lee A, et al. A body image scale for use with cancer patients. Eur J Cancer. 2001;37(2):189–97.

Chapter 17
MRI-Guided Focused Ultrasound Surgery of Breast Cancer

Hidemi Furusawa

17.1 Introduction

High-intensity focused ultrasound (HIFU) has been recognized to do some damage to the various tissues of the livings. MRI-guided focused ultrasound surgery (MRgFUS) is one of the thermal ablations to make the living tissue be in coagulation under the real-time MR image guidance.

Although radio frequency ablation (RFA) or cryoablation aims the cancer cell killing to surround them with the regular large volume like a fireball or an ice ball, MRgFUS takes a quite different principle to perform thermal coagulation of the cancerous tumor. That is, the target is coagulated thermally by 40–60 overlapped spindle spots which are various small volumes resulted from focused ultrasound beams.

17.2 Breast Application of MRgFUS

In Japan, US, and European countries, MRgFUS has been clinically applied in treatment of uterine fibroid, brain tumor, bone tumor, essential tremor, and breast cancer. The ability of MRI to visualize breast cancer (i.e., spatial resolution) is discussed separately. The ExAblate (InSightec Ltd, Tirat HaCarmel, Israel) therapeutic system is used in our hospital. The ExAblate treatment table (bed) uses the same gantry connectors as in 1.5/3.0 tesla MRI (GE Healthcare, Milwaukee, USA), enabling convenient and easy connecting and disconnecting operations. During the

H. Furusawa (✉)
Department of Breast Surgical Oncology, Kawaguchi Kogyo General Hospital, 1-18-15, Aoki, Kawaguchi 3320031, Japan
e-mail: hidemi.furusawa@kogyohsp.gr.jp

T. Kinoshita (ed.), *Non-surgical Ablation Therapy for Early-stage Breast Cancer*,
DOI 10.1007/978-4-431-54463-0_17

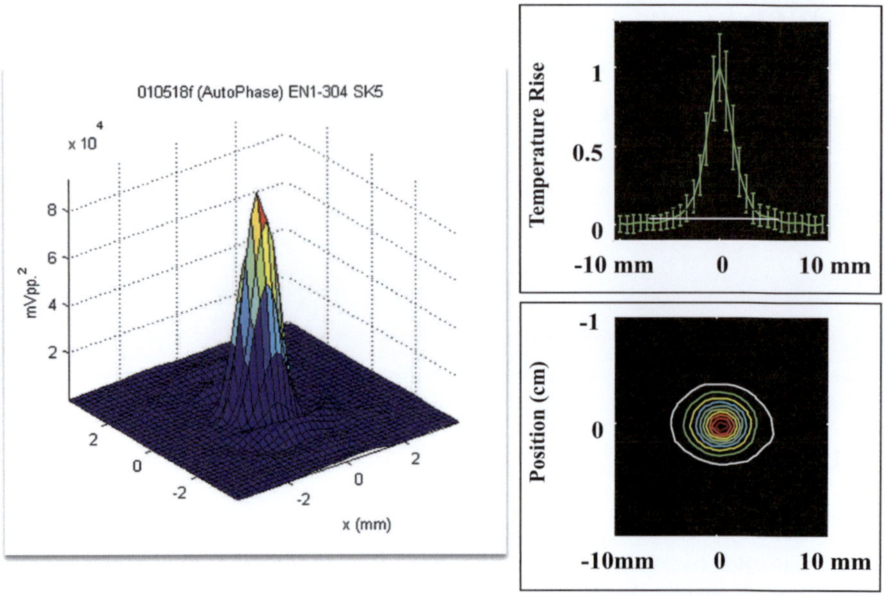

Fig. 17.1 Relation between the focal point and distance (as of September 2013)

treatment, the patient is placed in prone position with her affected breast inside the treatment coils, which are filled with cooled degassed water.

These treatment coils can help generate significantly clearer diagnostic images due to their compact design and thus closer contact with the breasts. During the treatment, the transducer emits ultrasound beams from 208 elements, which focus in the targeted volume, creating thermal coagulative necrosis in three-dimensional spindle-shaped volumes. Movement of the transducer and repeated energy emission allows sculpturing of the therapeutic lesion in size and shape.

The temperature increase is nearly zero at a distance of 1 cm from the target (Fig. 17.1). Although there are 14 types of spots of different diameters and length, a unique breast dedicated "weighted elongated spot" type is used for the treatment in our hospital for improved safety and accuracy, thanks to the advanced treatment software. By using this specific spot, the focal point will move horizontally from the major pectoral muscle side to the skin side during a sonication (i.e., energy emission) time of 40 s. Focused ultrasound energy of the spot [joules] is calculated by multiplying the ultrasound power [watts] and sonication time [seconds]. A built-in safety system is designed to automatically terminate the sonication to prevent burns once the calculated energy density on the skin exceeds 750 J. The entire treatment process is electronically recorded for reproducibility, making it possible to confirm the efficacy and adverse reactions even in posttreatment review of the procedure. This is a significant benefit of MRgFUS that none of the traditional surgical options can offer except endoscopic and robotic surgery.

17.3 MRI versus Ultrasound Guidance

Breast surgeons review usually the preoperative images obtained by different modalities to confirm the scope of involvement and ensure pathologically negative surgical margins during the operation, so that they can completely remove the both invasive and intraductal lesion of the breast.

For better identification of the cancer spreading inside the breasts including intraductal progression (spatial resolution of the breast cancer), the contrast MRI with gadolinium is the best modality as the clinicians and providers in concern with breast cancer know. However, contrast ultrasound using microbubble supersonic contrast medium (perflubutane: Sonazoid™) introduced in August 2012 is also expected to have a strong spatial resolution.

As focused ultrasound treatment is based on thermal coagulation to achieve denaturation of the proteins in the tumor cells and their components, continuous temperature monitoring of the sonicated volume is essential to understand the treatment effect in real time.

The system monitors temperature changes at the target and surrounding area, by taking real-time MR images every 3 s during sonication (Fig. 17.2), and provides the operator with this data in the form of a temperature graph (upper row). During

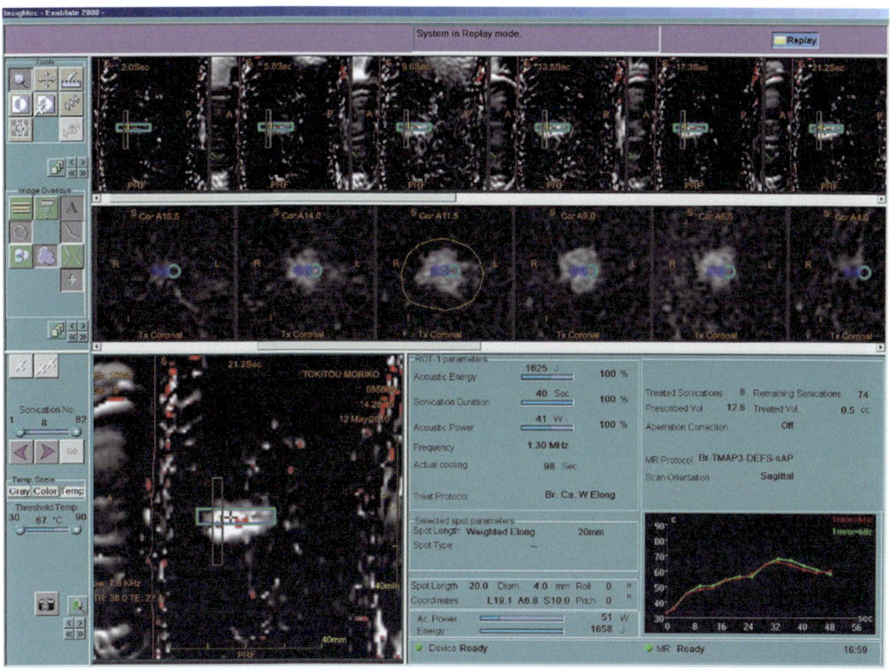

Fig. 17.2 ExAblate 2000™ console monitor (as of September 2013)

treatment, the therapeutic efficacy achieved in each spot can be confirmed based on the monitored temperature (lower right) and the reflection graph on the ultrasonically irradiated area. Based on the above, the MRI-guided treatment is generally preferred to the ultrasound-guided ablation techniques.

17.4 Clinical Research

We conducted a Phase II clinical study to evaluate the efficacy and safety of focused ultrasound treatment with 30 breast cancer patients who underwent surgical lumpectomy or mastectomy after MRgFUS treatment from February to September 2004 in Breastopia Namba Hospital in Miyazaki, Japan [1]. In the excised lumpectomy specimens after the focused ultrasound treatment, mean necrosis of the targeted breast tumors was 96.9 ± 4 % (median 100 %, range 78–100 %) [1] area in the prepared glass slides. Although the target lesion was indeed treated only 50 % in one case, the pathological treated area was 78 %.

One patient had a small residual untreated tumor adjacent to the major pectoral muscle, and one patient had a third-degree burn. These events led to the introduction of the abovementioned breast-dedicated weighted elongated spot.

Immediately after the completion of the treatment and resection study, a Phase III excisionless clinical trial has begun and is still ongoing (as at April 2014), aimed to enroll 100 subjects. In this study, no resection is performed after MRgFUS, and only adjuvant radiation (whole breast + boost) is provided to monitor the efficacy of this treatment modality. The primary endpoint is 5-year local recurrence rate and safety confirmation. The major criteria of enrollment of cases are shown in Table 17.1.

First, to identify any lymph node metastasis, we perform an anterior level I axillary lymph node sampling cranial to the third intercostobrachial nerve and the ventral to the second intercostobrachial nerve or sentinel lymph node biopsy.

Upon confirming the negativity of lymph node metastasis, we initiate MRgFUS treatment. The treatment area in the breast is manually drawn around the contrast-enhanced tumor in coronal view, with a 5 mm margin (Fig. 17.2, orange line in the middle).

Table 17.1 Major inclusions and exclusions

Inclusions	Exclusions
Tumor size $\leq$1.5 cm	Prior chemotherapy
Well-demarcated mass on MRI	Pure-type mucinous carcinoma
Confirmed by needle biopsy	Invasive micropapillary carcinoma
HER-2, ER, PgR status	Treatment team decision
Positive node	

Upon confirmation of targeted treated area, the device software automatically develops the treatment plan including the number of spots, ultrasound power, sonication time, and cooling time. Each of these factors can also be adjusted by the user at his/her own discretion.

A lesion area of approximately 10 mm in size requires about 40 spots and 80 min for the treatment (sonication duration 40 s and cooling duration 80 s per one spot.). The therapy effect is determined via contrast MRI immediately after treatment and pathological confirmation of no residual viable tumor cells by HE staining and single-strand-DNA immunohistochemical staining of postoperative needle biopsies after about 2–3 weeks. After this, the patient is referred for adjuvant radiation therapy.

The 5 mm free margin and limitation of tumor diameters to within 15 mm were set in order to confine the entire treatment duration to within 2 h. This has been demonstrated by the retrospective study on cases undergoing surgery in our hospital as what is required in order to achieve an average intraductal progression of 4 mm for invasive ductal carcinoma of 20 mm or smaller based on preoperative imaging evaluation (mainly via MRI). Patients with proven metastases were excluded because of the probable administration of postoperative chemotherapy, which would confound the local ultrasonic therapeutic effect. The ground for the exclusion standard will be discussed later in the corresponding sections. So far, we have enrolled 80 cases and excluded 14 in our excisionless study. Sixty-six patients completed the serial local treatment (MRgFUS + radiation therapy). Among the excluded patients, seven were positive for lymph metastases.

The average age was 57 (range 29–79) years, the mean of the largest tumor diameter 11.0 (5–15) mm, average treatment time 124 (41–246) minutes, and the median follow-up period 63 (4–91) months. No local recurrence, remote recurrence, or severe adverse reaction was detected in the 35 patients who were followed up for 60 months or longer.

After the breast-conserving surgery, sclerosis may develop with time to replace the space that had been occupied by the tumor, though no scar or deformation of breasts will appear, which is an advantage of this approach. In addition, even when selection bias is taken into account, patients in the MRgFUS group still presented significantly better outcomes compared with the 419 patients of invasive ductal carcinoma smaller than 15 mm in size, who underwent breast-conserving surgery without radiation therapy in our hospital during the same period. Five-year disease-free survival and 5-year survival rate were, respectively, 100 % and 100 % in the former and 97.2 % and 99.3 %, respectively, in the latter group.

The patients are followed up every 3 months for 1 year after the procedure and every 6 months after that, using mainly MRI and mammography (Figs. 17.3 and 17.4). Ultrasound follow-up is not recommended as it tends to exaggerate the efficacy and recurrence rate.

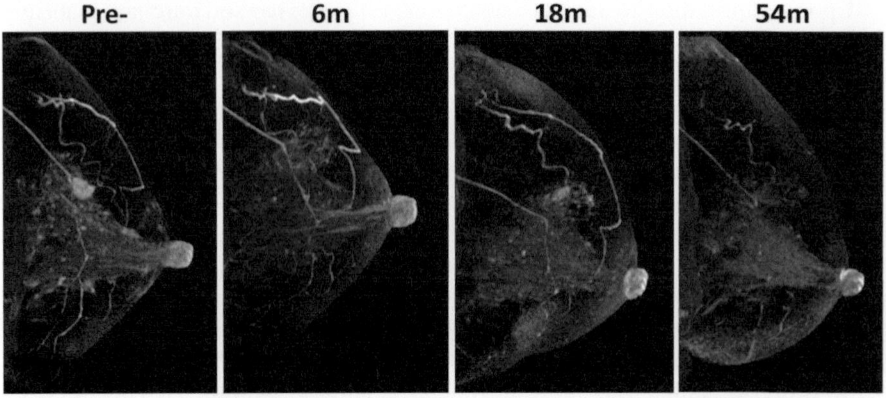

Fig. 17.3 A case of average postoperative progress on MRI (as of September 2013)

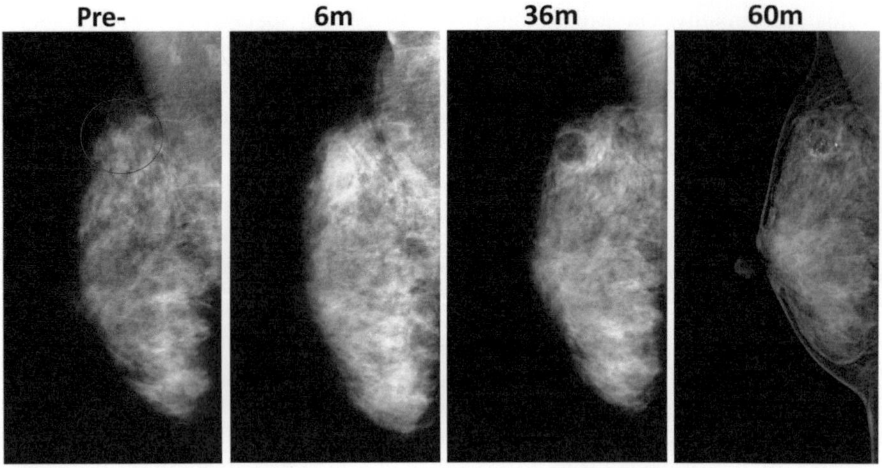

Fig. 17.4 A case of average postoperative progress mammography (*Red circle* marks the targeted tumor) (as of September 2013)

17.5 Unresolved Issues

As mentioned in the exclusion criteria, one of the unresolved issues with this therapy is that although MRI is useful in detecting tumors following preoperative chemotherapy on invasive lesions, it is not as effective in detecting local and intraductal components in a macular cancer nest, making it difficult to determine the areas to be treated. This is the same case in usual breast-conserving surgery as well.

Different from other tissue subtypes, pure-type mucinous carcinoma is composed of gelatinous substance with much water, resulting in excessively high permeability of ultrasound beams and consequent difficulty of focusing inside the tumor. Hence, achieving heat coagulation by focused ultrasound is ineffective in this case, as it will fail to achieve sufficient temperature rise inside the tumor. In addition, invasive micropapillary carcinoma, associated with a high risk of dissemination (cancer cell displacement) during needle biopsies, is also excluded in our study, as MRI cannot detect the affected area in this condition. More importantly, there is an issue regarding the interface between local cancer nest and normal tissues (glands, collagenous stroma, and fat) in the breast. These issues are related to the accuracy of the real-time imaging. In other words, although the angle of the MR image slicing remains the same – in both sagittal and axial orientations – throughout the treatment, when the angle of a certain sonication, particularly this angle, is very large, the accuracy of the MRI thermometry may be compromised. This is because real-time oblique imaging capability is not available for adjusting to the sonication angle. Therefore, in actual treatment, sonication has to be performed with the smallest angle possible. In addition, possible reflection of ultrasound at various tissue interfaces inside the breast may lead to reduced therapeutic efficacy, and in some cases, the sonication may not even effectively reach the target lesion.

The issue of the treatment area and the ultrasound energy cannot be ignored, either, particularly in fatty breasts where there is often a considerable difference between the planned area of treatment and the actual treatment area, resulting in a strong tendency of overtreatment and delayed healing of scars in the treatment area (Fig. 17.5).

The issue of energy thus is represented by the duration of the treatment. With safety as the top priority at present, the radiation for each spot lasts for 2 min in a cycle of treatment, including 40 s of radiation and 80 s of cooling, which is two times the former. Therefore, the cooling time is the rate-determining step throughout the treatment.

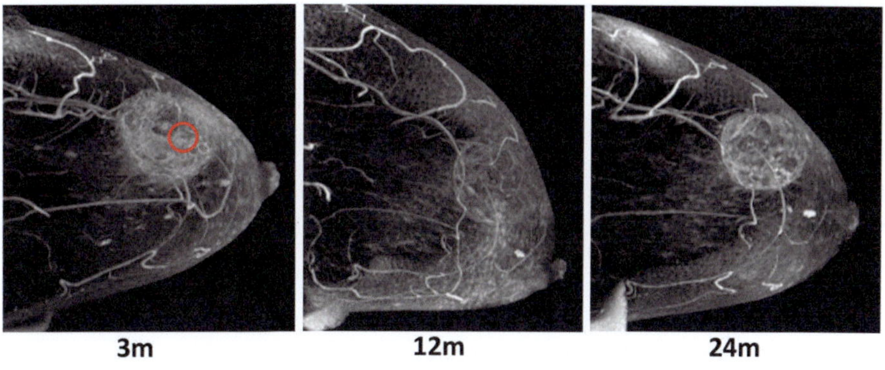

Fig. 17.5 A case of postoperative development of the fatty breast, shown by MRI. A 3 m. B 12m. C 24 m. The white spot in the left image is the target tumor and an example of overtreatment (as of September 2013)

17.6 Prospects

In view of emerging solutions for the above issues and the fact that both MRI technology and the treatment device are making continuous advancement, the future of this treatment is promising. For example, there is a new approach to dealing with mucinous carcinoma by injecting micro-(nano)-bubble into the tumor to increase the ultrasonic absorbency (i.e., to decrease the permeability). With a new estimation technique developed via the collaboration with the Department of Technology, Tokyo University, the issue concerning diffused reflection can be predicted before surgery. Meanwhile, in this early stage of the treatment for breast cancer, we are looking mostly at complete coagulation of cancer nests (as if making a hard-boiled egg). Based on the fact that a fertilized egg cannot be hatched even after half-boiled, it is highly possible that denaturing an individual cell into a "half-boiled egg" will suffice to deactivate the entire local tumor lesion. In this way, all parameters involved in the treatment may be downscaled, such as the sound energy and the planned treatment area, contributing to improved safety and reduced treatment time. An effective treatment can also be achieved at a lower temperature using a chemotherapy agent (ThermoDox™) to seal the thermal-sensitive liposome. Incidentally, ultrasonic treatment has been applied in treating not only local breast cancer but also breast cancer-related treatments. Bone metastases are common in patients with breast cancer or prostatic carcinoma.

Investigators in the USA and Europe have reported satisfying results of pain relief for patients with bone metastasis in relevant clinical studies.

In addition, a clinical study is underway in the USA to treat patients with neurological disorders such as essential tremor and tremor-dominant Parkinson's disease, which employs the same principles as Gamma Knife and CyberKnife. Furthermore, another study is also in progress to destroy the blood-brain barrier by opening up small holes.

17.7 Conclusion

Data on breast cancer local treatment using MR-guided focused ultrasound surgery (MRgFUS) are accumulating, and the MRI systems used for treatment are being improved.

The mortality of breast cancer has not been decreasing in Japan, and this is believed to be associated with the low medical examination rate. We believe it is important to raise the awareness and understanding of Japanese women that the detection of a small tumor means the chance to save their lives and breasts and make efforts to increase the examination rate by 10 % or so, regardless of how we achieve this. As the rate of appropriate examination increases, the detection rate of cancer at an early stage will increase, and the death rate will be, in turn, reduced. We are confident that focused ultrasound therapy can be one of the contributing factors to this cycle.

17.8 Summary

MRI-guided focused ultrasound surgery for breast cancer that uses magnetic resonance imaging (MRI) is the best modality to know preoperatively breast cancer spreading in most of all patients. The prognosis of breast cancer patients does not depend on local treatment. Accordingly the aim of local therapy is to completely eradicate viable cancer cells in the breast. This means there is no need to adhere to the usual surgical procedures. MR-guided focused ultrasound surgery (MRgFUS) is a noninvasive local therapy of breast cancer using high-intensity ablation and thermal coagulation. The clinical studies in our facility have proved that this local treatment has the potential to take place of the surgery in some cases. Patients for MRgFUS must be strictly selected.

17.9 Postscript

I submitted this paper in April 2014. And then the excisionless study had continued and finished in March 2015 in breastopia Namba Hospital. I moved and belonged to Kawaguchi Kogyo General Hospital in June 2015

Acknowledgment I offer my heartfelt thanks to Mr.Shidooka, Ms.Hirabara, Ms Inomata and all teammates of Breastopia Namba Hospital.

Reference

1. Furusawa H, et al. Magnetic resonance-guided focused ultrasound surgery of breast cancer: reliability and effectiveness. J Am Coll Surg. 2006;203:54–63.

Chapter 18 Ultrasonography Guided Nonsurgical Cryoablation for Small Breast Cancer

Eisuke Fukuma

18.1 Background

Cryotherapy for the treatment of human disease has a long history dating back to the reported treatment of cancer by James Arnott in 1845 [1] and cryotherapy has been applied for various kinds of skin disease in the late nineteenth century and early twentieth century. Indication of cryotherapy was extended to other organs, including lung [2], kidney [3], and liver [4] amongst others [5] after the late twentieth century. The Japan Society for Low Temperature Medicine was established in 1974.

Cryotherapy for breast disease is divided into several treatments. One of those is nonsurgical cryoablation for malignant [6, 7] and benign breast disease [8]. Another treatment is palliative cryotherapy for intractable bleeding from ulcerative breast cancer and a third treatment is cryoablation-assisted lumpectomy (CAL) [9].

Nonsurgical cryoablation for small breast cancer is mentioned in this chapter.

18.2 Theory of Cryoablation

Two mechanisms of the tumour-killing effect of cryoablation are known as rapid cooling and slow cooling (Fig. 18.1a). Rapid cooling near the probe, used for cryoablation, causes intercellular freezing, followed by mechanical destruction of the cell membrane with ice crystals. Slow cooling happens several mm inside the ice ball from its edge. Destruction of the cancer cell is explained with mechanical stress from the ice crystals, chemical stress (increasing electrolyte concentration),

---

E. Fukuma (✉)
Breast Center, Kameda Medical Center, 929 Higashi-cho, Kamogawa City, Chiba Prefecture 296-8602, Japan
e-mail: efosea@gmail.com

T. Kinoshita (ed.), *Non-surgical Ablation Therapy for Early-stage Breast Cancer*,
DOI 10.1007/978-4-431-54463-0_18

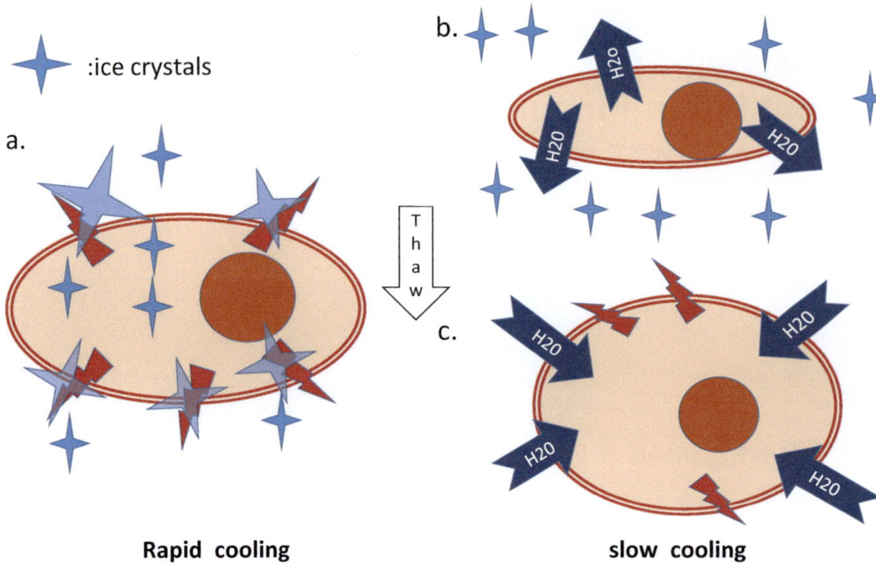

Fig. 18.1 Mechanism to destroy tumour cell with cryotherapy. (**a**) Rapid cooling (intracellular freezing): ice crystals are formed inside and outside tumour cells destroying the cell membrane directly (mechanical stress). (**b**, **c**) Slow cooling (extracellular freezing). (**b**) Flow of intracellular fluid to extracellular space causes shrinkage of the cells. (**c**) During time of thaw, influx of H2O from extracellular space to inside of the cell results in overexpansion of the cell, followed by mechanical stress and destruction of cell membrane. Outflow and influx of H2O in the cell causes rapid change of osmotic pressure and concentration of electrolytes (osmotic and chemical stress)

and osmotic stress (high osmotic pressure inside the cell caused by shrinkage of cells; Fig. 18.1b). Death of tumour cells is expected at less than −40 °C and this death varies according to the kind of cells Total death of tumour and normal cells is expected 5–8 mm away from the edge of the ice ball.

18.3 Equipment for Cryoablation of Breast Cancer

Freezing of breast cancers is achieved with insertion of the probe into the mass. The probe is expected to reach to −120–170 °C. Achieved lowest temperature varies according to the machines for freezing. Machines for cryotherapy for breast disease are divided into two different principles of freezing: argon-gas–based technology and liquid-nitrogen–based technology. CryoHit (Galil Medical C.C) and Visica I (Sanarus C.C, Fig. 18.2a not commercially available at present) are based on principle of the Joule and Thomson phenomenon with argon and helium gas. IceSense3 (IceCure C.C Fig. 18.2b) and Visica II (Sanarus C.C) depend on the freezing power of liquid nitrogen.

a. b.

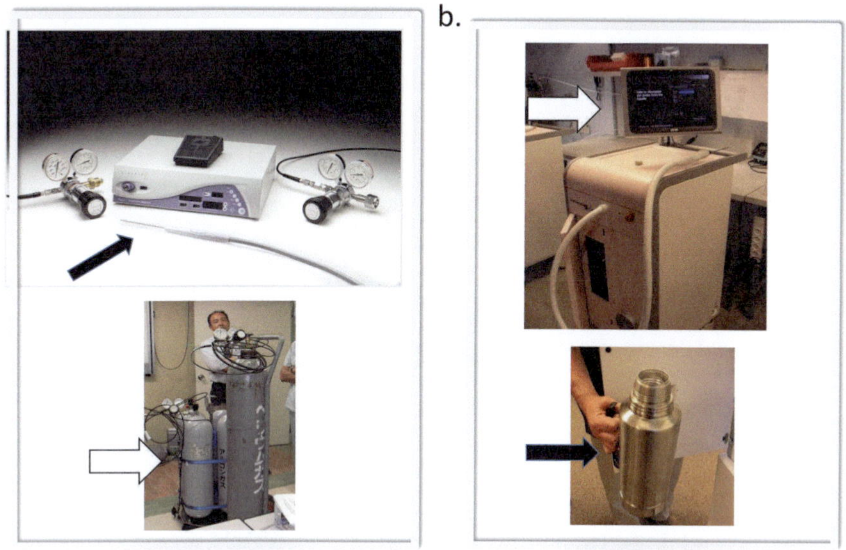

Fig. 18.2 Machine used for cryoablation for breast disease. (**a**) Visica I (Sanarus C.C) is based on Joule Thomson principle with high pressure argon and helium gas). Probe for insertion (*black arrow*). High pressure tanks are prepared for high pressure argon and helium gases. (**b**) IceSense3 (IceCure C.C) is based on cooling with liquid nitrogen. White arrow shows touch panel console on the top of the main body to control time of freezing, thaw, and warming. Also amount of flow volume to the probe is monitored with the console. Lower part of the main body store 2 l volume container of liquid nitrogen (*black arrow*)

IceSense3 has been used for nonsurgical cryoablation for small breast cancer at our institution since 2013. The main body of IceSense3 holds the container of two liters of liquid nitrogen, the console to regulate the inflow of liquid nitrogen into the probe and outflow of the gas nitrogen, and the conduit of liquid nitrogen from the main body to the probe. The probe is disposable and attached to the conduit in screwed attaching fashion. The diameter of the probe is 3.4 mm with a sharp tip and the active freezing zone is 20 mm and 40 mm of small and large probes each; the active freezing zone of the probe creates −170 °C at the lowest temperature (Fig. 18.3).

18.4 Indication of Nonsurgical Cryoablation

The size of the ice ball formed with IceSense3 reaches from 35 mm to more than 45 mm transversely to the probe and 40–50 mm longitudinally. The size of the cell death effect is expected within 5–8 mm away from the edge of ice ball (Fig. 18.4). If formed, the transverse size of the ice ball is 40 mm; within 24 mm in transverse size is expected to achieve cell destruction. Longitudinally, the size of ice ball reaches to

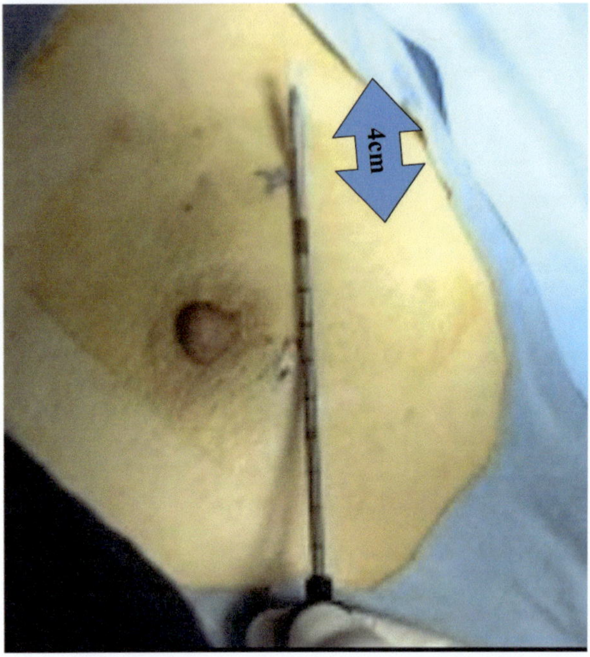

Fig. 18.3 Probe of IceSense 3 system. Probe of IceSense 3 system is 3.4 mm in diameter and active zone of freezing is 4 cm long (*white arrow*)

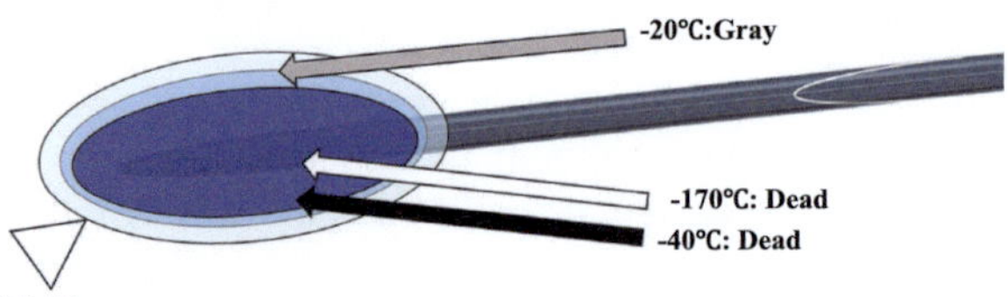

Fig. 18.4 Temperature gradient from the probe, which reaches to −170 °C. From the probe (*white arrow*) to −40 °C zone (*black arrow*) death of the tumour is expected. Death of the tumour cell from −40 to −20°C zone is gray and tumour-killing effect depends on type of cancer (*gray arrow*). Cancer cell is alive around the ice ball edge (0°C: *white arrow head*)

more than 40 mm when a large probe is used. The probe should be inserted along the longest diameter of the lesion and the direction of the longest diameter of the lesions is achieved along the radial direction from the nipple in most occasions. Lesion size should be measured with mammography, ultrasonography, and breast MRI and size of the lesions should be less than 10 mm (Figs. 18.5 and 18.6) because of the limited cell-destroying zone within the formed ice ball and the safety margin, 3–5 mm, from the targeted lesion to achieve local control of the cancer.

At present, biology of the cancer is important to choose the candidate for nonsurgical cryoablation and other than Luminal A-like lesions should be excluded as candidates. Moreover, a negative of sentinel node metastasis and distant metastasis are crucial for indication of nonsurgical cryoablation.

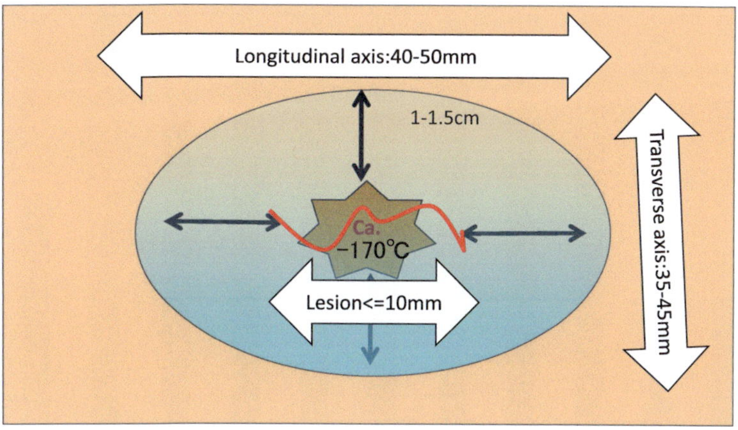

Fig. 18.5 Indication of nonsurgical cryoablation for small breast cancer. Size of formed ice ball with IceSense3 is 35–45 mm in transverse axis of the probe and 40–50 mm in longitudinal axis. Transversely 40-mm sized ice ball expects 24-mm sized area to destroy cancer lesion. The lesion, including mass and DCIS, have to be less than 10 mm

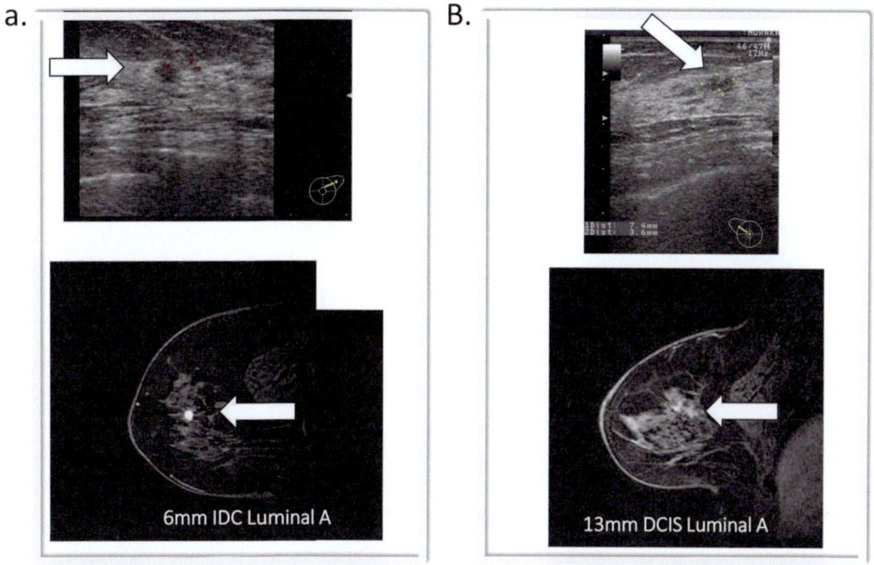

Fig. 18.6 Candidates are selected with breast imaging. (**a**) Candidate. Both ultrasonography and breast MRI showed localised lesion less than 10 mm (*white arrows*). (**b**) Not candidate. Although the lesion was less than 10 mm with ultrasonography (*white arrow*), breast MRI disclosed 13 mm long lesion

Based on inclusion criteria and longstanding experience of nonsurgical cryoablation, the number of nonsurgical cryoablations is increasing in a number of patients having local control, mastectomy, breast conservative surgery, and nonsurgical cryoablation for breast cancer (Fig. 18.7).

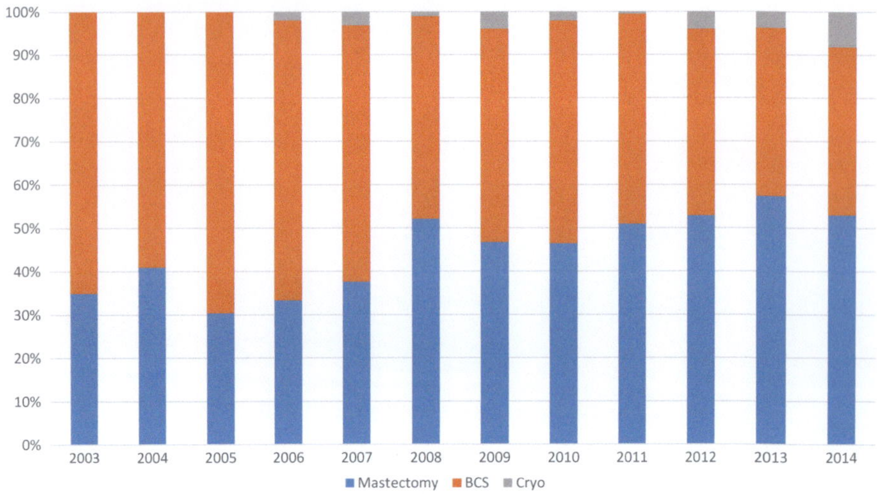

Fig. 18.7 Serial change of breast surgery at Kameda Medical Center. Nonsurgical cryoablation for breast cancer among breast surgeries has been increasing in numbers since 2006 and 8.2 % of surgery is done with nonsurgical cryoablation in 2014

18.5 Evaluation Before the Procedure and Follow-Up After the Procedure

Before the decision of indication, physical examination, ultrasonography, mammography, and/or breast MRI are performed to know the lesion size. A PET scan is mandatory, according to the staging of breast cancer. Also vacuum assisted biopsy (VAB) or core needle biopsy (CNB) has to be performed to learn the pathology and subtype of the breast cancer. VAB is recommended because of the larger amount of the specimen. Sentinel node biopsy (SNB) is needed to know the nodal state of the patient with invasive breast cancer, which is disclosed by VAB or CNB. SNB is able to be eliminated for the patient with DCIS, the lesion of which is nearly or totally excised with VAB.

The first step for successful cryoablation is a breast MRI to learn the proper targeting of the lesion after 1 or 1.5 months after the cryoablation. If calcification of the lesion is identified with mammography before cryoablation, mammography is added to learn the proper targeting at the first postprocedural breast imaging. And then 6 and 12 months after the procedure, a breast MRI and other modalities of breast imaging are performed to learn in-breast tumour recurrence (IBTR).

After identifying the proper targeting of the lesion, whole breast irradiation and hormonal therapy are scheduled.

18.6 Practice of Nonsurgical Cryoablation

Nonsurgical cryoablation can be performed under local anesthesia and with day surgery. Setting up of the procedure is simple: 20 cc of 1% lidocaine with epinephrine and 23 G needle, scalpel, and normal saline to prevent thermal injury of the skin from ice ball (Fig. 18.8a, b). Four liters of liquid nitrogen are needed for 20-min freezing time.

The patient lies down on the back and an intravenous line inserted. In most patients, the site of insertion of the probe is the periareolar region. In some patients with the cancer in the lower part of the breast, a skin incision is added along the inframammary fold. The skin incision should be selected to achieve penetration of the probe along the longest caliber of the lesion (Fig. 18.9).

Before adding the skin incision, local anesthesia is injected into the incised site, needle tract, subcutaneous area, and behind the major pectral fascia. When the

a.

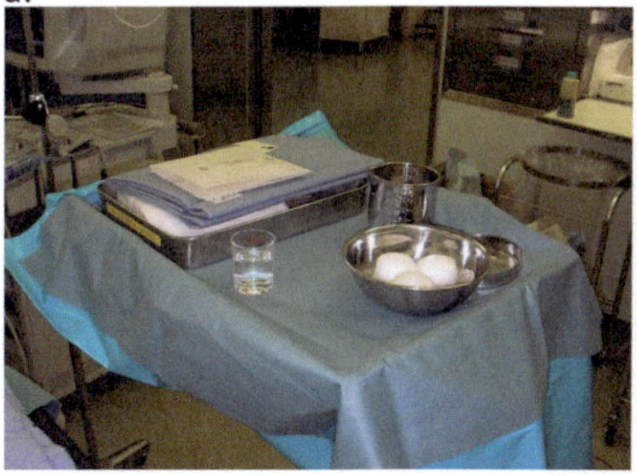

b.

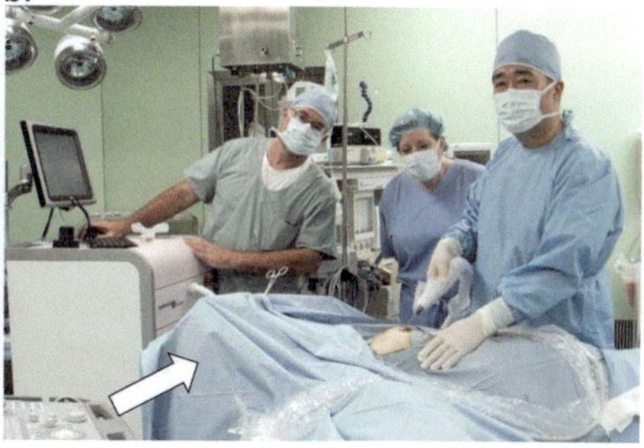

Fig. 18.8 Setup for nonsurgical cryoablation. (**a**) Preparation. 20 cc of 1% lidocaine with epinephrine. 23G needle. Scalpel. Normal saline. Dressing. Gauze. Material and instruments for one stitch closure. Pean. (**b**) Staff and positioning. One surgeon, medical engineer, and circulating nurse are enough for the procedures. Head of the patient is indicated with *white arrow*

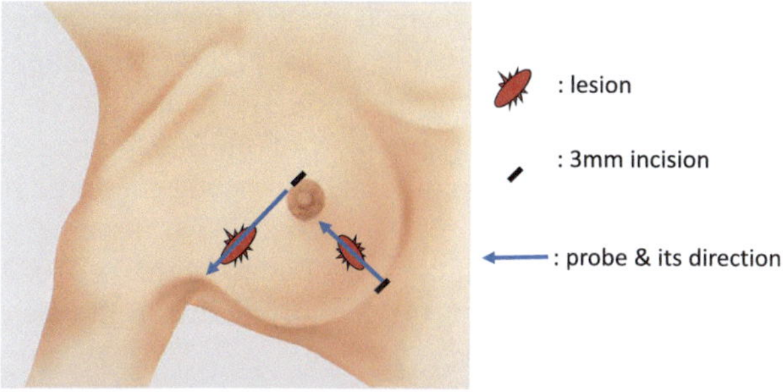

Fig. 18.9 Selection of incision site. Site of incision is selected according to relative location of the lesion and longitudinal axis direction of the lesion

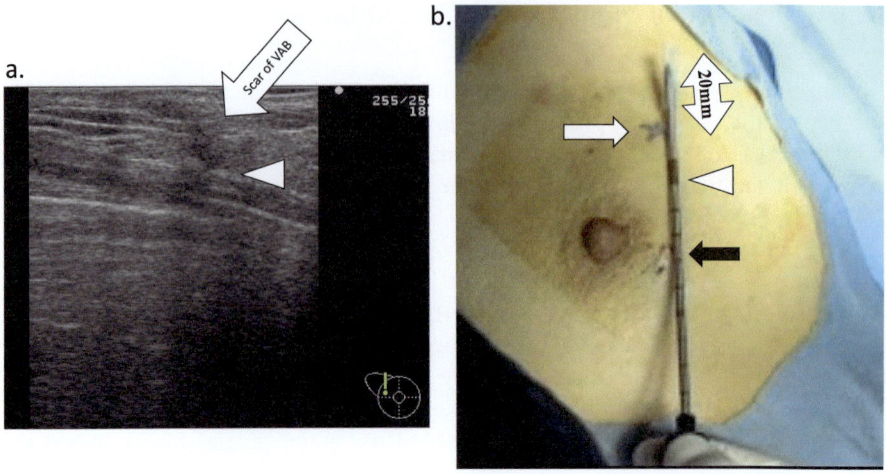

Fig. 18.10 Evaluation of the lesion and the breast before adding incision. (**a**) Evaluation with ultrasonography. The lesion is barely identified with ultrasonography (*white arrow*) in thin thickness breast. Injection of local anesthesia should be given in the space below the pectral major fascia (*white arrow head*). After penetration of the lesion with the probe, local anesthesia is administered under the skin. (**b**) Proper incisional site. Location of the skin surface mark above the lesion (*white arrow*) is 20 mm away from tip of the probe. Incision site (*black arrow*) should be more than 10 mm away from active freezing zone (*white arrow head*)

lesion is hardly identified because of a small lesion or postbiopsy state, injection of that should be after penetration of the lesion with the probe (Fig. 18.10a).

Through a 3 mm long skin incision, a large probe is inserted along the longest lesion site.

The distance from the tip of the probe to the mid portion of the lesion should be around 20 mm because the lowest temperature is expected at that point (Fig. 18.10b). In most cases, the probe penetrates the centre of the lesion. When the size of the breast with the lesion is not thick, the probe is inserted into the relatively dorsal part of the lesion. In the case of mucinous cancer, penetration of the lesion is avoided as much as possible.

IceSense3 has a programmed and manual mode of freezing, thaw, and warming. One treatment session with IceSense3 consists of first freezing, thaw, second freezing, and warming (double-freezing method). The manual mode of the program is frequently used because adjusting the size of the ice ball is easier than the programmed mode. Although the longitudinal axis along the large probe becomes larger than 40 mm, the size of the ice ball along the transverse axis should be controlled by measuring its size with ultrasonography (Fig. 18.11). The transverse axis diameter is decided according to the size of the lesion, breast thickness, and location of the probe inside the lesion.

After the cryoablation finished, the probe is extracted. The incision is closed with absorbable suture in one stitch. The incision is covered with a few sheets of

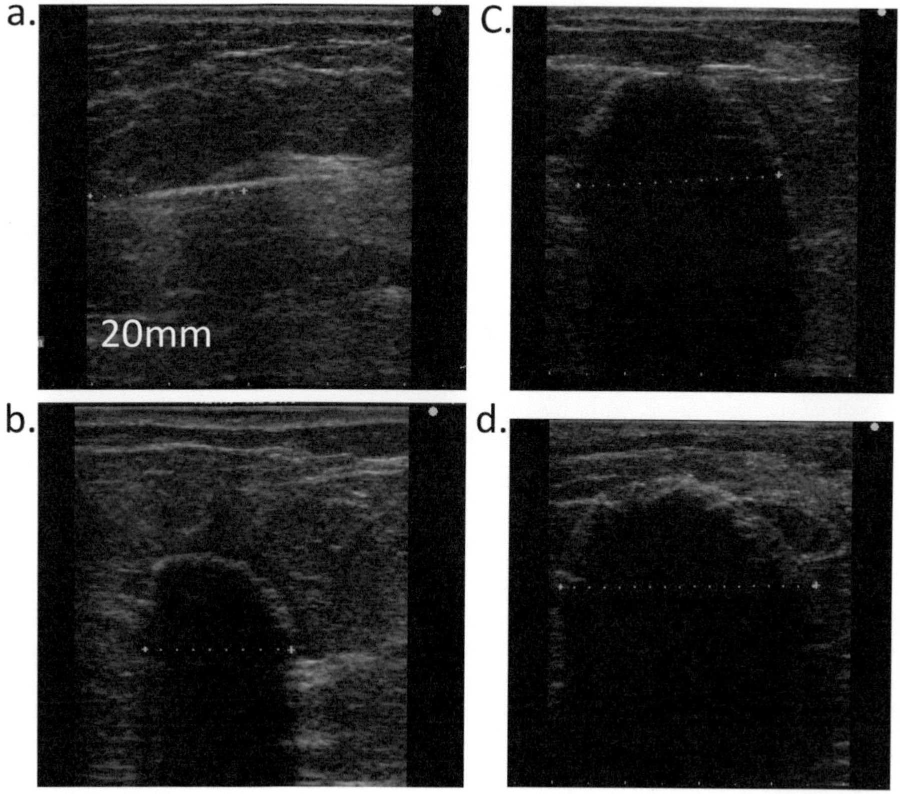

Fig. 18.11 Observing growing ice ball with ultrasonography. (**a**) Distance from tip of the probe to the lesion is 20 mm along longitudinal axis of the probe. (**b–d**) Measurement of growing ice ball along transverse axis of the probe is easy with ultrasonography. The ablated zone can be controlled well with these procedures

gauze but do not compress too much to avoid pressure necrosis. The total time of the whole session takes 60–70 min, but the actual freezing time is 12–22 min (double-freezing method) and 6–10 min thaw time.

One day after cryoablation, the patient visits as an outpatient to remove the dressing and check the treated breast.

18.7 Technique of to Achieve Successful Cryoablation Anywhere and Any Size of the Breast

Breast size among Asian women is smaller than that of Caucasian women and thickness of the breasts is different according to location of the lesions. The size of the ice ball is expected to be larger than 35 mm to destroy the cancer cells of 10-mm

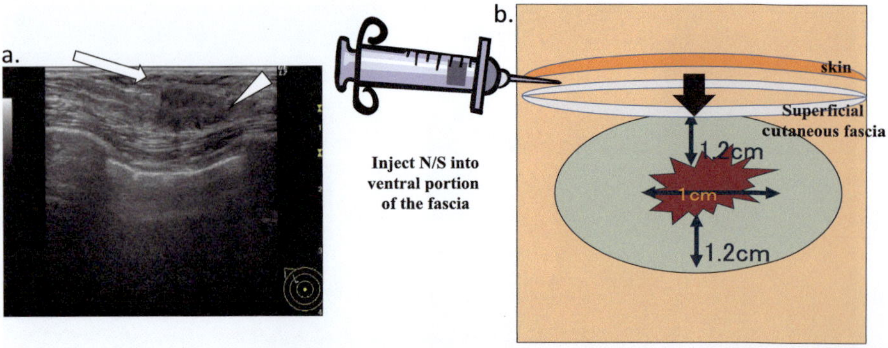

Fig. 18.12 Protecting the skin is achieved by injecting saline in the space between the skin and the superficial cutaneous fascia. (**a**) Image with ultrasonography. Although the lesion is closed, the injection made the gap between the skin and the superficial subcutaneous fascia. This lesion is a candidate because the gap could be expanded with injecting saline. (**b**) The space between the skin and the subcutaneous fascia can be expanded by injecting saline. The ice ball engulfs the fascia

size lesions even though thickness of the breast, where the lesion is located, is less than 15 mm. If cryoablation is applied for all candidates who satisfy the inclusion criteria, a cautious approach is demanded to avoid thermal injury of the skin and the chest wall, especially among patients with thin breasts. During the freezing procedure, the probe is lifted up and shaken to prevent thermal injury to the chest wall. Injection of normal saline to the space between the skin and the subcutaneous fascia is carried out to avoid thermal injury to the skin (Fig. 18.12a, b). The gap between the skin and the fascia is expanded enough to prevent thermal injury by injecting saline. Saline should be injected accurately into the adjacent area under the skin with an ultrasonography-guided procedure.

Destroying the cancer cells can be achieved even though the lesion is adjacent to the subcutaneous fascia with injecting saline when the distance from the fascia to the edge of ice ball beyond the fascia (Fig. 18.13a–d). The volume of saline into the gap is unlimited and the several patients who received more than 350 cc of saline injection to avoid thermal injury to the skin were experienced.

18.8 Serial Change of Breast Imaging After Nonsurgical Cryoablation

It is important to know the serial change of breast imaging after cryoablation to distinguish inflammatory change after cryoablation from IBTR. A breast MRI one or 1.5 months after cryoablation, aimed to discover the proper targeting of cryoablation, shows granulation formed at the ablated area (Fig. 18.14a, b) and peripheral enhancement around the granulation is observed. Peripheral

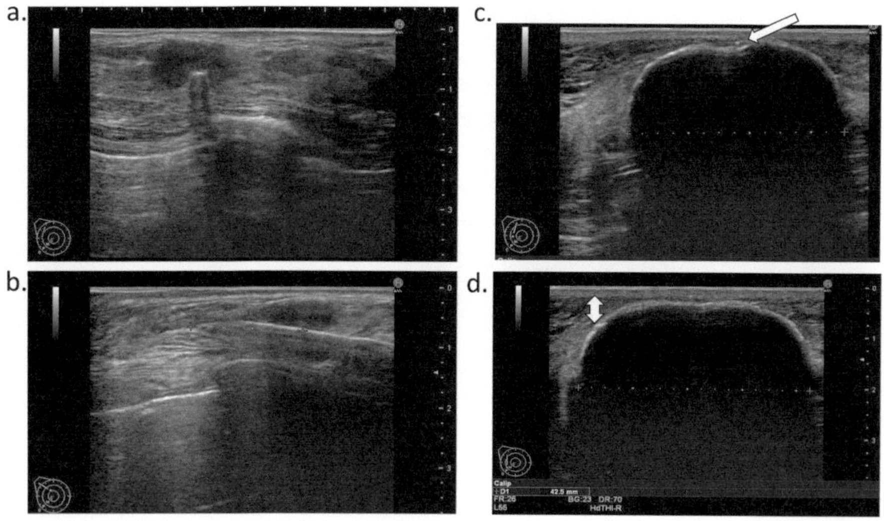

Fig. 18.13 Finding a way to perform cryoablation in thin thickness breasts. (**a**) Ultrasonography with transverse axis of the probe before freezing. The probe was inserted into the dorsal part of the lesion because of assurance of cancer extirpation of dorsal part. (**b**) Ultrasonography with longitudinal axis of the probe before freezing. The probe was inserted into the dorsal part of the lesion because of assurance of cancer extirpation of dorsal part. (**c**) Ultrasonography with transverse axis of the probe after freezing. Growing ice ball adjacent to the skin was accurately observed. 23G needle, injecting saline, was identified (*white arrow*). (**d**) Ultrasonography with transverse axis of the probe after freezing. End of second freezing. Size of the ice ball along transverse axis was 42.5 mm. Gap between the skin and the fascia is more than 5 mm

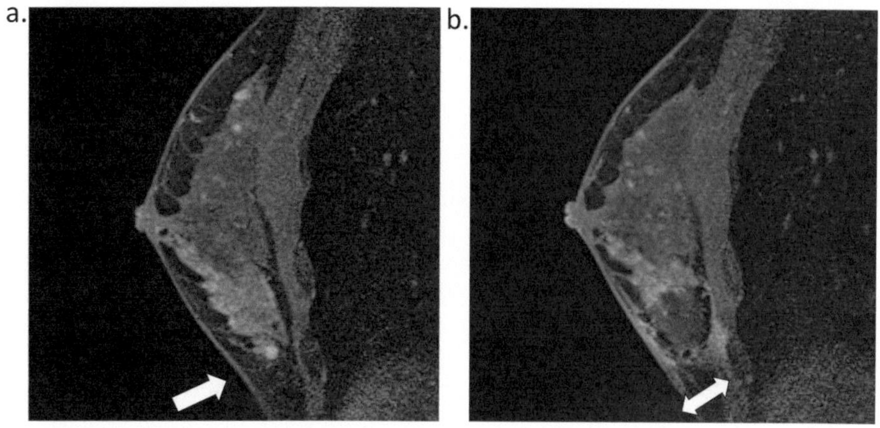

Fig. 18.14 Breast MRI 1–1.5 months after cryoablation to know accurate targeting of the lesion. (**a**) The lesion before cryoablation (*white arrow*). (**b**) After cryoablation, targeting the lesion was performed well. Ablated area from the skin and part of the muscle was observed. No thermal injury of the skin is observed

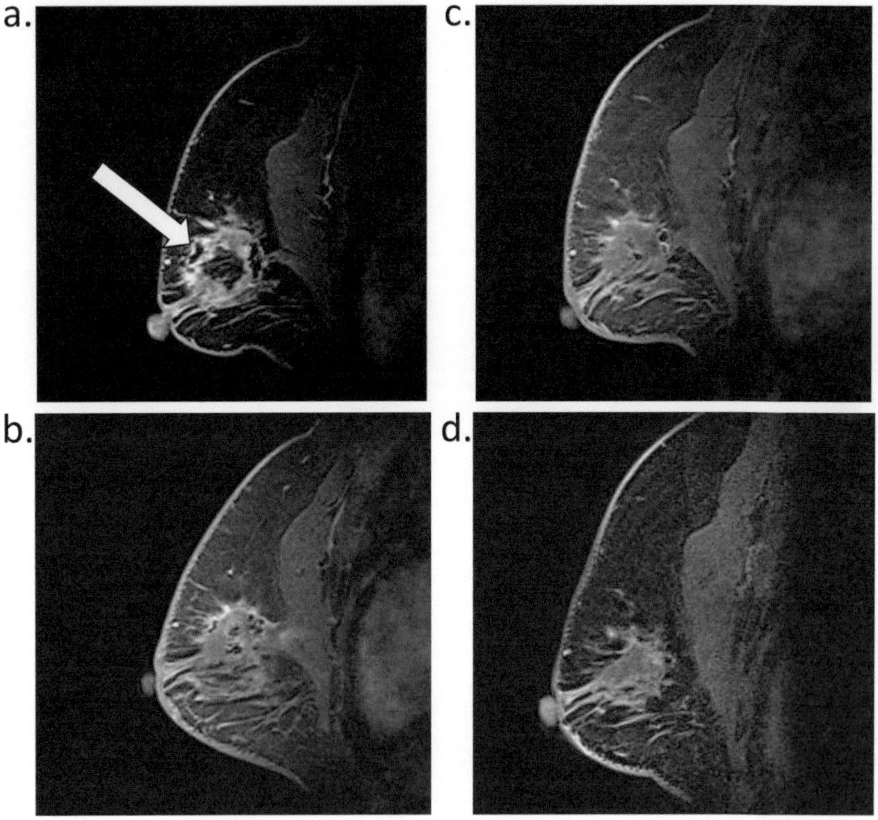

Fig. 18.15 Serial changes of breast MRI after cryoablation. (**a**) One month after: peripheral enhancement around the granulation was noted (*white arrow*). (**b**) Six months after: peripheral enhancement subsided. (**c**) Eleven months after. (**d**) Thirty-three months after: peripheral enhancement was diminished. Granulation was smaller than before

enhancement is subsided serially after 6 months and then it is speculated to be able to diagnose IBTR (Fig. 18.15a–d).

Although the density of the ablated area of the breast is high after cryoablation, calcification remaining in the breast after cryoablation is easily identified with mammography. Mass lesion or distortion is hardly recognised with mammography (Fig. 18.16a–c).

Granulation formed after cryoablation, identified with ultrasonography, also gradually grows smaller in size (Fig. 18.17a–d). Imaging inside the granulation varies.

One IBTR after nonsurgical cryoablation is experienced. IBTR was developed 5 years after cryoablation for T1a Luminal A invasive breast cancer. Although it was recognised with breast MRI and mammography, ultrasonography failed to find the lesion. MR-guided VAB disclosed DCIS in the lesion (Fig. 18.18).

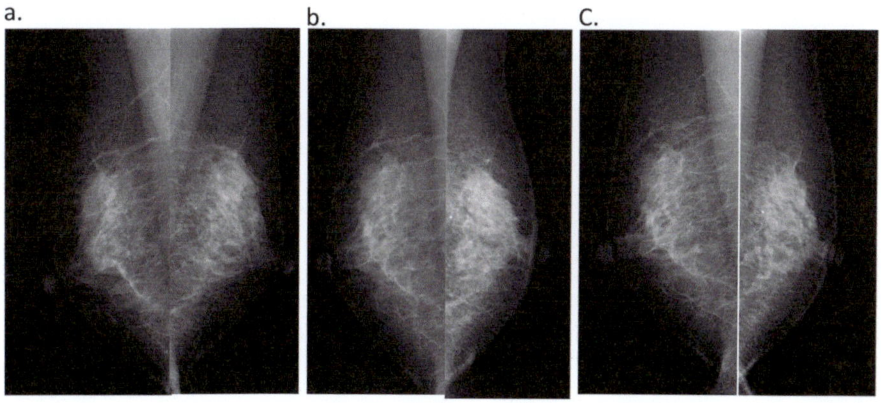

Fig. 18.16 Serial changes of mammography after cryoablation. (**a**) Preoperative mammography: cancer was in upper region of left breast. (**b**) Eleven months after cryoablation: High density was noted at the ablated area. (**c**) Thirty-three months after: area of high density was smaller

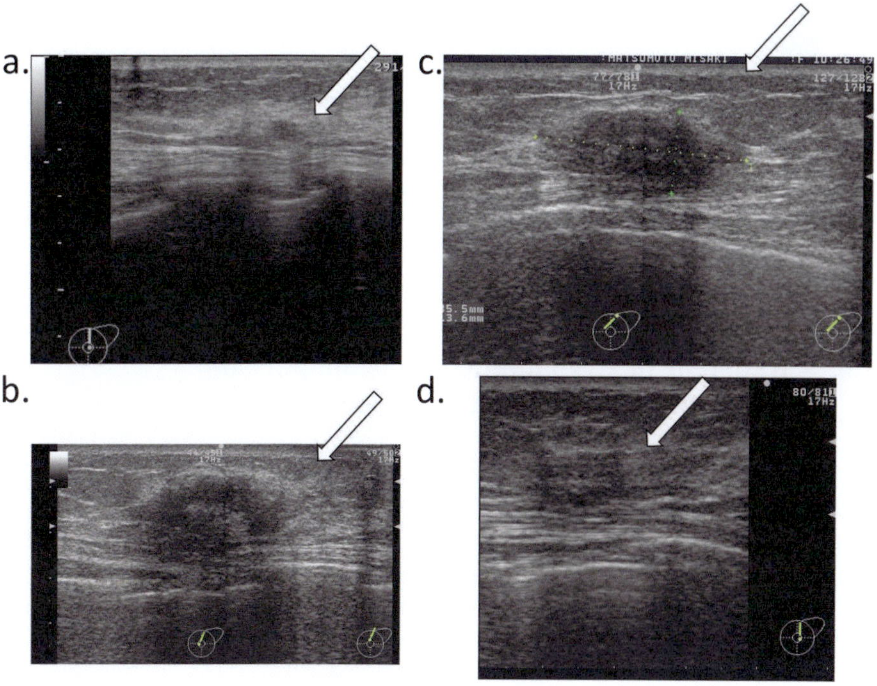

Fig. 18.17 Serial changes of ultrasonography after cryoablation. (**a**) Preoperative ultrasonography: the lesion was indicated with *white arrow*. (**b**) Six months after cryoablation: granulation was indicated with *white arrow*. (**c**) Fifteen months after cryoablation: Granulation is smaller than at 6 months. (**d**) Forty-seven months after cryoablation: granulation was smaller than at 15 months but still there

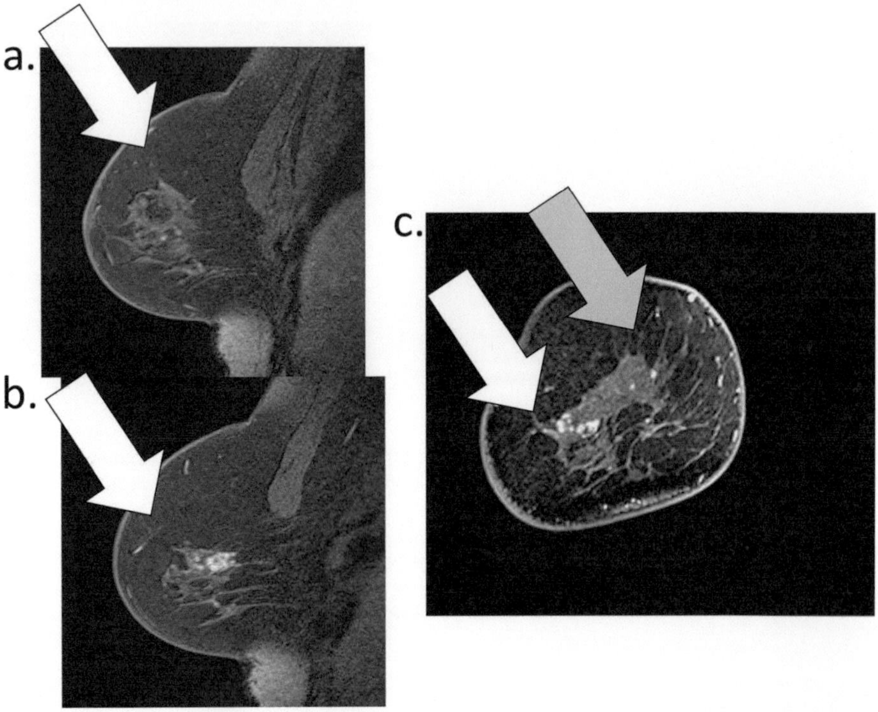

Fig. 18.18 IBTR after nonsurgical cryoablation with breast MRI. (**a**) Ablated area (*white arrow*) on sagittal section. (**b**) IBTR (*white arrow*) in right outer region on sagittal section. (**c**) IBTR (*grey and white arrow*) was caudal to ablated area on coronal section

18.9 Rationale of Cryoablation and Comparison with Breast Conservative Surgery

Small breast cancer, which is less than 10 mm as lesion size, Luminal A and sentinel node negative, is known as a favorable type of breast cancer. Local control with breast conservative surgery is expected to have a low IBTR rate. The IBTR rate after breast conservative surgery is less than 1% at our institution. One patient developed IBTR among 150 patients with nonsurgical cryoablation and this result of the procedure is comparable with that of breast conservative surgery (Fig. 18.17). No thermal injury to the patients has been observed.

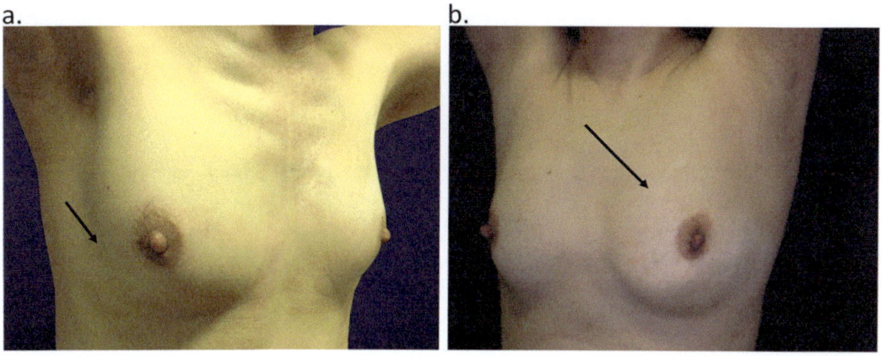

Fig. 18.19 Cosmetic effect after nonsurgical cryoablation for small breast cancer. (**a**) Thirty-two months after cryoablation in marginal area of right lower outer quadrant. (**b**) Fifty-nine months after cryoabaltion in left upper inner quadrant

18.10 Cosmetic Outcome and Long-Term Results

Cosmetic outcome after nonsurgical cryoablation is excellent (Fig. 18.19). Although induration caused by destroying the lesion and normal breast tissue is palpable for a longer time period, its size grows gradually smaller. In most patients, induration is palpable less than index finger tip size.

18.11 Conclusion

Nonsurgical cryoablation is comparable local treatment with conservative breast surgery for favorable-type small breast cancer and expansion of indication should be followed in the near future.

References

1. Gage AA. History of cryosurgery. Semin Surg Oncol. 1998;14(2):99–109.
2. Inoue M, Nakatsuka S, Yashiro H, Ito N, Izumi Y. Percutaneous cryoablation of lung tumors: feasibility and safety. J Vasc Interv Radiol. 2012;23(3):295–302.
3. Miki K, Shimomura T, Yamada H. Percutaneous cryoablation of renal cell carcinoma guided by horizontal open magnetic resonance imaging. Int J Urol. 2006;13(7):880–4.
4. Ei S, Hibi T, Tanabe M, Itano O, et al. Cryoablation provides superior local control of primary hepatocellular carcinomas of >2 cm compared with radiofrequency ablation and microwave coagulation therapy: an underestimated tool in the toolbox. Ann Surg Oncol. 2015;22 (4):1294–300.
5. Igarashi K, Yamamoto N, Shirai T, Hayashi K. The long-term outcome following the use of frozen autograft treated with liquid nitrogen in the management of bone and soft-tissue sarcomas. Bone Joint J. 2014;96-B(4):555–61.

6. Sabel MS. Nonsurgical ablation of breast cancer: future options for small breast tumors. Surg Oncol Clin N Am. 2014;23(3):593–608.
7. Sabel MS, Nehs MA, Su G, Lowler KP, et al. Immunologic response to cryoablation of breast cancer. Breast Cancer Res Treat. 2005;90(1):97–104.
8. Kaufman CS, Littrup PJ, Freeman-Gibb LA, et al. Office-based cryoablation of breast fibroadenomas with long-term follow-up. Breast J. 2005;11(5):344–50.
9. Tafra L, Fine R, Whitworth P, et al. Prospective randomized study comparing cryo-assisted and needle-wire localization of ultrasound-visible breast tumors. Am J Surg. 2006;192(4):462–70.

Chapter 19
Importance of Breast Imaging Before and After Nonsurgical Ablation Therapy

Mitsuhiro Tozaki

19.1 Terminology

"Nonsurgical ablation therapy" is a frequently used term in Japan. Performing cancer therapy without performing surgery (nonsurgical) is emphasized by this term, and it means that the technique is ablation. However, the term "image-guided tumor ablation" instead of "nonsurgical ablation" is usually used abroad [1]. The term "image-guided tumor ablation" does not include any mention of whether the breast cancer therapy is surgical or nonsurgical, and since the term simply means performing ablation during imaging, "image-guided tumor ablation" precisely expresses the fact that the technique is ablation. In Japan, an attempt to determine whether "image-guided tumor ablation" is a method of treatment that can replace current breast cancer surgery is being conducted by breast surgeons at several institutions. Consequently, the term "nonsurgical ablation" is being preferentially used in Japan for treatment in which surgery is not performed.

In this article we will explain breast tumor ablation using the term "image-guided tumor ablation" that is being used abroad.

19.2 Definition of "Image-Guided Tumor Ablation"

The term "tumor ablation" is defined as the direct application of chemical or thermal therapies to a specific focal tumor (or tumors) in an attempt to achieve eradication or substantial tumor destruction [1]. The term "direct" aims to

M. Tozaki (✉)
Department of Radiology, Sagara Hospital Affiliated Breast Center, 3-28 Tenokuchi-cho, Kagoshima city, Kagoshima, Japan 892-0845
e-mail: e-tozaki@keh.biglobe.ne.jp

T. Kinoshita (ed.), *Non-surgical Ablation Therapy for Early-stage Breast Cancer*,
DOI 10.1007/978-4-431-54463-0_19

distinguish chemical and thermal therapies used for tumor ablation from therapies that are administered orally or via an intra-arterial or peripheral venous route. Image guidance is critical to the success of direct tumor ablation therapies. Since most of direct tumor ablation therapies can be performed by using any of several imaging modalities, i.e., ultrasonography (US), computed tomography (CT), magnetic resonance imaging (MRI), fluoroscopy, and positron emission tomography (PET), unless a particular imaging modality is mandated as part of the technique, the more general term **image guidance** is preferred instead of using the name of a particular imaging modality. Theoretically, however, virtually all available ablation techniques can be used with more than one modality.

19.3 Five Steps Involved in Image-Guided Tumor Ablation

Five steps are involved in image-guided tumor ablation: planning, targeting, monitoring, controlling, and assessing treatment response [1]. Planning is the step that is performed before the ablation procedure, and assessing the response to ablation is performed after the procedure has been completed. Targeting, monitoring, and controlling are all performed during the procedure.

Planning
Imaging techniques, including US, CT, MRI, and, more recently, PET, are being used to help determine whether patients are suitable candidates for an ablation procedure. Imaging tasks that are particularly important consist of determining tumor size and shape, number, and location within the organ relative to blood vessels, as well as critical anatomical structures that might be at risk for injury during an ablation procedure.

Targeting
The term "targeting" is used to describe the step during an ablation procedure that involves placement of an applicator, e.g., a radiofrequency (RF) electrode or cryoprobe, into the tumors. While much of the current image-guided tumor ablation literature describes the use of modalities such as US and CT to target tumors for the purpose of ablating them, targeting is only one aspect of intraprocedural image guidance. The qualities of an ideal targeting technique are clear delineation of the tumor(s) and the surrounding anatomy, coupled with real-time imaging and multiplanar and interactive capabilities.

Monitoring
The term "monitoring" is used to describe the process by which the effects of therapy are viewed during a procedure. Changes in images that occur during a procedure are used to assess the effects of treatment. Important functions of monitoring include determining how well the tumor and/or target is being covered

by the ablation zone and whether any adjacent normal structures are being affected. MRI is currently the only modality with well-validated techniques for real-time temperature monitoring [2–5]. The term "monitoring" is not used for the step in which the response to treatment is assessed; that step is called "assessing response to treatment."

Controlling
This term is used to describe the intraprocedural tools and techniques that are used to control the treatment. To control an image-guided ablation procedure, the treatment should be monitorable, such so that the operator can utilize the image-based information obtained during monitoring to control it.

Assessing Treatment Response
Imaging used to assess an image-guided tumor ablation procedure is performed after the ablation procedure is completed, and this step is explained below in the "Terminology Used in Relation to Postprocedural Imaging" section.

19.4 Limitation of US for Image-Guided Tumor Ablation

In recent years, the effectiveness of image-guided tumor ablation of breast cancer has been reported [6–22]. Procedures such as radiofrequency ablation (RFA) [6–8] and high-intensity focused ultrasound (HIFU) [9–11] destroy tumor cells by heating. In contrast, cryoablation destroys cancer cells by cooling them with a cryoprobe [12–22]. Both thermal therapies are theoretically acceptable but still undergoing clinical investigation.

Regarding imaging modalities for image-guided tumor ablation of breast cancer, MRI is helpful for therapy planning, temperature monitoring, the delineation of the ablation zone, the detection of residual disease (assessing treatment response), and follow-up after treatment [8, 18, 22]. On the other hand, the widely adopted US-guided tumor ablation is most effective for only the targeting step.

One disadvantage of US-guided tumor ablation is the difficulty in visualizing the ablation zone. For instance, visualizing the area behind the ice ball is difficult in performing US-guided cryoablation because of acoustic shadowing. Only the surface of the ice ball facing the transducer can be delineated using US, possibly limiting evaluations of whether the tumor has been completely encased [17]. For these reasons, MRI-guided ablation may be more excellent than US-guided ablation. Particularly the inability to use it to evaluate the ablation zone (assessing treatment response) immediately after tumor ablation must be said to be the greatest shortcoming of US-guided tumor ablation in regard to cancer therapy. However, because of the technical convenience of US-guided needle insertion and limitations in the availability of MR-compatible devices, US-guided RFA or US-guided cryoablation is more commonly performed.

19.5 Importance of MRI for Image-Guided Tumor Ablation

Manenti et al. [8] reported that postablation MR images after RFA were strongly correlated with the results of histological analyses. Postablation MR images are helpful for measuring the ablation zone and evaluating the presence of any residual tumor. In addition, the ablation of appropriate margins beyond the borders of the tumor is necessary to achieve complete tumor destruction. Postablation MR images are also helpful for measuring the ablative margin.

19.5.1 MRI-Guided Tumor Ablation (Cryoablation): Articles in the World

As for MRI-guided cryoablation, only two papers have been published [19, 20]. Morin et al. [19] studied the use of MRI-guided cryoablation for 25 invasive cancers (range, 12–60 mm; mean, 30 mm). They used a 0.5-T open-configuration MR system, and MR images were acquired with a standard transmit-receive linear surface square coil placed directly over the treated breast. The authors found that MRI was very adequate for discriminating between the tumor and the ice ball, and no viable tumor cells were found in any of the pathologic region covered by the ice ball. However, the MRI protocol used in their study, which lacked a dedicated breast coil, utilized a supine patient position, and a relatively thick imaging slice (5 mm) was insufficient for demonstrating the utility of MRI, compared with the current standard MRI protocol for the breast. High-resolution MR images using a dedicated breast coil may be even more helpful for therapy planning and verification of the nonsurgical ablation of breast cancer.

In another study on MRI-guided cryoablation, Pusztaszeri et al. [20] treated 11 patients with invasive breast cancers less than 25 mm in size. The treatment was unsuccessful in one case because of technical problems, and the tumor was found adjacent to the ablation zone during a histopathological examination in this case. However, the MRI sequences, MR coils, and technical details of cryoprobe insertion were not mentioned in their paper. In addition, skin ulceration and/or necrosis was observed in five patients. To avoid frostbite of the skin, the injection of saline under the skin near the ice ball has been reported to be useful [18].

19.5.2 MRI-Guided Cryoablation: Initial Experience in Kameda Hospital (Figs. 19.1, 19.2, and 19.3)

The cryoablation system and US were set up outside the MR room (Fig. 19.1). A 1.5-Tesla MR unit (Avanto; Siemens Medical Solutions, Erlangen, Germany) and

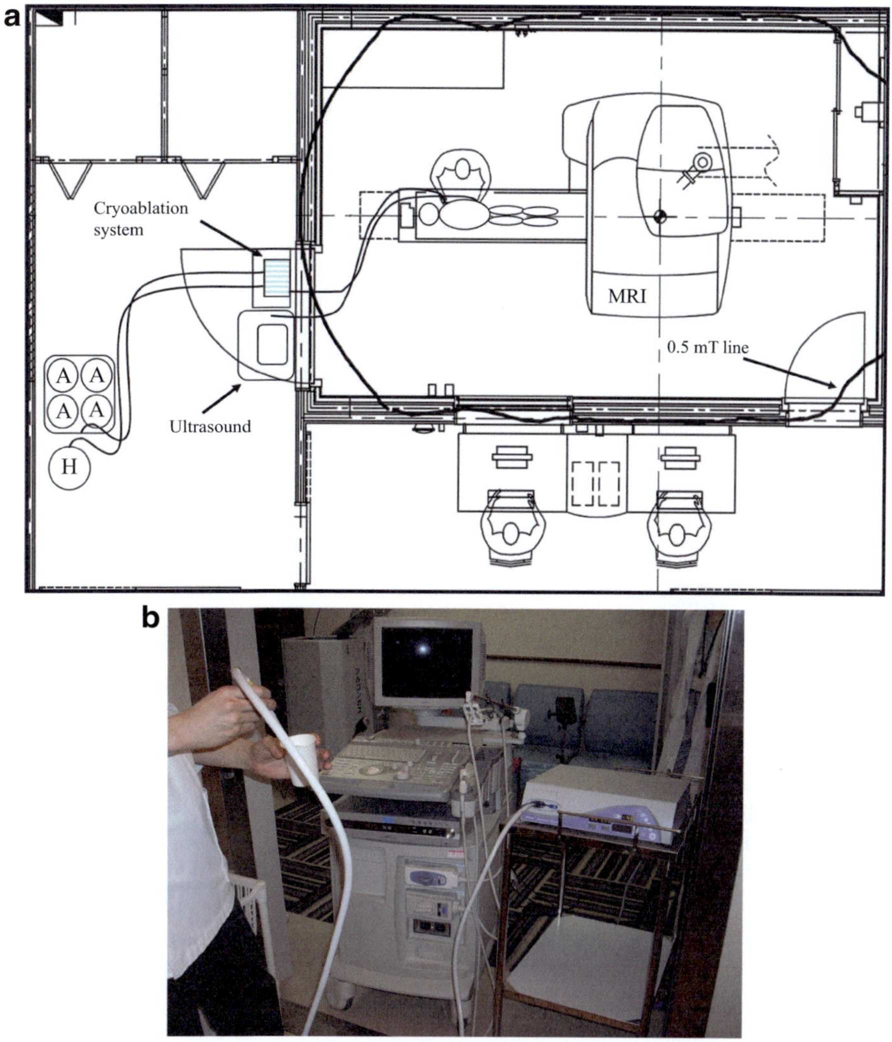

Fig. 19.1 Illustration (**a**) and picture (**b**) of the cryoablation system. Ultrasound, helium, (H) and argon (A) gas canisters and a tabletop cryoablation system were set up outside the magnetic resonance (MR) room

dedicated breast coil (7-channel or 4-channel breast biopsy coil; Siemens Medical Solutions, Erlangen, Germany) were used. US (SSD-4000; Aloka, Tokyo, Japan) with a 10-MHz linear probe was performed before and during the cryoablation.

The actual procedure consisted of the following steps:

Therapy Planning

1. The patient was placed in a prone position over the coil, and the breast was moderately compressed using the compression plates (Fig. 19.2a).

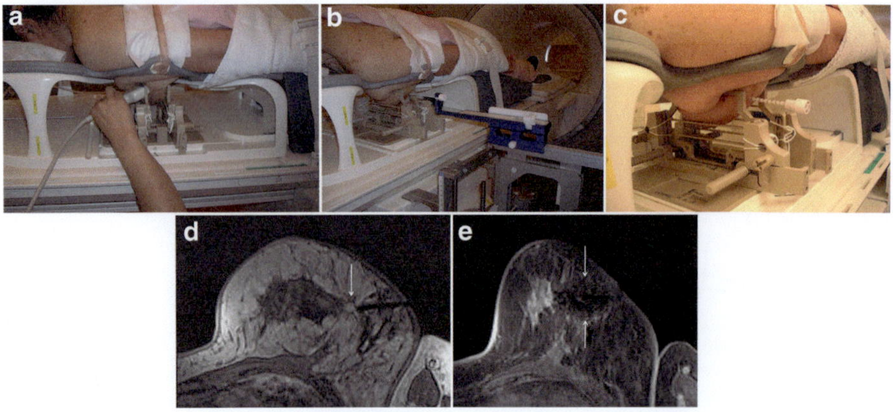

Fig. 19.2 MRI-guided cryoablation (case 1). (**a**) The breast was moderately compressed using the compression plates. (**b**) Using the same technique of MRI-guided breast biopsy, the MR-compatible puncture needle was advanced to the appropriate depth. (**c**) The plastic tube of the puncture needle was left in the breast. (**d**) Transverse contrast-enhanced T1-weighted MR image shows an enhanced tumor (*arrow*) and the inserted plastic tube. (**e**) Transverse contrast-enhanced, fat-suppressed T1-weighted MR image shows that tumor is completely encased within the ablation zone (*arrows*)

2. Before the injection of the contrast material, sagittal and transverse three-dimensional volumetric interpolated breath-hold examination (3D-VIBE) sequences without fat suppression were performed (TR/TE, 4.3/1.4; flip angle, 15°; field of view, 16 cm; matrix size, 192 × 192; slice thickness, 1 mm; time of acquisition, 61 s).
3. After the intravenous injection of 10 mL of Gd-DTPA from a 20-mL syringe (Magnevist®, Bayer Yakuhin Ltd., Japan), sagittal and transverse 3D-VIBE sequences with fat suppression were performed (TR/TE, 4.3/1.4; flip angle, 15°; field of view, 16 cm; matrix size, 192 × 192; slice thickness, 1 mm; time of acquisition, 66 s).
4. The distances between the tumor margin and the surrounding tissue (skin and thoracic muscle) were calculated using three perpendicular planes (sagittal, transverse, and coronal multiplanar reconstruction images).

Targeting

5. The patient was removed from the magnet.
6. After cleansing the skin, a local anesthesia was applied and a skin nick was made with a scalpel. Using the same technique of MRI-guided breast biopsy [23], the MR-compatible puncture needle was advanced to the appropriate depth (Fig. 19.2b), and the plastic tube of the puncture needle was left in the breast (Fig. 19.2c).

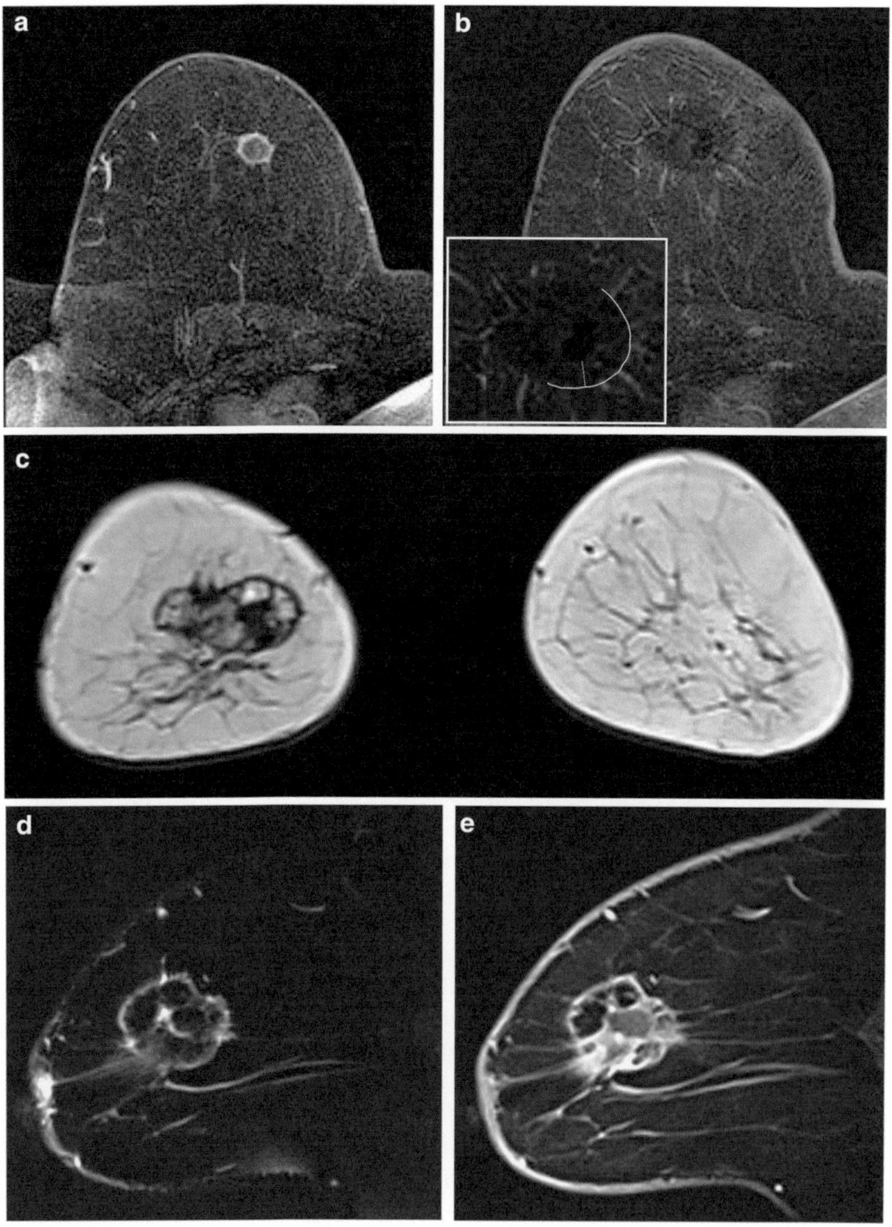

Fig. 19.3 MRI-guided cryoablation (case 2). (**a**) Transverse contrast-enhanced fat-suppressed T1-weighted MR image demonstrates a 12 mm-sized enhanced mass without surrounding intraductal extension. (**b**) Transverse contrast-enhanced fat-suppressed T1-weighted MR image shows that the non-enhanced tumor is completely encased within the ablation zone. Inset shows the border of the ablation zone (*solid line*), and the minimum ablative margin (*dotted line*) is 6.5 mm. (**c**) Coronal T1 weighted MR image obtained 9 weeks after cryoablation demonstrates the well-delineated ablation zone. (**d**) Sagittal fat-suppressed T2-weighted MR image obtained 9 weeks after cryoablation demonstrates the hypointense tumor encased within the ablation zone. (**e**) Sagittal contrast-enhanced fat-suppressed T1-weighted MR image obtained 9 weeks

7. After verifying the appropriate location of the plastic tube (Fig. 19.2d), the cryoprobe was advanced into the tumor under US guidance.
8. Central placement within the tumor was confirmed using two orthogonal planes.

Cryoablation

9. Immediately after creation of the ice ball, breast compression was removed.
10. We performed cryoablation using a double-freeze-thaw protocol. A passive thaw lasting 10 min was interposed between the two high freeze cycles, and an active thaw with helium gas was performed after the second freeze.
11. During cyroablation, saline was injected under the skin near the ice ball as required to avoid causing frostbite on the skin.
12. The cryoprobe was removed during the active thaw with helium gas.

Verification of Treatment

13. After the completion of cryoablation, the patient was moved into the magnet again.
14. Sagittal and transverse fat-suppressed T2-weighted images (TR/TE, 8750/94; field of view, 16 cm; matrix, 179 × 256; slice thickness, 3 mm; and time of acquisition, 79 s) were obtained. After verifying the creation of the ice ball (Fig. 19.2e), 3D VIBE sequence with fat suppression was performed before and after intravenous injection of the remaining 10 mL of Gd-DTPA in the 20-mL syringe.

One advantage of performing MRI immediately before cryoablation is therapy planning. MRI can be used to predict sites in danger of coming into contact with the increasing ice ball using three perpendicular images. In our protocol, the breast was temporarily compressed using compression plates to facilitate the insertion of the cryoprobe into the tumor. However, the breast compression was removed immediately after creation of the ice ball. Another advantage of MRI was the ability to verify the site of cryoablation. MR images obtained immediately after cryoablation are thought to be useful to both the operators and the patients.

Regarding cryoprobe insertion into the tumor (targeting), Morin et al. [19] reported that the breast was transfixed with an 18-gauge puncture needle through the long axis of the tumor under US guidance. Considering the indications of cryoablation, i.e., a small size (<15 mm) and localized tumor without surrounding DCIS, cryoprobe insertion under US guidance may be easier and safer than insertion under MRI guidance for US-visible breast cancers.

We used the MRI-guided breast biopsy technique to insert an MR-compatible puncture needle as far as the tumor margin. We then inserted the cryoprobe into the trocar, and inserted the cryoprobe inside the tumor, guided by US. The combination of needle insertion into the tumor under US guidance with therapy planning and verification of cryoablation using MRI may be a feasible and promising treatment

Fig. 19.3 (continued) after cryoablation demonstrates a 12 mm-sized non-enhanced mass in the ablation zone with peripheral enhancement (benign periablational enhancement)

protocol. If the MR-compatible cryoablation system is approved under the Pharmaceutical Affairs Act in Japan in the future, MRI-guided cryoablation may become more widely adopted. Moreover, this is an age when multiple cryoprobes are being used, and time and energy are being wasted by using a single cryoprobe as in this technique. Performing MRI-guided cryoablation with more than one cryoprobe in the future is definitely not a dream. When it becomes a reality, even broader indications are anticipated, and we hope that the number of breast cancer patients who receive the benefits of nonsurgical cryoablation will increase.

19.6 Terminology Used in Relation to Postprocedural Imaging

Ablation Zone

The term “ablation zone” is used to describe the radiologic region or zone where the effect of the ablation is visible, i.e., the area of gross tumor destruction visualized by imaging.

Ablative Margin

The term “ablative margin” is used for the margin beyond the border of the tumor that needs to be destroyed in order to achieve complete tumor destruction (Fig. 19.3b). For highly vascular organs, such as the kidney and liver, creation of an ablative margin results in low attenuation and absent perfusion zones that extend into the parenchyma.

Benign Periablational Enhancement

“Benign periablational enhancement” is a transient finding that is seen during both pathology examinations and contrast-enhanced imaging examinations, and its presence suggests a benign physiologic response to thermal injury in the form of reactive hyperemia initially and fibrosis and a giant cell reaction later [24]. Depending on the protocol used for contrast-enhanced imaging, i.e., the injection rate and scanning delay, benign periablational enhancement is seen immediately after the ablation procedure and may persist for as long as 6 months. It usually appears in the form of a penumbra, or a thin rim peripheral to the zone of ablation (Fig. 19.3e), that typically measures up to 5 mm acutely but most often measures 1–2 mm. It is a relatively concentric, symmetric, and uniform zone with smooth inner margins, and it needs to be differentiated from “irregular peripheral enhancement.”

Irregular Peripheral Enhancement

The term “irregular peripheral enhancement” is used to describe the imaging findings that are seen when residual tumor is present at the margin of the ablation zone. Residual unablated tumor often grows in a scattered, nodular, or eccentric pattern. Irregular peripheral enhancement indicates incomplete local treatment, i.e., the presence of residual unablated tumor. If left untreated, the residual tumor tends to continue to grow. Because of the delayed enhancement characteristics of many hypovascular tumors, this finding is often best appreciated by comparing delayed images with the baseline images.

19.7 Conclusion

In this article we have explained the importance of breast imaging before and after nonsurgical ablation therapy. First, we provided a simple explanation of the difference in the meaning of the term “nonsurgical ablation” in Japan and abroad. Next, we described the advantages and limitations of ultrasonography during the performance of nonsurgical ablation therapy, and we explained the usefulness of MRI. We have also stated our personal opinions regarding the current status and future prospects for MRI-guided tumor ablation, and we have interspersed our experience with cryoablation at our own institution into our explanation. Finally, we have explained the proper terminology that should be used in regard to imaging after performing nonsurgical ablation. Needless to say, “imaging” both before and after image-guided tumor ablation plays a very important role. We hope that this article will be useful in the proper popularization of image-guided tumor ablation.

References

1. Goldberg SN, Grassi CJ, Cardella JF, et al. Image-guided tumor ablation: standardization of terminology and reporting criteria. Radiology. 2005;235:728–39.
2. Silverman SG, Tuncali K, Adams DF, et al. MR imaging-guided percutaneous cryotherapy of liver tumors: initial experience. Radiology. 2000;217:657–64.
3. Quesson B, de Zwart JA, Moonen CT. Magnetic resonance temperature imaging for guidance of thermotherapy. J Magn Reson Imaging. 2000;12:525–33.
4. Lewin JS, Connell CF, Duerk JL, et al. Interactive MRI-guided radiofrequency interstitial thermal ablation of abdominal tumors: clinical trial for evaluation of safety and feasibility. J Magn Reson Imaging. 1998;8:40–7.
5. Vogl TJ, Muller PK, Hammerrstingl R, et al. Malignant liver tumors treated with MR imaging-guided laser-induced thermotherapy: technique and prospective results. Radiology. 1995;196:257–65.
6. Fornage BD, Sneige N, Ross MI, et al. Small (< or = 2-cm) breast cancer treated with US-guided radiofrequency ablation: feasibility study. Radiology. 2004;231:215–24.
7. Oura S, Tamaki T, Hirai I, et al. Radiofrequency ablation therapy in patients with breast cancers two centimeters or less in size. Breast Cancer. 2007;14:48–54.
8. Manenti G, Bolacchi F, Perretta T, et al. Small breast cancers: in vivo percutaneous US-guided radiofrequency ablation with dedicated cool-tip radiofrequency system. Radiology. 2009;251:339–46.
9. Wu F, Wang ZB, Cao YD, et al. A randomised clinical trial of high-intensity focused ultrasound ablation for the treatment of patients with localised breast cancer. Br J Cancer. 2003;89:2227–33.

10. Gianfelice D, Khiat A, Amara M, Belblidia A, Boulanger Y. MR imaging-guided focused US ablation of breast cancer: histopathologic assessment of effectiveness- initial experience. Radiology. 2003;227:849–55.
11. Furusawa H, Namba K, Thomsen S, et al. Magnetic resonance-guided focused ultrasound surgery of breast cancer: reliability and effectiveness. J Am Coll Surg. 2006;203:54–63.
12. Rand RW, Rand RP, Eggerding FA, et al. Cryolumpectomy for breast cancer: an experimental study. Cryobiology. 1985;22:307–18.
13. Staren ED, Sabel MS, Gianakakis LM, et al. Cryosurgery of breast cancer. Arch Surg. 1997;132:28–33.
14. Pfleiderer SO, Freesmeyer MG, Marx C, Kühne-Heid R, Schneider A, Kaiser WA. Cryotherapy of breast cancer under ultrasound guidance: initial results and limitations. Eur Radiol. 2002;12:3009–14.
15. Pfleiderer SO, Marx C, Camara O, Gajda M, Kaiser WA. Ultrasound-guided, percutaneous cryotherapy of small (< or = 15 mm) breast cancers. Invest Radiol. 2005;40:472–7.
16. Sabel MS, Kaufman CS, Whitworth P, et al. Cryoablation of early-stage breast cancer: work-in-progress report of a multi-institutional trial. Ann Surg Oncol. 2004;11:542–9.
17. Roubidoux MA, Sabel MS, Bailey JE, Kleer CG, Klein KA, Helvie MA. Small (<2.0-cm) breast cancers: mammographic and US findings at US-guided cryoablation-initial experience. Radiology. 2004;233:857–67.
18. Ozaki S, Fukuma E, Tozaki M, et al. The use of non-surgical cryoablation for minimal breast cancer. J Jpn Surg Assoc. 2008;69:3038–47. (Japanese with English abstract).
19. Morin J, Traoré A, Dionne G, et al. Magnetic resonance-guided percutaneous cryosurgery of breast carcinoma: technique and early clinical results. Can J Surg. 2004;47:347–51.
20. Pusztaszeri M, Vlastos G, Kinkel K, Pelte MF. Histopathological study of breast cancer and normal breast tissue after magnetic resonance-guided cryotherapy ablation. Cryobiology. 2007;55:44–51.
21. Littrup PJ, Jallad B, Chandiwala-Mody P, D'Agostini M, Adam BA, Bouwman D. Cryotherapy for breast cancer: a feasibility study without excision. J Vasc Interv Radiol. 2009;20:1329–41.
22. Tozaki M, Fukuma E, Suzuki T, Hoshi K. Ultrasound-guided cryoablation of invasive ductal carcinoma inside the MR room. Magn Reson Med Sci. 2010;9:31–6.
23. Tozaki M, Yamashiro N, Sakamoto M, Sakamoto N, Mizuuchi N, Fukuma E. MR-guided vacuum-assisted breast biopsy: results in 100 Japanese women. Jpn J Radiol. 2010;28:527–33.
24. Goldberg SN, Gazelle GS, Compton CC, Mueller PR, Tanabe KK. Treatment of intrahepatic malignancy with radiofrequency ablation: radiologic-pathologic correlation. Cancer. 2000;88:2452–63.

Chapter 20
Future and Development of Nonsurgical Ablation of Breast Cancer

Shoshu Mitsuyama

20.1 Introduction

Breast cancer is the most frequently occurring female cancer, and the highest cause of mortality from cancer in women worldwide. In Japan, breast cancer is increasing, and at present, approximately 70,000 patients a year contract the disease, making it the top-ranking female cancer. Mammography (MMG) screening for breast cancer started in Japan in 2000. Thereafter, the frequency of Stage 0 and I in 2011 became 19.2 %, approximately two times that in 2004, and the rate is expected to continue to increase in the near future if the checkup rate for breast cancer screening rises the same as in the United States of America (USA) and European countries. Basically, treatment of breast cancer is a surgical therapy. A big clinical trial conducted by Fisher et al. [1, 2] revealed that breast-conserving surgery (BCS) followed by radiotherapy is equivalent to a mastectomy in the long-term survival rate of patients in the USA.

Therefore, BCS is mostly performed in patients with early-stage breast cancer worldwide, and the rate of BCS is approximately 60 % in Japan now [3]. The main goals of breast-conserving therapy (BCT), which includes BCS combined with radiotherapy, are cosmetically acceptable preserved breasts and favorable results of long-term survival and in-breast recurrence (IBR). However, breast cancer patients are not fully satisfied with the cosmetic results after BCT, and it occasionally causes patients' complaints and anxiety. Patients in Asian countries who have smaller breasts are the most likely to be dissatisfied with the cosmetic outcome after BCT. Therefore, oncoplastic surgery to fill the defects of the preserved breast after BCS is warranted in this population. Two kinds of techniques are commonly used for good

S. Mitsuyama (✉)
Kitakyushu Municipal Medical Center, 2-1-1 Bashaku, Kokurakita-ku, Kitakyushu, Fukuoka 802-0077, Japan
e-mail: shomi@crest.ocn.ne.jp

T. Kinoshita (ed.), *Non-surgical Ablation Therapy for Early-stage Breast Cancer*,
DOI 10.1007/978-4-431-54463-0_20

cosmetic results with a volume displacement or volume replacement method. Autologous fat grafting as a lipofilling [4] might also represent an important role to fill up a deformity after BCT.

Endoscopic BCS is a new minimally invasive technique. Some clinical studies [5–7] have shown that it is safe and has good cosmetic outcome. It is getting popular now in Japan, but to excise a tumor it needs two skin incisions and two-port method; one is in the axilla and the other is in the areolar region. On the other hand, Yamashita et al. [8] reported good cosmetic results using a one-port method in the axillary region as an excellent endoscopic BCS.

Based on this background, minimally invasive therapy (MIT), especially nonsurgical ablation (NSA) therapy, has been explored with the intention of achieving equivalent efficacy but with improved cosmetic results compared to standard BCT. By using either a percutaneous or extracorporeal approach, a targeted breast tumor is destroyed, while a destructive energy is transmitted into the breast mass instead of surgical removal. Various kinds of energy are employed to raise temperature or to drop temperature to the heating or freezing point in the targeted mass. Several modalities, such as radiofrequency ablation (RFA), high-intensity focused ultrasound (HIFU) surgery, cryoablation (CA), laser ablation, and microwave ablation, have been investigated for this purpose. The RFA, HIFU, and CA as MIT for breast cancer are attractive and popular in Japan. Each method has unique characteristics in thermal ablation technique, as summarized in Table 20.1.

As for heavy ion radiotherapy, a preliminary clinical trial was started in Japan in 2013 for breast cancer patients more than 60 years old with tumor size less than 2.0 cm, but there is no available data about it yet.

The movement to MIT in breast cancer treatment is expanding to axillary lymph node dissection now. The lymph node dissection can be omitted for patients with negative node or micro-metastasis less than 2 mm by a sentinel lymph node biopsy

Table 20.1 Comparison of thermal ablation techniques for breast cancer

Thermal ablation methods	Radiofrequency ablation (RFA)	Cryoablation (CA)	High-intensity focused ultrasound surgery (HIFU)
Energy conduction and ablation	Heat, not conformal	Cold, not conformal	Heat, conformal
Energy delivery through skin	Percutaneous, with an electrode probe	Percutaneous with an applicator	Transcutaneous with no probe insertion
Imaging guidance	Ultrasound	Ultrasound	Ultrasound, MRI
Ablation time (varies with tumor size)	10–30 min	15–30 min	30–120 min
Complete ablation	76–100 %	36–83 %	20–100 %
Side effects after ablation	Moderate discomfort, skin burn	Minimal discomfort	Moderate discomfort, skin burn
Required anesthesia	IV sedation, general, local	Local	IV sedation, general

IV intravenous

Modified from Z. Zhao. F.Wu/EJSO36 (2010) 1150

Table 20.2 Questions related to nonsurgical ablation therapy

1. Proper indication
Tumor size
Distance between tumor and skin, nipple, and underlying muscle layer
Accurate diagnostic modality for EIC
Nonpoor prognostic and predictive factors:
ER negativity, HER2 positivity, high Ki-67 value
Invasive lobular carcinoma
Neoadjuvant therapy
Multicentricity
BRCA positivity
2. Kind of device, method, and maneuver
3. Appropriate time for SNB and indication for SN-positive patient
4. Method for judgment of effectiveness
Appropriate time
Image modality
Place of CNB performed
Appropriate histopathological staining method (HE, NADH, ssDNA)
Standard criteria for judgment
5. Radiation therapy
Indication of hypofractionated radiotherapy
Need of boost irradiation
6. Adverse events
7. Evaluation of cosmetic result
8. Long-term in-breast recurrence and overall survival rate

(SNB) [9], and it is becoming globally accepted that axillary dissection can be safely omitted in patients with one or two positive sentinel nodes when whole breast radiation is planned followed BCS [10, 11]. Compared with conventional BCS, the main advantages of NSA are that it is much less invasive because of no incision, less scarring, less pain, and shorter recovery time. NSA combined with no axillary lymph node dissection is ideal for breast cancer patients as a benefit of early detection of small breast cancer.

With the widespread application of screening MMG for breast cancer, the detected cancer continues to decrease in size. Therefore, the need for a nonsurgical therapy (NST) using RFA, HIFU, and CA without axillary dissection for early-stage small breast cancer is strongly emphasized. The ultimate goal of NST is not to be inferior in long-term safety, such as IBR and overall survival (OS), but to be superior in cosmetic outcome compared to the standard BCT. But there are no available data of long-term results, and many questions remain to be resolved.

The aim of this paper is to review published data of MIT, especially RFA, HIFU, and CS, and to propose many kinds of questions to be resolved, as shown in Table 20.2, for patients with early-stage small breast cancer by some prospective clinical trials in the future.

20.2 Radiofrequency Ablation (RFA)

The first study of RFA for breast cancer was performed by Jeffrey et al. [12] in 1999, and a complete ablation was found by resected specimens in four of five enrolled patients without complication. Subsequently, several feasibility studies in the world were conducted to evaluate the effectiveness of RFA followed by surgical resection for small breast cancer [13–23]. These studies suggested that RFA could be effective for local control of small, well localized breast cancer, with less complication. It was reported that the average rate of complete coagulation necrosis and skin burn as complication was 87 % and 3 % for tumors less than 2.0 cm in diameter, respectively [14–18, 20, 22, 23]. Based on the good results of these feasibility studies, several trials for RFA have been performed without surgical excision, and the reported effectiveness of RFA was that no IBR was encountered for tumors less than 2.0 cm in diameter between follow-up of 2 and 82 months [24–28]. Head et al. [29] reported that three of five elderly patients with non-palpable cancers were treated and followed for up to 7 years and no IBR occurred without resection after RFA.

In Japan, there are several excellent data of RFA with and without resection.

Oura et al. [24] performed RFA followed by radiation therapy in 52 patients with a localized tumor less than 2.0 cm in diameter, and no patient had viable cancer cells in the ablated lesion on postoperative cytological assessment. No recurrence encountered at a mean follow-up of 15 months after RFA. Noguchi et al. [30] conducted RFA followed by an ultrasound (US)-guided mammotome biopsy for 18 patients with 2.0 cm in greatest diameter and reported that a complete response was histologically observed only in 8 of 18 cases (44 %), but NADH-diaphorase and ssDNA dying did not demonstrate any viable tumor cells in the ablated lesions. There was no case of local recurrence at a mean follow-up of 60 months. Kinoshita et al. [21] finished a clinical trial of Phase I/II for 50 breast cancer cases with tumor diameter less than 3.0 cm to evaluate the usefulness of RFA followed by resection as a substitute treatment of BCS in 2006 and reported that the complete ablation rate was 83 % and 85 % for tumor diameter less than 2.0 cm and for that of without extensive intraductal components (EIC) by a histopathological examination, respectively.

As a next step, Kinoshita et al. conducted a prospective multicenter clinical study called Radiofrequency Ablation Therapy for Early Breast Cancer as Local Therapy (RAFAELO) in 2013 to evaluate the efficacy and to standardize RFA without resection for early-stage breast cancer. The inclusion criterion was mainly ductal carcinoma with tumor diameter less than 1.5 cm on MMG, US, and MRI. The primary endpoint is a 5-year IBR rate, and the secondary endpoints are incomplete ablation rate, OS, disease-free survival (DFS), and adverse events (AE).

In 2005, the Breast Cancer Society for Minimally Invasive Therapy was founded in Japan for the purpose of contributing to the welfare of breast cancer patients, and many members have reported several feasibility or observational studies on the use of RFA. As a preliminary investigation for the next multi-institutional clinical trial,

520 cases of RFA therapy with no resection performed were accumulated from ten main institutions to clarify the safety and AE. The report revealed that 25 patients (4.8 %) developed IBR at a mean follow-up of 45 months, and the IBR-free survival rate in patients with tumor diameter less than 2.0 cm was significantly superior to that in patients with tumor more than 2.1 cm [unpublished data]. The risk factors for IBR were revealed as follows: ER negativity, HER2 positivity, lymph node metastases, no radiation therapy, adjuvant chemotherapy after RFA, and neoadjuvant treatment. In addition, the rate of RFA-induced nipple damage and skin burn was 1.3 % and 2.9 %, respectively. Persistent induration in the ablated lesion was observed in 193 cases (37 %). Finally, breast cancer less than 2.0 cm in diameter without high risk factors was recommended to be suitable as an appropriate candidate for RFA in Japan, and induration formation was regarded as an important complication.

Thereafter, a prospective multi-institutional Phase II clinical trial for nonsurgical RFA was started in 2012 in Japan based on these preliminary results. The inclusion criteria are ductal breast cancer with Stage 0 or Stage I, non-macrometastasis by SNB, and non-EIC. The primary endpoint is complete ablation rate on histopathological evaluation, and the secondary endpoints are safety, cosmetic result, 10 years recurrence-free survival (RFS), and OS. MRI and a US-guided (USg) core needle biopsy (CNB) are planned at 4 weeks after RFA, and multi-biopsied specimens are performed by histopathological evaluation using HE and NADH dying, and if judged there is no residual cancer, patients are going to be followed for 10 years after adjuvant therapy and breast irradiation, but surgical resection is enforced for patients with residual cancer. Cosmetic outcome is evaluated every year using criteria of the Japanese Breast Cancer Society. These two prospective clinical trials have already started in Japan, and many of the questions in Table 20.2 are expected to be resolved from the results of these clinical trials. Many results in Japan and foreign countries have revealed that tumor more than 2.1 cm in diameter is significantly higher than tumor of 2.0 cm or less in the IBR rate, and tumor size less than 2.0 cm is thought to be a proper candidate for RFA. Two prospective clinical trials are now ongoing for tumors less than 2.0 cm in diameter and 1.5 cm in Japan.

It is mandatory to ablate to 1.0 cm a normal breast tissue together with a tumor in successful RFA. Therefore, a minimum distance of at least 1.0 cm between tumor and skin, nipple, and pectoral muscle will be necessary for NSA.

EIC is reported to be a predictive factor for IBR, and a special radiologist, especially for MRI, should be involved in accurate evaluation on MMG, US, and MRI.

ER negativity, HER2 positivity, and high Ki-67 value might be excluded for their poor prognostic factor, but the conclusion will be delivered many from ongoing trials.

Invasive lobular carcinoma should be excluded because of difficulty to identify the extent of the disease, both clinically and histopathologically.

In addition, the cases after performance of neoadjuvant therapy should enter the exclusion criteria because many IBRs have occurred in this population in Japanese surveys, but in the future, some selected cases with a small, well defined tumor after neoadjuvant therapy might be candidates for RFA.

So-called luminal A-like breast cancer with less than 2.0 cm in diameter and no EIC is considered to be a proper candidate for RFA without resection.

Multifocal breast cancer is usually thought to be noncandidate for RFA. Breast cancer patients with BRCA positive seem to have a tendency of multifocal lesion in the breast, and total mastectomy is recommended internationally at present [31], even if it is possible to perform BCS. Therefore, the BRCA-positive patients might be excluded from RFA.

Many reports have already been published about devices, methods, and maneuvers.

A cool-tip radiofrequency needle electrode is generally used and inserted into the center of a tumor. The method and maneuver are standardized to some extent now, but the procedure should be performed by an operator who is fully trained and experienced in interventional breast US, because the operator must push forward the tip of the needle into the center of the tumor to achieve complete ablation and prevention of complications, such as skin and underlying muscle burns. In one Japanese trial, RFA was strictly restricted to institutions in which more than five cases have been experienced. It is desirable that a metallic marker be left in the center of the ablated tumor to facilitate evaluation of the effectiveness with imaging after RFA.

SNB is essential at present, but abbreviation might be possible in the future if an evaluation of axillary lymph node status is enabled exactly with an improved or a newly developed image modality. As for an appropriate time for SNB, there are two kinds of method. One is that the SNB is performed on the same day just before RFA, and the other is to perform SNB on a day before RFA. Their benefits and disadvantages should be discussed and resolved. In addition, many panelists in the consensus meeting of St. Gallen 2013 [11] believed that the axillary dissection could be safely omitted in patients with one or two positive sentinel nodes when whole breast radiation therapy following BCS is planned. No dissection for patients with micro-metastasis less than 2 mm is accepted internationally now [9]. These concepts are adapted only for BCS at present, but could expand to NSA in the future.

An evaluation of complete ablation is difficult after RFA without resection. Evaluation by MMG, US, MRI, and PET is required, and Vilar et al. [32] reported that MRI is effective in detecting residual lesions after RFA. But the judgment should be entrusted to an experienced radiologist for MRI because the image is thought to be difficult to evaluate after RFA and radiation. Therefore, the assessment of the efficacy of RFA always requires not only an image by MRI but also histopathological confirmation [33]. MRI-guided CNB is desirable for an abnormal lesion detected by MRI, but the available facilities are limited.

When and where a tissue biopsy should be performed after RFA is an important issue. In clinical trials, some kinds of CNB methods are recommended for the ablated lesion included in the center and marginal place of an ex-tumor at 1 or 3 months after RFA, together with image evaluation.

But a conventional histopathological evaluation by H&E staining for the ablated tissue shows a spectrum of changes ranging from necrosis to nearly normal tissue after RFA. The H&E staining alone is not always reliable in demonstrating the viability of cancer cells. A useful NADH-diaphorase staining has been introduced to evaluate the effectiveness [34, 35], but it needs a tissue to be snap-frozen immediately in liquid nitrogen, and it is difficult to cut a frozen section when the tissue consists predominantly of adipose tissue. But both H&E and NADH-diaphorase staining are still essential to evaluate tumor cell viability for successful RFA. Motoyoshi et al. [36] reported that ssDNA staining might be useful for assessment of cell viability when there is some interval after RFA. The development of excellent staining is further expected for the evaluation of viable cancer cells. In addition, histopathological criteria are necessary to clarify the complete ablation with no remnant viable cancer cells. In near future, the criteria for effectiveness after RFA should be ruled out by pathologists specialized in breast cancer, and a central histopathological committee should judge the effectiveness based on the rule in clinical trials.

Conventional radiation therapy is essential after RFA, the same as after BCS. But a hypofractionated radiotherapy such as 40 Gy in 15 or 42.5 Gy in 16 fractions is supported by a big clinical trial [37] for selected early-staged breast cancer patients after BCS, and this short course whole breast radiation therapy has advantages in terms of cost patients' convenience. This useful modality will be applicable for patients more than 60 years old with early-stage breast cancer after RFA. A need for boost irradiation is unknown after RFA.

The cosmetic result and AE are as important issues as curability for breast cancer, but RFA itself has hardly any problems because the wound is inconspicuous without resection, but it is important to consider complications, particularly skin burn, that could spoil the cosmetic result. The burn rate is very low, as many investigators have shown, but the induration in the ablated breast causes patients' dissatisfaction and anxiety. Therefore, if the induration remains for a long time, its removal by some device should be considered for the relief and evaluation of remnant or recurrent breast cancer. Oura et al. [24] showed that cosmetic results after RFA were excellent in 83 %, good in 12 %, and fair in 6 % with a mean follow-up of 15 months. Noguchi et al. [28] reported that cosmetic results were assessed as excellent in 95 % after RFA followed by mammotome biopsy at a median follow-up of 60 months, and most patients were satisfied with the cosmetic results of the preserved breast. But there is no data of a long-term (more than 5 years) cosmetic result yet. An excellent long-term cosmetic result could be revealed in ongoing clinical trials with fair evaluation.

Long-term results, such as IBR and OS rates, are the most important items. Ito et al. [38] showed that a tumor less than 2.0 cm in diameter is considered to be comparable to that of BCS in terms of IBR rate from multi-institutional retrospective accumulated data for RFA without surgical excision for a mean follow-up of 50 months in Japan, but long-term follow-up data is still unknown. In the future, an excellent result of IBR and OS rate could be expected by nonsurgical RFA for a localized tumor with less than 2.0 cm, non-EIC, node negative, and no poor-risk biomarker.

New Challenges for RFA as a Promising Strategy

1. Rechallenge for IBR after RFA
2. RFA for IBR after BCT
3. Aged patients with advanced disease

The treatment or management for IBR after RFA depends on the recurrence site (ablated or other site) and type (solitary or multiple). No data for management is available, but rechallenge of RFA might be thought possible if the patient desired RFA instead of a surgical treatment.

Mastectomy is a standard treatment for IBR or a new cancer in the ablated breast after BCT at present, but whether or not RFA therapy is suitable for such cases is an interesting question and should be resolved.

Susini et al. [39] reported a result of RFA for three elderly patients with inoperable breast cancer, and no evidence of local recurrence was found by MRI and CNB after a follow-up of 18 months. Marcy et al. [40] also reported a result of RFA after hormonal therapy for four inoperable elderly patients, and no breast recurrence was encountered in three of the patients with a median follow-up of 15 months. The follow-up periods were too short to allow investigation of the effectiveness for elderly patients with advanced disease, but RFA is promising as a local therapy for aged patients with advanced disease or severe morbidity.

20.3 High-Intensity Focused Ultrasound Surgery (HIFU)

This treatment is the most noninvasive approach in MIT for breast cancer at present. It employs an extracorporeal ultrasound energy to ablate a targeted tumor at depth, without any needle insertion. Two kinds of modalities, MRI and US, are available as image guidance.

Ultrasound-Guided HIFU (USgHIFU)
Wu et al. [41] reported a good result from a prospective Phase III clinical trial. USgHIFU was performed for 22 patients with breast cancer followed by chemotherapy, radiation therapy, and tamoxifen treatment. Five-year DFS and RFS rates were 95 % and 89 %, respectively, and the cosmetic result was judged to be good to excellent by 94 % of the patients.

MR-Guided HIFU (MRgHIFU)
A contrasting MRI is a standard superior modality for diagnosis of the extent of breast cancer, and MRgHIFU causes thermocoagulation and fusion necrosis of target tissue with the advantage of not having any influence on neighboring normal tissue. The software of the treatment instrument has been improved with more safety and accuracy now. Therefore, MRgHIFU can precisely deliver energy to a given point in soft tissue, accurately within 1 mm, without interrupting skin integrity, and changes of temperature around the treated region are consecutively fed back to an operator in detail during MRgHIFU, which gives the operator precise

information fully for control of the induced thermal effect. However, MRgHIFU is painful to patients because it needs a long time to heat gradually, and patients have to remain in an abdominal position during treatment. The cost of the instrument is very expensive, but an international multi-institutional clinical trial called the American College of Radiology Imaging Network (ACRIN) study has already been started for the advantages of MRgHIFU in the USA, Canada, and Japan. In addition, a Phase III clinical trial for MRgHIFU without resection is now ongoing by Furusawa et al. because a 97 % cure rate of tumor volume was gotten histopathologically in their Phase II study [42]. The criteria are intended for low-risk breast cancer such as tumor less than 1.5 cm in diameter, no lymph node metastasis, and well localized tumor. The method for evaluation of the effectiveness includes a contrasting MRI as image and HE and ssDNA staining as a histopathological evaluation by core needle biopsy specimen at 2 weeks after MRgHIFU. An intermediate analysis using 34 cases with more than 24 months following has shown that there is no local recurrence, distant recurrence, or serious AE in median follow-up of 44 months. Pure mucinous cancer should be excluded to cover the disadvantage of MRgHIFU, and a 5 mm safety margin to tumor in all directions will be compulsory to ensure complete ablation. A safe margin to skin is required to prevent skin burn, too.

There are many unsolved questions, as shown in Table 20.2, but most should be resolved with improvement of the instrument and treatment method. MRgHIFU will be one of the excellent modalities to satisfy both diagnosis and treatment among NSA procedures because of its extracorporeal approach. Excellent long-term follow-up data is expected in international and Japanese clinical trials.

20.4 Cryoablation (CA)

CA is an alternative procedure that uses an extreme freeze for a targeted tumor in the form of an "ice ball". CA for breast cancer has been restricted to patients with advanced disease and benign fibroadenoma, but has also been tried for small breast cancers in pilot and feasibility studies using US or MRI as image guidance. Surgical resection was performed for all patients after CA, and the complete ablation rate as confirmed by a histopathological evaluation was reported to range from 36 % to 83 % [43–46]. Sabel et al. [47] reported a result in a multi-institutional study that 29 patients with early breast cancer less than 2.0 cm were treated with CA followed by surgical resection 1–4 weeks later, and CA successfully destroyed 100 % of cancers less than 1.0 cm, but there is no reliable data for tumors larger than 1.5 cm in terms of complete ablation. Therefore, CA is a good candidate for patients with invasive ductal carcinoma less than 1.5 cm without EIC. It is a simpler and easier method than other NSA treatments, because it can be performed on an outpatient basis under a local anesthesia for minimal pain, side effects, and discomfort. In addition, an indirect anticancer effect due to embolus of the surrounding blood vessels and a potential immunological benefit is expected by CA, too. Fukuma et al. [48] reported that USgCA without resection was performed for eight patients with small breast cancer (mean size 7.6 mm), and a short-term follow-up (mean 10.5 months) failed to reveal any local recurrence at the ablated sites. The indication from published clinical trial data seems to be patients with invasive ductal cancer less than 1.5 cm in diameter and little intraductal component. Invasive lobular cancer, colloid cancer, and cancer with EIC should be excluded because of their high potentiality of IBR. A follow-up by MRI is required, but there are some problems to be settled. An image specialist of breast disease should perform CA because it is difficult to observe the chest wall side by US due to "ice ball" during CA therapy, and it is essential to insert a probe tip exactly in the center of the tumor to prevent incomplete ablation and skin frostbite. One more reason is that residual cancer or recurrence in the ablated site may be underestimated in the evaluation using a contrasting MRI for return disorder due to blood vessel embolus from freezing. There is no available data of clinical trials yet; therefore, not only further improvement of the MRI apparatus but also accumulated data of image and histopathological data of biopsied specimens are expected in international and Japanese clinical trials in the near future. However, nonsurgical CA therapy could become a safe and useful treatment for selected patients with small breast cancer due to the ease of maneuvering and the QOL of patients.

20.5 Conclusion

A good aesthetic outcome of breast cancer treatment correlates with good psychological recovery from breast cancer treatment.

RFA and MRgHIFU are thought to be comparable to BCT from many data in the short-term follow-up results of IBR, OS, and cosmetic outcome. After long-term follow-up data is reported to be comparable to BCT in prospective international and Japanese multi-institutional clinical trials with good quality, these therapies will be beneficial for breast cancer patients with small tumor less than 2.0 cm. The checkup rate for breast cancer screening in Japan is extremely low compared to in the USA and European countries at present, and the mortality rate also has not improved, but these NSA treatments for early-stage breast cancer could contribute to an increase in the checkup rate in the future because of non-resection therapy and excellent outcome, both safety and cosmetic results.

CA is thought to be inferior to BCT, too, but a prospective clinical trial is expected to start for clarification of its effectiveness in the near future.

Not only curability and excellent cosmetic result but also a functional and psychological benefit is a final goal of breast cancer treatment. Many efforts to satisfy these issues for breast cancer patients are tried now, using NSA or oncoplastic surgery, such as autologous fat graft, endoscopic breast surgery, and reconstruction method, for example, volume displacement or replacement, but NSA therapies will become the best choice among them because of no prominent skin incision. They will contribute to the well-being of most patients with breast cancer within 2.0 cm in diameter. Therefore, the two ongoing prospective trials of nonsurgical RFA in Japan should yield an excellent result as soon as possible, and NSA therapy in breast cancer could be standardized as an ultimate breast-conservative therapy, the so called cure with no incision, and bring breast cancer patients many benefits.

In an era where more and more women with early-stage breast cancer survive, all medical staff (breast and plastic surgeons, radiologists, etc.) should focus on safety and acceptable excellent cosmetic results for well-being, especially for women in Asian countries with smaller breasts.

References

1. Fisher B, Bauer M, Margolese R, Poisson R, Pilch Y, Redmond C, et al. Five-year results of a randomized clinical trial comparing total mastectomy and segmental mastectomy with or without radiation in the treatment of breast cancer. N Engl J Med. 1985;312(11):665–73.
2. Fisher B, Anderson S, Bryant J, Margolese RG, Deutsch M, Fisher ER, et al. Twenty-year follow-up of a randomized trial comparing total mastectomy, lumpectomy, and lumpectomy plus irradiation for the treatment of invasive breast cancer. N Engl J Med. 2002;347 (16):1233–41.
3. Saji S, Hiraoka M, Tokuda Y, Fukui N, Ikeda T. Trends in local therapy application for early breast cancer patients in the Japanese Breast Cancer Society Breast Cancer Registry during 2004–2009. Breast Cancer. 2012;19:1–3. doi:10.1007/s12282-011-0308-z.
4. Kolle SF, Fisher-Nielsen A, Mathiasen AB, Eiberg JJ, Oliveri RS, Glovinski PV, et al. Enrichment of autologous fat grafts with ex-vivo expanded adipose tissue-derived stem cells for graft survival: a randomized placebo-controlled trial. Lancet. 2013;382 (9898):1113–20. doi:10.1016/S0140-6736(13)61410-5.
5. Fukuma E. Endoscopic breast surgery for breast cancer. Nihon Geka Gakkai Zasshi. 2006;107 (2):64–8. (In Japanese with English summary).
6. Saimura M, Mitsuyama S, Anan K, Koga K, Watanabe M, Toyoshima S, et al. Endoscopy-assisted breast – conserving surgery for early breast cancer. Asian J Endosc Surg. 2013;6 (3):203–8. doi:10.1111/ases.12018.Epub2013Feb1.
7. Park HS, Lee JS, Lee JS, Park S, Kim SI, Park BW. The feasibility of endoscopy-assisted breast conservation surgery for patients with early breast cancer. J Breast Cancer. 2011;14 (1):52–7. doi:10.4048/bc.2011.14.152. Epub2013Mar31.
8. Yamashita K, Shimizu K. Transaxillary retromammary route approach of video-assisted breast surgery enables the inner-side breast cancer to be resected for breast conserving surgery. Am J Surg. 2008;196(4):578–81. doi:10.1016/j.amjsurg.2008.06.028.
9. Galimberti V, Cole BF, Zurrida S, Viale G, Luni A, Veronesi P, et al. Axillary dissection versus no axillary dissection in patients with sentinel-node micrometastases (IBCSG23-01): a phase 3 randomized controlled trial. Lancet Oncol. 2013;14(4):297–305. doi:10.1016/S1470-2045(13)70035-4.Epub2013Mar11.
10. Giuliano AE, Hunt KK, Ballman KV, Beitsch PD, Whitworth PW, Blumencranz PW, et al. Axillary dissection vs no axillary dissection in women with invasive breast cancer and sentinel node metastasis: a randomized clinical trial. JAMA. 2011;305(6):569–75. doi:10.1001/jama.2011.90.
11. Goldhirsch A, Winner EP, Coates AS, Gelber RD, Piccart-Gebhart M, Thurlimann B, et al. Personalizing the treatment of women with early breast cancer: highlights of the St Gallen International Expert Consensus on the Primary Therapy of Early Breast Cancer 2013. Ann Oncol. 2013;00:1–18. doi:10.1093/annonc/mdt303.

12. Jeffrey SS, Birdwell RL, Ikeda DM, Daniel BL, Nowels KW, Dirbas FM, et al. Radiofrequency ablation of breast cancer: first report of an emerging technology. Arch Surg. 1999;134:1064–8.
13. Izzo F, Thomas R, Delrio P, Rinaldo M, Vallone P, DeChiara A, et al. Radiofrequency ablation in patients with primary breast carcinoma. a pilot study in 26 patients. Cancer. 2001;92 (8):2036–44.
14. Burak WE, Angese DM, Povoski SP, Yanssens TL, Bloum KJ, Wakely PE, et al. Radiofrequency ablation of invasive breast carcinoma followed by delayed surgical excision. Cancer. 2003;98(7):1369–76.
15. Singletary SE. Feasibility of radiofrequency ablation for primary breast cancer. Breast Cancer. 2003;10(1):4–9.
16. Hayashi AH, Silver SF, van der Westhuizen NG, Donald JC, Parker C, Fraser S, et al. Treatment of invasive carcinoma with ultrasound-guided radiofrequency ablation. Am J Surg. 2003;185(5):429–35.
17. Noguchi M, Earashi M, Fujii H, Yokoyama K, Harada K, Tsuneyama K. Radiofrequency ablation of small breast cancer followed by surgical resection. J Surg Oncol. 2006;93 (2):120–8.
18. Khatri VP, McGahan JP, Ramsamooi R, Griffey S, Brock J, Cronan M, et al. A phase II trial of image-guided radiofrequency ablation of small invasive breast carcinoma: use of saline-cooled tip electrode. Ann Surg Oncol. 2007;14(5):1644–52. Epub2007Feb15.
19. Medina-Franco H, Soto-Germes S, Ulloa-Gomez JL, Romero-Trejo C, Uribe N, Ramirez-Alvarado CA, et al. Radiofrequency ablation of invasive breast carcinoma: a phase II trial. Ann Surg Oncol. 2008;15(6):1689–95. doi:10.1245/s10434-008-9875-4. Epub 2008 Mar 25.
20. Imoto S, Wada N, Sakemura N, Hasebe T, Murata Y. Feasibility study on radiofrequency ablation followed by partial mastectomy for stage I breast cancer patients. Breast. 2009;18 (2):130–4. doi:10.1016/j.breast.2009.02.008. Epub 2009 Mar 26.
21. Kinoshita T, Iwamoto E, Tsuda H, Seki K. Radiofrequency ablation as local therapy for early breast carcinoma. Breast Cancer. 2011;18(1):10–7. doi:10.1007/s12282-009-0186-9. Epub 2010 Jan14.
22. Hung WK, Mak KL, Ying M, Chan M. Radiofrequency ablation of breast cancer: a comparative study of two needle designs. Breast Cancer. 2011;18(2):124–8. doi:10.1007/s12282-009-0181-1. Epub 2009 Nov27.
23. Ohtani S, Kochi M, Ito M, Higaki K, Takada S, Matsuura H, et al. Radiofrequency ablation of early breast cancer followed by delayed surgical resection – a promising alternative to breast-conserving surgery. Breast. 2011;20(5):431–6. doi:10.1016/j.breast.2011.04.007. Epub 2011 Jun8.
24. Oura S, Tamaki T, Hirai I, Ohta F, Nakamura R, et al. Radiofrequency ablation therapy in patients with breast cancer two centimeters or less in size. Breast Cancer. 2007;14(1):48–54.
25. Nagashima T, Sakakibara M, Sangai T, Kazama T, Fujimoto H, Miyazaki M. Surrounding rim formation and reduction in size after radiofrequency ablation for primary breast cancer. Jpn J Radiol. 2009;27(5):197–204. doi:10.1007/s11604-009-0322-7. Epub2009Jun25.
26. Yamamoto N, Fujimoto H, Nakamura R, Arai M, Yoshii A, Kaji S, et al. Pilot study of radiofrequency ablation therapy without surgical excision for T1 breast cancer: evaluation with MRI and vacuum-assisted core needle biopsy and safety management. Breast Cancer. 2011;18(1):3–9. doi:10.1007/s12282-010-0197-6. Epub2010Mar4.
27. Yoshinaga Y, Enomoto Y, Fujimitsu R, Shimakura M, Nabeshima K, Iwasaki A. Image and pathological changes after radiofrequency ablation of invasive breast cancer: a pilot study of nonsurgical therapy of early breast cancer. World J Surg. 2013;37(2):356–63. doi:10.1007/s00268-012-1820-9.
28. Noguchi M, Motoyoshi A, Earashi M, Fujii H. Long-term outcome of breast cancer patients treated with radiofrequency ablation. Eur J Surg Oncol. 2012;38(11):1036–42. doi:10.1016/j.ejso.2012.08.006. Epub2012Sep2.

29. Head JF, Elliot RL. Stereotactic radiofrequency ablation: a minimally invasive technique for nonpalpable breast cancer in postmenopausal patients. Cancer Epidermiol. 2009;33 (3–4):300–5. doi:10.1016/j.canep.2009.07.007. Epub 2009 Aug20.
30. Noguchi M, Motoyoshi A, Earashi M, Fuzii H. Long-term outcome of breast cancer patients treated with radiofrequency ablation. EJSO. 2012;38:1036–42.
31. National Comprehensive Cancer Network. NCCN clinical practice guidelines in oncology. Breast Cancer. ver2. 2011.
32. Villar VS, Goldman SM, Ricci MD, Pincerato K, Oliveira H, Abud TG, et al. Analysis by MRI of residual tumor after radiofrequency ablation for early stage breast cancer. AJR. 2012;198 (3):W285–91. doi:10.2214/AJR.10.5581.
33. Nakamura S, Ishiyama M, Tsunoda-Shimizu H. Magnetic resonance mammography has limited ability to estimate pathological complete remission after primary chemotherapy or radiofrequency ablation therapy. Breast Cancer. 2007;14(2):123–30.
34. Seki K, Tsuda H, Iwamoto E, Kinoshita T. Histopathological effect of radiofrequency ablation therapy for primary breast cancer, with special reference to changes in cancer cells and stromal structure and a comparison with enzyme histochemistry. Breast Cancer. 2011;18(1):18–23. doi:10.1007/s12282-010-0215-8. Epub2010Aug4.
35. Tsuda H, Seki K, Hasebe T, Sasajima Y, Shibata T, Iwamoto E, Kinoshita T. A histopathological study for evaluation of therapeutic effects of radiofrequency ablation in patients with breast cancer. Breast Cancer. 2011;18(1):24–32. doi:10.1007/s12282-010-0222-9. Epub2010Sep23.
36. Motoyoshi A, Noguchi M, Earashi M, Zen Y, Fujii H. Histopathological and immunohistochemical evaluations of breast cancer treated with radiofrequency ablation. J Surg Oncol. 2010;102:385–91.
37. START Trialists' Group, Bentzen SM, Agrawal RK, Aird EG, Barrett JM, Barett-Lee PJ, Bentzen SM, et al. The UK Standardisation of Breast Radiotherapy (START) Trial B of radiotherapy hypofractionation for treatment of early breast cancer: a randomized trial. Lancet. 2008;371(9618):1098–107. doi:10.1016/S0140-6736-(08)60348-7. Epub 2008Mar 19.
38. Ito T, Oura S, Yamamoto N, Nagamine S, Takahashi M, Tanino H, Mitsuyama S, et al. Radiofrequency ablation (RFA) of breast cancer: a multicenter retrospective analysis. 2012ASCO Abstract #97433.
39. Susini T, Nori J, Olivieri S, Livi L, Bianchi S, Mangialavori G, et al. Radiofrequency ablation for minimally invasive treatment of breast carcinoma, a pilot study in elderly inoperable patients. Gynecol Oncol. 2007;104(2):304–10. Epub 2006 Oct27.
40. Marcy PY, Magne N, Castadot P, Bailet C, Namer M. Ultrasound-guided percutaneous radiofrequency ablation in elderly breast cancer patients: preliminary institutional experience. Br J Radiol. 2007;80(952):267–73. Epub 2006Oct26.
41. Wu F, Wang ZB, Cao YD, Chen WZ, Bai J, Zou JZ, et al. A randomised clinical trial of high-intensity focused ultrasound ablation for the treatment of patients with localized breast cancer. Br J Cancer. 2003;89(12):2227–33.
42. Furusawa H, Namba K, Thomsen S, Akiyama F, Bendet A, Tanaka C, Yasuda Y, et al. Magnetic resonance-guided focused ultrasound surgery of breast cancer: reliability and effectiveness. J Am Coll Surg. 2006;203:54–63.
43. Morin J, Traore A, Dionne G, Dumont M, Fouquette B, Dufour M, et al. Magnetic resonance-guided percutaneous cryosurgery of breast carcinoma: technique and early clinical results. Can J Surg. 2004;475(5):347–51.
44. Roubidoux MA, Sabel MS, Bailey JE, Kleer CG, Klein KA, Helvie MA. Small (<2.0-cm) breast cancers: mammographic and US findings at US-guided cryoablation-initial experience. Radiology. 2004;233(3):857–67.
45. Pfleiderer SO, Marx C, Camara O, Gajda M, Kaiser WA. Ultrasound-guided, percutaneous cryotherapy of small (< or=15mm) breast cancer. Invest Radiol. 2005;40(7):472–7.

46. Pusztaszeri M, Vlastos G, Kinkel K, Pelte MF. Histopathological study of breast cancer and normal breast tissue after magnetic resonance-guided cryotherapy ablation. Cryobiology. 2007;55(1):44–51. Epub2007Jun2.
47. Sabel MS, Kaufman CS, Whitworth P, Chang H, Stocks LH, Simmons R, et al. Cryoablation of early-stage breast cancer: work-in-progress report of a multi-institutional trial. Ann Surg Oncol. 2004;11(5):542–9.
48. Fukuma E, Ozaki S, Tozaki M, Sakamoto N, Abe S, Kurihara T, et al. Cryosurgery for breast disease. Jpn J Interv Radiol. 2008;23:260–6. (In Japanese with English summary).

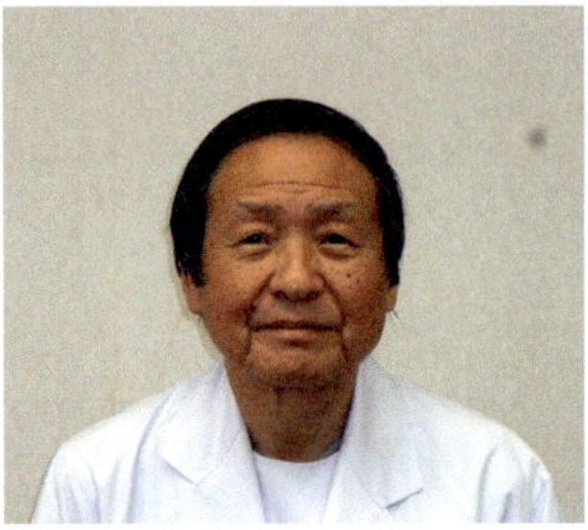

Shoshu Mitsuyama

MIX
Papier aus verantwortungsvollen Quellen
Paper from responsible sources
FSC® C105338

If you have any concerns about our products,
you can contact us on
ProductSafety@springernature.com

In case Publisher is established outside the EU,
the EU authorized representative is:
Springer Nature Customer Service Center GmbH
Europaplatz 3, 69115 Heidelberg, Germany

Printed by Libri Plureos GmbH
in Hamburg, Germany